Automation and Validation of Information in Pharmaceutical Processing

DRUGS AND THE PHARMACEUTICAL SCIENCES

DRUGS AND THE PHARMACEUTICAL SCIENCES

A Series of Textbooks and Monographs

1. Pharmacokinetics, *Milo Gibaldi and Donald Perrier*
2. Good Manufacturing Practices for Pharmaceuticals: A Plan for Total Quality Control, *Sidney H. Willig, Murray M. Tuckerman, and William S. Hitchings IV*
3. Microencapsulation, *edited by J. R. Nixon*
4. Drug Metabolism: Chemical and Biochemical Aspects, *Bernard Testa and Peter Jenner*
5. New Drugs: Discovery and Development, *edited by Alan A. Rubin*
6. Sustained and Controlled Release Drug Delivery Systems, *edited by Joseph R. Robinson*
7. Modern Pharmaceutics, *edited by Gilbert S. Banker and Christopher T. Rhodes*
8. Prescription Drugs in Short Supply: Case Histories, *Michael A. Schwartz*
9. Activated Charcoal: Antidotal and Other Medical Uses, *David O. Cooney*
10. Concepts in Drug Metabolism (in two parts), *edited by Peter Jenner and Bernard Testa*
11. Pharmaceutical Analysis: Modern Methods (in two parts), *edited by James W. Munson*
12. Techniques of Solubilization of Drugs, *edited by Samuel H. Yalkowsky*
13. Orphan Drugs, *edited by Fred E. Karch*
14. Novel Drug Delivery Systems: Fundamentals, Developmental Concepts, Biomedical Assessments, *Yie W. Chien*
15. Pharmacokinetics: Second Edition, Revised and Expanded, *Milo Gibaldi and Donald Perrier*
16. Good Manufacturing Practices for Pharmaceuticals: A Plan for Total Quality Control, Second Edition, Revised and Expanded, *Sidney H. Willig, Murray M. Tuckerman, and William S. Hitchings IV*
17. Formulation of Veterinary Dosage Forms, *edited by Jack Blodinger*
18. Dermatological Formulations: Percutaneous Absorption, *Brian W. Barry*
19. The Clinical Research Process in the Pharmaceutical Industry, *edited by Gary M. Matoren*
20. Microencapsulation and Related Drug Processes, *Patrick B. Deasy*
21. Drugs and Nutrients: The Interactive Effects, *edited by Daphne A. Roe and T. Colin Campbell*

22. Biotechnology of Industrial Antibiotics, *Erick J. Vandamme*
23. Pharmaceutical Process Validation, *edited by Bernard T. Loftus and Robert A. Nash*
24. Anticancer and Interferon Agents: Synthesis and Properties, *edited by Raphael M. Ottenbrite and George B. Butler*
25. Pharmaceutical Statistics: Practical and Clinical Applications, *Sanford Bolton*
26. Drug Dynamics for Analytical, Clinical, and Biological Chemists, *Benjamin J. Gudzinowicz, Burrows T. Younkin, Jr., and Michael J. Gudzinowicz*
27. Modern Analysis of Antibiotics, *edited by Adjoran Aszalos*
28. Solubility and Related Properties, *Kenneth C. James*
29. Controlled Drug Delivery: Fundamentals and Applications, Second Edition, Revised and Expanded, *edited by Joseph R. Robinson and Vincent H. Lee*
30. New Drug Approval Process: Clinical and Regulatory Management, *edited by Richard A. Guarino*
31. Transdermal Controlled Systemic Medications, *edited by Yie W. Chien*
32. Drug Delivery Devices: Fundamentals and Applications, *edited by Praveen Tyle*
33. Pharmacokinetics: Regulatory • Industrial • Academic Perspectives, *edited by Peter G. Welling and Francis L. S. Tse*
34. Clinical Drug Trials and Tribulations, *edited by Allen E. Cato*
35. Transdermal Drug Delivery: Developmental Issues and Research Initiatives, *edited by Jonathan Hadgraft and Richard H. Guy*
36. Aqueous Polymeric Coatings for Pharmaceutical Dosage Forms, *edited by James W. McGinity*
37. Pharmaceutical Pelletization Technology, *edited by Isaac Ghebre-Sellassie*
38. Good Laboratory Practice Regulations, *edited by Allen F. Hirsch*
39. Nasal Systemic Drug Delivery, *Yie W. Chien, Kenneth S. E. Su, and Shyi-Feu Chang*
40. Modern Pharmaceutics: Second Edition, Revised and Expanded, *edited by Gilbert S. Banker and Christopher T. Rhodes*
41. Specialized Drug Delivery Systems: Manufacturing and Production Technology, *edited by Praveen Tyle*
42. Topical Drug Delivery Formulations, *edited by David W. Osborne and Anton H. Amann*
43. Drug Stability: Principles and Practices, *Jens T. Carstensen*
44. Pharmaceutical Statistics: Practical and Clinical Applications, Second Edition, Revised and Expanded, *Sanford Bolton*
45. Biodegradable Polymers as Drug Delivery Systems, *edited by Mark Chasin and Robert Langer*
46. Preclinical Drug Disposition: A Laboratory Handbook, *Francis L. S. Tse and James J. Jaffe*

47. HPLC in the Pharmaceutical Industry, *edited by Godwin W. Fong and Stanley K. Lam*
48. Pharmaceutical Bioequivalence, *edited by Peter G. Welling, Francis L. S. Tse, and Shrikant V. Dinghe*
49. Pharmaceutical Dissolution Testing, *Umesh V. Banakar*
50. Novel Drug Delivery Systems: Second Edition, Revised and Expanded, *Yie W. Chien*
51. Managing the Clinical Drug Development Process, *David M. Cocchetto and Ronald V. Nardi*
52. Good Manufacturing Practices for Pharmaceuticals: A Plan for Total Quality Control, Third Edition, *edited by Sidney H. Willig and James R. Stoker*
53. Prodrugs: Topical and Ocular Drug Delivery, *edited by Kenneth B. Sloan*
54. Pharmaceutical Inhalation Aerosol Technology, *edited by Anthony J. Hickey*
55. Radiopharmaceuticals: Chemistry and Pharmacology, *edited by Adrian D. Nunn*
56. New Drug Approval Process: Second Edition, Revised and Expanded, *edited by Richard A. Guarino*
57. Pharmaceutical Process Validation: Second Edition, Revised and Expanded, *edited by Ira R. Berry and Robert A. Nash*
58. Ophthalmic Drug Delivery Systems, *edited by Ashim K. Mitra*
59. Pharmaceutical Skin Penetration Enhancement, *edited by Kenneth A. Walters and Jonathan Hadgraft*
60. Colonic Drug Absorption and Metabolism, *edited by Peter R. Bieck*
61. Pharmaceutical Particulate Carriers: Therapeutic Applications, *edited by Alain Rolland*
62. Drug Permeation Enhancement: Theory and Applications, *edited by Dean S. Hsieh*
63. Glycopeptide Antibiotics, *edited by Ramakrishnan Nagarajan*
64. Achieving Sterility in Medical and Pharmaceutical Products, *Nigel A. Halls*
65. Multiparticulate Oral Drug Delivery, *edited by Isaac Ghebre-Sellassie*
66. Colloidal Drug Delivery Systems, *edited by Jörg Kreuter*
67. Pharmacokinetics: Regulatory • Industrial • Academic Perspectives, Second Edition, *edited by Peter G. Welling and Francis L. S. Tse*
68. Drug Stability: Principles and Practices, Second Edition, Revised and Expanded, *Jens T. Carstensen*
69. Good Laboratory Practice Regulations: Second Edition, Revised and Expanded, *edited by Sandy Weinberg*
70. Physical Characterization of Pharmaceutical Solids, *edited by Harry G. Brittain*
71. Pharmaceutical Powder Compaction Technology, *edited by Göran Alderborn and Christer Nyström*

72. Modern Pharmaceutics: Third Edition, Revised and Expanded, *edited by Gilbert S. Banker and Christopher T. Rhodes*
73. Microencapsulation: Methods and Industrial Applications, *edited by Simon Benita*
74. Oral Mucosal Drug Delivery, *edited by Michael J. Rathbone*
75. Clinical Research in Pharmaceutical Development, *edited by Barry Bleidt and Michael Montagne*
76. The Drug Development Process: Increasing Efficiency and Cost Effectiveness, *edited by Peter G. Welling, Louis Lasagna, and Umesh V. Banakar*
77. Microparticulate Systems for the Delivery of Proteins and Vaccines, *edited by Smadar Cohen and Howard Bernstein*
78. Good Manufacturing Practices for Pharmaceuticals: A Plan for Total Quality Control, Fourth Edition, Revised and Expanded, *Sidney H. Willig and James R. Stoker*
79. Aqueous Polymeric Coatings for Pharmaceutical Dosage Forms: Second Edition, Revised and Expanded, *edited by James W. McGinity*
80. Pharmaceutical Statistics: Practical and Clinical Applications, Third Edition, *Sanford Bolton*
81. Handbook of Pharmaceutical Granulation Technology, *edited by Dilip M. Parikh*
82. Biotechnology of Antibiotics: Second Edition, Revised and Expanded, *edited by William R. Strohl*
83. Mechanisms of Transdermal Drug Delivery, *edited by Russell O. Potts and Richard H. Guy*
84. Pharmaceutical Enzymes, *edited by Albert Lauwers and Simon Scharpé*
85. Development of Biopharmaceutical Parenteral Dosage Forms, *edited by John A. Bontempo*
86. Pharmaceutical Project Management, *edited by Tony Kennedy*
87. Drug Products for Clinical Trials: An International Guide to Formulation • Production • Quality Control, *edited by Donald C. Monkhouse and Christopher T. Rhodes*
88. Development and Formulation of Veterinary Dosage Forms: Second Edition, Revised and Expanded, *edited by Gregory E. Hardee and J. Desmond Baggot*
89. Receptor-Based Drug Design, *edited by Paul Leff*
90. Automation and Validation of Information in Pharmaceutical Processing, *edited by Joseph F. deSpautz*
91. Dermal Absorption and Toxicity Assessment, *edited by Michael S. Roberts and Kenneth A. Walters*

ADDITIONAL VOLUMES IN PREPARATION

Preparing for FDA Pre-Approval Inspections, *edited by Martin D. Hynes III*

Polymorphism in Pharmaceutical Solids, *edited by Harry G. Brittain*

Automation and Validation of Information in Pharmaceutical Processing

edited by
Joseph F. deSpautz
INCODE Corp.
Herndon, Virginia

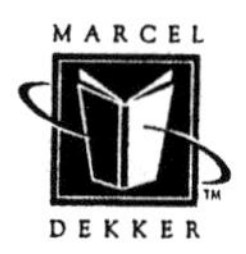

Marcel Dekker, Inc. New York • Basel

Library of Congress Cataloging-in-Publication Data

Automation and validation of information in pharmaceutical processing/edited by Joseph F. deSpautz.
p. cm.—(Drugs and the Pharmaceutical sciences: v.90)
Includes bibliographical references and index.
ISBN 0-8247-0119-4 (alk. paper)
1. Pharmaceutical industry—Automation. 2. Pharmaceutical technology—Automation. 3. Information technology. I. deSpautz, Joseph F. II. Series.
RS192.A94 1998
615'.39'0285—dc21

98-21356
CIP

This book is printed on acid-free paper.

Headquarters
Marcel Dekker, Inc.
270 Madison Avenue, New York, NY 10016
tel: 212-696-9000; fax: 212-685-4540

Eastern Hemisphere Distribution
Marcel Dekker AG
Hutgasse 4, Postfach 812, CH-4001 Basel, Switzerland
tel: 44-61-261-8482; fax: 44-61-261-8896

World Wide Web
http://www.dekker.com

The publisher offers discounts on this book when ordered in bulk quantities. For more information, write to Special Sales/Professional Marketing at the headquarters address above.

Current printing (last digit):
10 9 8 7 6 5 4 3 2

PRINTED IN THE UNITED STATES OF AMERICA

Preface

How will pharmaceutical manufacturers adapt to the business drivers of the next five to ten years? Prognosticators envision an industry of a small number of dominant companies, with the remainder being either acquired or incorporated into these global supply chain giants. Globalization of markets and facilities are increasing at the same or faster pace as at the end of the 1980s.

Companies are integrating downstream and upstream processes to form vertical market organizations to control entire product development and distribution cycles. Cost reductions, rationalization of facilities, simplification of process lines, and unique distribution initiatives are being planned and developed for all pharmaceuticals, over the counter (OTC) products, ethicals, biologics, implants, and devices. These initiatives involve organizational change, use of information technology (IT), and a greater awareness of manufacturing processes to achieve business goals. The United States and international regulatory agencies are increasing their mandated watch on the industry to have providers maintain and increase their compliance of regulatory practices and guidelines. As product manufacture uses more IT, this scrutiny will increase. In order to maintain high-quality products as well as high-quality documentation, managers and workers all along the supply chain need to be aware of the activities of their upstream suppliers and downstream customers.

This book is designed for readers involved in the development, manufacture, and distribution of regulated products who manage issues in automation. They may be specialists in manufacturing products for research and clinical trials, pilot plant scale-up, or commercial product manufacture who need to define their requirements for automated equipment. They may be material planners, purchasing directors, production schedulers, document developers, or quality control technicians trying to make complementary changes in their paperbound domains. As information systems become more aligned with functional areas, program managers, system managers, software developers, and analysts must become familiar with end-user activities, system validation concepts, and desktop integration requirements for 24-hours-a-day, 7-days-a-week operations. As computer-based systems become more prolific in operations, specialists and nonspecialists will need to understand the organizational, technological, and business perspectives of pharmaceutical manufacturing automation.

Industry issues make the application of automation complex and expensive. Regulatory compliance makes the impact of automation far-reaching throughout the supply chain. Automation project teams need to contain cross-functional skills and direction. No longer can a manager or project team be concerned solely with hardware, software, and equipment interfaces. They must address how a system will increase their own productivity and impact other supply-chain functions. The overall objective of this book is to help present and future managers better prepare themselves and their organizations to deal with automation.

Information technology provides the building blocks for automation. Education and training in the pharmaceutical workplace make workers a valuable asset. Organizational change, reengineering, and worker performance become important for project success. The business and information processes are the third and perhaps the most important perspective. Only by incorporating the company's business strategies into the project will the resulting automation solution become a competitive advantage. These perspectives are complementary, and may all be relevant to a specific automation project. They are the framework to describe the state of the art of pharmaceutical manufacturing automation.

The U.S. Food and Drug Administration (FDA) has published good manufacturing process (GMP) guideline changes to support electronic identification (eID) and electronic signatures for batch record recording. How will these guideline changes alter the manufacturing environment? How will the leading-edge companies use these changes to gain a competitive advantage? Is the present technology for electronic batch records, document management and image storage, and retrieval systems capable of supporting reliable, validated operations? This book communicates how these guidelines and technologies will influence manufacturing automation, cause change in organizations, and require a differently trained work force.

Business process reengineering, worker knowledge development, and total quality programs are being planned and implemented to ensure that the people are capable of using and accepting these new systems. Topics described include how human resource programs maximize productivity gains for automation initiatives. Distributed information and documentation for regulatory compliance are essential for manufacturing automation. The reader will understand the need and challenge of computer system validation as automated systems use networks, data center operations, and software management practices.

Contributors to this book are domain experts through their activities in academia, consulting, system integration, and pharmaceutical manufacturing. An attribute common to all is their dedication to quality and excellence in pharmaceutical operations. The contributors come from manufacturing organizations, automation vendors, software providers, consulting companies, research firms, and computer vendors. This book would not be possible without their dedicated efforts to develop the materials and add their insights and experiences. The staff of Marcel Dekker, Inc., made it all possible by their dedication to developing and producing this book.

Joseph F. deSpautz

Contents

Contributors

David J. Adler Eli Lilly & Company, Indianapolis, Indiana

Frederick R. Bickel Kineticon Group, Inc., Loveland, Colorado

Richard E. Blanchette Green Mountain Technology Inc., Boulder, Colorado

Mark Castro* Pfizer Pharmaceutical Group, Groton, Connecticut

Jack Conaway Winners Consulting Group, Amherst, New Hampshire

Joseph F. deSpautz INCODE Corp., Herndon, Virginia

Anthony R. Gonzalez* Pfizer Pharmaceutical Group, Brooklyn, New York

Jeffrey S. Gramm Glaxo Wellcome Inc., Research Triangle Park, North Carolina

Joseph A. Hercamp Eli Lilly & Company, Indianapolis, Indiana

Baha Korkmaz[†] The Foxboro Company, Foxboro, Massachusetts

Kenneth S. Kovacs Bailey Controls Company, Wickliffe, Ohio

Joseph J. Kowalski Capitol Management Consulting, Inc., Hopewell, New Jersey

---

*Formerly with BW Manufacturing, Inc., West Greenwich, Rhode Island
[†]*Current affiliation*: Automation Vision, Inc., Wrentham, Massachusetts

Sean M. Megley‡ PerSeptive Biosystems, Cambridge, Massachusetts

Colman O'Murchu SmithKline Beecham Pharmaceuticals, King of Prussia, Pennsylvania

Teri Stokes GXP International, Acton, Massachusetts

Teddy H. Tom Moore Products Co., Spring House, Pennsylvania

James L. Vesper LearningPlus, Rochester, New York

Steven B. Williams Eli Lilly & Company, Indianapolis, Indiana

‡*Current affiliation*: Vanstar, Jamestown, Rhode Island

1

Introduction

Joseph F. deSpautz

INCODE Corp., Herndon, Virginia

Pharmaceutical manufacturers have achieved significant benefits using automated systems over the years. Reference 1 is a collection of papers from conferences and symposia defining automation projects in the early 1980s. These systems are typically automating a single-unit operation, such as a solid dosage unit operation, laboratory testing, and robotics. In the ensuing years pharmaceutical products have become more complex and clinical trials more lengthy, with greater population samples and regulatory compliance more extensive and important.

Pharmaceutical manufacturers have continued to make high-quality products, generate high-quality documentation, and develop competent knowledge workers to maintain the processes and computer systems used in manufacturing. As products and processes have become more complex, so have the systems to support the processes. Unit operational systems are still in wide use and they are expanding into complete plant floor systems. Integration to enterprise-level business systems for planning, scheduling, and management is now commonplace. The manufacturing environment is being united to the business and the wider enterprise of suppliers and customers. Information about processes is needed to support the requirements of all these different groups. Recording of real-time data to support the actual manufacturing processes for manufacturing support, optimization, and batch record recording still have to be done and to a greater degree of accuracy and timeliness. In solid dosage operations, biotechnology, and devices operations, systems are being planned and implemented for

1. Manual and semiautomatic operations
2. Stand-alone and integrated unit operations
3. Complete material, equipment, and sampling traceability across product lines
4. Multiplant and multinational rollouts of common systems
5. Integrating supplier and customer information into manufacturing systems for planning and scheduling, monitoring and control, and quality management

Some companies have implemented ''paperless or paper-light environments'' using electronic batch record systems to create a competitive advantage. One company has a multisite implementation of an electronic batch record system (2). Others have electronic batch record systems in the planning and construction stages. The U.S. FDA has published its guidelines in 21 CFR part 11, *Electronic Records: Electronic Signatures* in March 1997 (3). By issuing the guidelines, the U.S. FDA has eliminated the uncertainty for making paperless automation an attainability reality.

Different research companies have defined many models that have expanded and contracted the three principal manufacturing domains—planning and scheduling, execution, and process control. Independent of the model, the elements of the system in view must perform their tasks to support the business processes using trained and empowered workers to produce high-quality products according to their predetermined specifications and quality standards and capture the information about the process and products in a validated system.

From a technology perspective these systems involve the computer control of hardware, software, interfaces to other application systems, and special devices and document management. Systems now use PC-based workstations and servers as well as minicomputers and small mainframes. Client-server technology is becoming the standard for the technology platforms using the new operating systems.

As newer technology is introduced to automate the more advanced functionality, regulatory compliance has had to keep pace with the complexity of the information technology used in these systems. The FDA definition of process validation is contained in the *General Principles of Validation* guideline (4) as

> establishing documented evidence which provides a high degree of assurance that a specific process will consistently produce a product meeting its predetermined specifications and quality attributes.

This definition applies to computer-based systems as well as to the process. The Pharmaceutical Research and Manufacturers Association (PhARMA; formerly the PMA) developed a life cycle approach to computer-related system validation (5). The Parenteral Drug Association (PDA) Committee on Validation of Computer-Related Systems report (6) defined a method emphasizing comprehensive computer-related system requirements (functional and design specifications), computer system construction, implementation, and qualification.

An Advanced Manufacturing Research (AMR) survey (7) on business barriers to Computer Integrated Manufacturing (CIM) concluded that system solutions must address more than information technology. An overwhelming 70 percent stated that people, as well as training, organizations, and changes in culture, need to be included in any systemic solution. The human component in systems design and implementation has often been overlooked. With the investments in people, the human asset has become one of the most important in the pharmaceutical manufacturing environment.

The focus of this book is on computer-based systems for automation and information integration. The book is organized into a number of sections spanning automation initiatives throughout the supply chain functions and the use of Information Technology (IT) for pharmaceutical process automation. The sections are as follows:

- Systems Planning for Automation
- Implementating Automation
- Computer Systems Validation
- Supply Chain Automation

The first three sections present IT initiatives that are common across different automation and integration projects in pharmaceutical manufacturing. The themes of regulatory compliance and system development life cycle are constant, as would be expected for projects in regulated industries. Examples of supply chain projects using these techniques are presented in Section IV. Any text on this very large subject will not cover all of the facets of automation and validation in pharmaceutical manufacturing. Our intent is to provide the reader with a view of the state of the art in automation of pharmaceutical systems and be a reference for future projects.

REFERENCES

1. D. J. Fraade, ed., *Automation of pharmaceutical operations,* Pharmaceutical Technology Publications, Springfield, Oregon, 1983.
2. C. Anthony and S. Lucash, A multisite implementation of an electronic batch record system, *Pharm. Tech. 21* (4), (April 1997).
3. Federal Register, Thursday, March 20, 1997, Volume 62, No. 54, Rules and Regulations, 21 CFR Part 11, Electronic Records; Electronic Signatures, Final rule.
4. *General Principles of Validation*, Food and Drug Administration, Center for Drug Evaluation and Research, Rockville, Maryland, May 1987.

5. Validation concepts for computer systems used in the manufacture of drug products, PMA's Computer Systems Validation Committee, PMA Proceedings: Concepts and Principles for Validation of Computer Systems Used in the Manufacturing and Control of Drug Products, Chicago, 1986. Reprinted in Pharm. Tech. (May 1986).
6. Validation of computer-related systems, technical report no. 18, PDA *J. Pharm. Sci. Tech.*, supplement, *49* (S1), (1995).
7. Integrated Manufacturing: Barriers and Opportunities in the Fortune 500, AMR Report, Advanced Manufacturing Research, Inc., Boston, MA, April 1990.

2

Information Systems Planning

Colman O'Murchu

SmithKline Beecham Pharmaceuticals, King of Prussia, Pennsylvania

I. INTRODUCTION

The purpose of this section of the chapter is to describe some of the issues pertinent to information systems (IS) planning, and outline one pharmaceutical company's approach to assembling and implementing such plans. Future IS planning will revolve around systems integration, and this section describes the planning of such activities. The section's objectives can be summarized as follows:

- Define IS and systems integration
- Discuss why systems integration is important
- Outline some of the benefits of systems integration
- Describe the main characteristics of IS plans
- Provide a methodology for preparing and implementing a plan
- Give some examples of existing plans
- Compare and contrast these plans
- Arrive at some conclusions

The type of planning discussed here refers to standalone pharmaceutical manufacturing plants only. This section does not address the type of multienterprise, often international IS planning required to link entire pharmaceutical companies' R&D, manufacturing, and marketing operations together in the 1990s. Reference will be made to such companywide systems, however, where they link in with plant information systems.

Information systems planning should take account of every computer interface in a manufacturing plant, present and future. This section will describe ways of ensuring that each important piece of computer infrastructure is taken into account.

II. SOME BACKGROUND

In 1994, SmithKline Beecham (SB) was a $12 billion/year pharmaceutical company based in the United Kingdom with over seventy manufacturing plants throughout the world. The manufacturing organization, called WSO (Worldwide Supply Organization) has an information resources group dedicated to supporting the plant network Information Resources (IR) needs. In addition, WSO has a central engineering department that has significant manufacturing process control expertise. The combination of these groups can provide the resources necessary to provide systems planning to sites worldwide.

Historically, process-associated computer systems at SB and other pharmaceutical companies have been implemented at manufacturing sites without a coherent strategy in place. Normally such systems are justified purely on a financial basis by demonstrating certain operating cost savings that can be gained from improved efficiency and repeatability. In many cases it is difficult to justify the significant additional expense of tying different process control systems together. Typically this has resulted in standalone process control or monitoring systems that have different platform needs.

System incompatibilities are frequently addressed by ensuring that the required process data from each system is written down on paper and entered in a manual document control system. No real effort is ever made to have systems communicate with one another so that data may be passed between systems electronically.

In the last five years, this has begun to change. Most pharmaceutical companies have begun to see that competitive advantage can be gained from properly the integration of process computer systems. Much effort has gone into quantifying this advantage; however, it is not an easy task. Many systems integration projects would never go ahead if justification was based on financial criteria alone. It requires much education and a management ''leap of faith'' in order to make such projects happen.

III. WHAT ARE "INFORMATION SYSTEMS" AND WHAT IS MEANT BY "INTEGRATION?"

A. Information Systems

Table 1 describes IS typically used in highly automated pharmaceutical plants. These are general descriptions and do not reflect specific facility applications.

Table 1 Information Systems Used in Automated Pharmaceutical Plants

System	Acronym	Description
Distributed control system	DCS	A process control computer system which, while functionally integrated, contains subsystems that may be physically separated from one another. It comprises operator consoles, a communications system and remote or local processor units performing control, logic, and calculation and measurement functions.
Programmable logic controller	PLC	A microprocessor-based controller, usually with multiple inputs and outputs, that contains an alterable program of instructions to implement I/O control, logic, timing, PID control, and communication.
Standalone preprogrammed controller		A controller with multiple I/O which contains instructions similar to a PLC, but whose program cannot be changed.
Supervisory control and data acquisition	SCADA	A system that uses the controller or computer program output of one system as an input to other (usually higher level) computer, in addition to monitoring and storing process data.
Lab information management system	LIMS	A computer system that obtains and manages anaytical data from laboratory instruments via a systemwide communications network. It can also interface with online process instrumentation.
Manufacturing executions system	MES	A PC or mainframe-based package that coordinates scheduling and execution of batch processes. In addition, it provides an electronic interface between lab information, document management, and manufacturing resource planning systems.
Inventory management system		A PC-based computer package that keeps track of incoming raw materials, in-process materials (and sometimes equipment), and material for shipment in a facility. Barcode readers are interfaced with the PC package to input data.

Table 1 Continued

System	Acronym	Description
Manufacturing resource planning	MRP 2	An extension of the inventory management system, it contains those features and also allows plant equipment resources to be scheduled and managed. It is frequently a mainframe computer application, permitting site-to-site electronic coordination of manufacturing resources.
Office systems/local area network	LAN	The connection of several data processing machines to share a suite of applications and data files such as word processors, spreadsheets, and electronic mail.
Automated maintenance system		A PC-based package that automatically tracks and schedules maintenance for instruments and other plant equipment.
Fieldbus communications protocol		An ISA standard under development for a bus to have two-way interconnection between process control sensors, actuators, and control devices.

B. What Is Meant by "Systems Intregation?"

Systems integration is the planning and implementation of unifying computer systems in the manufacturing facility toward the common strategic goal of that facility. It sets up the communications between individual systems so that critical data from one system are available in another where required. In addition, it is the planning required today so that future systems can be incorporated and upgraded while a coherent "whole" is maintained.

The end product of systems integration is a suite of key manufacturing software products in a facility that can communicate with one another if necessary. Also, it is important that communication between systems can be set up with minimum effort. Systems integration planning allows such factors to be taken into account.

Some examples of systems integration efforts typically found in pharmaceutical plants include the following:

1. Similar programmable logic controllers (PLCs) controlling different pieces of equipment. PLCs could be used to control similar pieces of equipment, such as reactor vessels or fermentors. These PLCs could be tied to-

gether across a communications highway to allow information to be passed back and forth (such as vessel availability information) between controllers.
2. A distributed control system (DCS) or PLC communicating with a lab information management system (LIMS). This type of integration could allow in-process lab analysis results to be communicated electronically from a LIMS to a plant process control system.
3. DCS or PLC communicating with an MES. This creates an environment in which the process control system is communicating with an array of applications through the MES, such as an MRP2 system, a document management system for potential electronic batch record production.

C. Why Is Systems Integration Important?

The benefits of automating equipment and information communications in new or existing pharmaceutical manufacturing plants are many. Typically, when justification is being sought for automation, the following criteria are used.

1. Operating Cost Savings

If an existing piece of manual plant is to be automated, cost savings can be anticipated in such areas as

1. More productive use of equipment.
2. Less manpower required to operate the equipment. (This can sometimes be offset by higher maintenance costs due to increased instrumentation.)
3. Less possibility of rejected material than in the manual operating state.
4. Possible faster cycle times, creating increased revenues if the product is in demand.

2. Improve Regulatory Compliance

A properly validated computer system controlling a piece of equipment will ensure that the material produced will always be within specification. In addition, the validated system can be certain of producing the correct documentation to support the Quality Assurance (QA) release of the finished product.

3. Product Consistency and Quality

A properly automated piece of equipment consistently mimics the performance of "the best operator on his best day." This means that the equipment should be capable of producing product of the highest possible quality on a consistent basis.

4. Process Security and Reliability

Automation of a process can lessen the possibility that process upsets occur. If they do occur, the process controller can ensure that the upset does not go undocumented.

It is incumbent on the persons justifying automation on a particular project to quantify the benefits from automation as outlined above.

This is not the whole story, however. The categories described above reflect automation of standalone pieces of equipment or processes. The integration of different systems into a coherent whole can provide benefits, in addition to those stated above, to operations far beyond what the individual "islands of automation" can do on their own.

Systems integration is of vital importance because it takes account of the overall business goals of the manufacturing facility. Its stated goal is usually to improve the facility bottom line over the long term by facilitating increases in revenues and decreases in costs. Individual islands of automation will deliver benefits to the areas being automated. Those benefits can be small in comparison to those delivered when such islands of automation begin to talk to one another.

IV. WHAT ARE THE BENEFITS OF SYSTEMS INTEGRATION?

Some of the benefits of automation have been outlined above. This section will address the additional benefits that a manufacturing site can gain from the proper implementation of integration between different systems.

1. Integrity of electronic communication of critical information between systems. Often it is vital that accurate information is communicated between two different systems. When this communication is performed manually (e.g., if an operator jots down information from one system and manually keys it into another), there is a good deal of scope for error. Good planning and integration of such systems can eliminate these errors, and the integrity of communication of these data can be maintained.
2. Improved regulatory compliance. If integrated systems are properly validated, it is possible to ensure that data passing between systems will always maintain their integrity. A manual transfer of data from one system to another may not stand up as easily to regulatory scrutiny. Manual Standard Operating Procedures (SOPs) must be adhered to at all times when data are being moved between standalone systems. Advance validation planning for systems integration, therefore, is the key to delivering systems integration capable of being fully validated.
3. Improvement in productivity over standalone systems. When data are transferred electronically between systems in a properly validated environment, enormous labor savings can result. There is no need to transfer the data manually between the systems using clipboards. There is no need to physically check that the data have been transferred, because

the system takes care of that. There is no need to manually execute an approval cycle to confirm the data transfer, as this can be done electronically. In addition, benefits can be gained in product cycle times. In some cases at SB, communication and approval of sample quality data from the process areas to a LIMS could take several days. With the implementation and validation of electronic data interchange between LIMS and a process DCS, the communication and approval cycle can be completed in a matter of minutes. When a product is in demand in the marketplace, this kind of systems integration can have a huge impact on the bottom line.

Sometimes, unexpected benefits can result from automation and systems integration. On one SB automation project, there was a significant product yield improvement from the newly automated process, even though the justification for the project was based on product quality and regulatory compliance. Fortunately, a sudden, significant increase in demand occurred for the product after project completion and the automated process was more than capable of absorbing it.

Nonetheless, the difficulty remains in justifying automation projects (and even more so systems integration projects) due to the sometimes high up-front costs. This is why it is important to have a coherent systems integration plan for a facility; this will allow systems integration to be developed carefully over time rather than having haphazard, possibly inefficient solutions at single points in the process.

V. WHAT ARE THE MAIN CHARACTERISTICS OF AN INFORMATION SYSTEMS PLAN?

This can be determined by obtaining answers to some pertinent questions, including those below.

A. What Is the Long-Term Business Plan of the Facility?

Both new and existing manufacturing facilities will have a long-term business plan. In SB this is called a 10 > 3/1 plan. It outlines where the facility would like to be in ten years and what needs to be accomplished in the medium term (three years) and the short term (one year) in order for the ten-year goal to become a reality. This plan addresses areas such as the following:

- Facility expansion
- Retrofits for new processes, based on anticipated changes in customer requirements
- Modifications to existing processes (e.g., combining steps)
- Projected facility and people requirements for existing and future products

- Cost reduction philosophy
- Product quality goals
- Continuous improvement goals

The IS plan must ultimately be in agreement with the 10 > 3/1 plan for the facility.

B. What Are the Regulatory Requirements of the Facility?

The validation requirements of the facility must be determined when embarking on an IS plan. Is this an FDA, CBER (Center for Biologicals Evaluation and Research), or CDER (Center for Drug Evaluation and Research) regulated facility? Authors of an IS plan must be aware of what processes are under regulatory control, and how information from those areas is processed in the development of batch reports. They should understand what the compliance issues are for a site to receive regulatory approval for computer systems controlling "Good Manufacturing Practices" (GMP) processes. In addition, future regulatory requirements (e.g., what the FDA rules will be for electronic batch records) must be anticipated.

C. What Information Systems Are Covered by the Scope of the Plan?

Some IS plans undertake more than others. It is important to develop the scope of the plan early in the undertaking. Some questions that should be asked include the following:

- What areas of the facility will be covered?
- Will it just be the processing areas or will all plant computer systems in the facility fall under the plan?
- What external systems are in place today that interface with the facility (e.g., companywide MRP2)?
- What external systems will be implemented/upgraded over the life of the plan and how should they be integrated?

In many cases today it is imperative to include all site computer systems in a single plan, because one day they may be all linked together somehow. However, it is also important to be realistic about what can be achieved with the available resources when putting together a plan.

D. What Is the Current Situation at an Existing Facility?

Of key importance is determining the current level of instrumentation in key process areas. In addition, the establishment of a baseline for computer systems at an existing facility is important.

1. For Instruments

- What is the current level of instrumentation in each area?
- What will be the level of instrumentation required to provide the most benefit to the plan?
- How soon should this be implemented?
- What are the budgetary constraints?
- What are the facility instrumentation constraints?

2. For Computers

- What current systems (if any) are in place on the plant floor?
- If there are any, are they standalone or integrated in any way?
- What brand names are they? Are they compatible?
- What information is required from and by such systems?
- How is information communicated to and from these systems?
- What office and mainframe applications interface with the manufacturing process?
- What other areas have computer applications? Warehouse? Maintenance? Effluent treatment?
- What outside systems (e.g., corporate mainframe) does the site interface with?

E. What Is the Systems Goal of the Facility?

Plant operations must agree where their facility would like to be in, say, ten years. Often it is the responsibility of the IS planners to initiate this step, because they will have a good understanding of future systems pathways. As with all technology, however (and particularly with computers), this involves a certain amount of risk. What future computer functionality will be available at that time is unknown, and no one wants to be tied down to ''archaic'' systems that seem state of the art today. A diagrammatic example of how a facility could formulate a ten-year plan is provided in Fig. 1 (discussed in Section VII. B).

F. What Are the High Priorities?

When a systems baseline for the facility has been established, it is possible to establish priorities. In fact, priorities usually become very obvious during discussions about the current situation of a facility. For example, if a plant process has very little instrumentation and plant management wants it to be fully automated in ten years, a strong, early emphasis on instrumentation becomes imperative. If, on the other hand, a facility contains a significant base of standalone PLCs, a priority might be to establish if the PLCs should talk to each other, and if they do, how to make it happen.

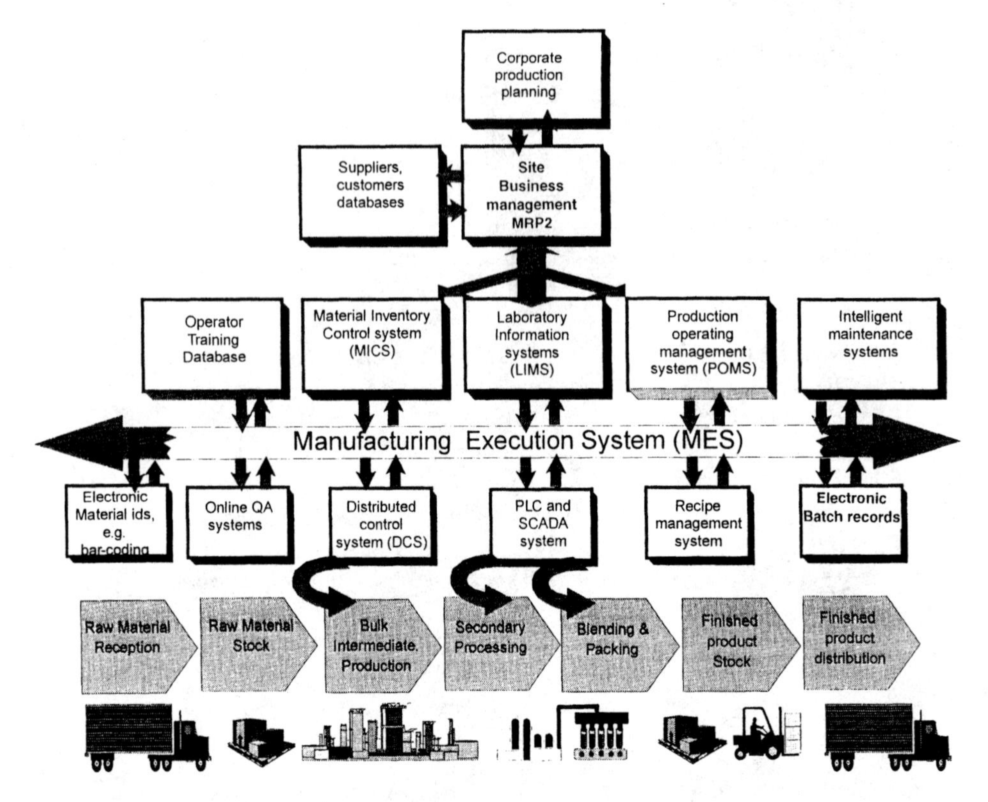

Fig. 1 Diagram of penicillin plant ten-year automation vision.

G. What Are the Low Priorities?

It is important to integrate into an IS plan those items that are not required immediately. One way to do this is to establish a "needs" and a "wants" list. The needs will appear in the list of high priorities. The wants should be categorized differently. The wants can be determined by analysis of the site master plan and future spending projections.

An example of a need versus a want in a facility might be the integration of a DCS and a LIMS. If a new, FDA-regulated manufacturing facility is being built, it is likely that for many reasons, DCS (or PLC/Sequential Control and Data Acquisition (SCADA)) control of the process would be seen as a need. In addition, justification could easily be found for the automated management of lab information at a new facility using a LIMS; hence it could be seen as a need.

The facility might find it desirable to have the DCS and the LIMS communicate electronically in a validated environment. The benefit would be the instantaneous transfer of process analysis information between the systems, quite possibly resulting in greater integrity and reduced batch cycle time. However, it would be more difficult to justify the integration of a DCS (or PLC/Sequential Control and Data Acquisition (SCADA)) and LIMS at this stage in the life of a facility. In addition to the expense, the work involved in the start-up could delay the project. If, however, the ultimate goal of the new facility is complete systems integration, it is important to state in the IS planning document how and when this will be done later. This will permit plant management to align future budgets and staff resources for such a project at a later date.

H. What Are the Hardware/Platform Issues?

One of the benefits of IS planning is that it provides an opportunity to plan for systems to be on similar hardware platforms. In many existing facilities, systems managers spend much of their time learning about different platforms, databases, and operating systems. Trying to integrate systems with such inherent differences can be a nightmare.

In a new facility or an expansion, IS planners may be able to determine up front if different systems can operate on the same operating platform. An example of this might be a DCS and a LIMS that operate in either an open VMS or a UNIX environment. It makes sense to decide early on in a project whether it is worthwhile that these two applications should be on the same platform. If according to the plan they are to be integrated later (so that the two systems can communicate electronically), then serious consideration should be given to having them on the same platform. This will save time, money, and headaches when the plan is being implemented later.

I. What Are the Budget and Resource Constraints?

As always, budgets and resources need to be given full consideration. The following questions should be asked of the site:

- Is there money to do the IS plan?
- Who will be the site contact?
- What is the capital budget strategy over the next ten years? Expansion? Consolidation?
- What level of capital spending has occurred in the last two to three years?

An IS plan must be aligned with the way a facility intends to manage its capital budget. Reviews of the IS plan should take place with this in mind (e.g., submit the plan for approval before the budget is "set in stone").

In addition, personnel and training requirements must be established. What training will staff need to come up to speed with all developments? Also, a human resources plan should be obtained to establish what the site philosophy will be over the next ten years (e.g., with regard to unions or how operators' duties will change with increasing technology).

VI. WHAT IS AN APPROPRIATE METHODOLOGY FOR PREPARING AND IMPLEMENTING AN INFORMATION SYSTEMS PLAN?

The following process is one that has been used successfully at SB. It assumes that sufficient money and resources have been made available to do the work.

A. Initiation

The following steps should be taken to initiate a study to develop a site IS plan.

1. *Meet with Site Leaders*

- Meet site management to explore its requirements.
- Document what it expects from an IS plan.
- Explain what will be required of it. (This is outlined further later in this section.)

2. *Plan a Site Visit*

- Plan a site "survey" visit to assess the current situation and prepare a detailed agenda for that visit.
- Agree with site personnel who the key people are for information gathering.
- Obtain the agreement of key people to participate in the study.
- Communicate to the site the intent of the survey and the plan.

B. The Site Survey

A typical site IS survey might proceed as follows.

1. *Conduct a Site Survey*

- Prepare a brief presentation to site management to kick off the visit
- Spend thirty to forty-five minutes with key personnel (as agreed with site) in the following areas:
- Production/operations
- Engineering
- Maintenance
- Environmental/safety
- Quality Control and Quality Assurance (QC/QA)
- Inventory management/warehouse
- Human resources
- Finance

The questions asked should be developed in advance for each area, using Section V as a guide.

2. *Prepare a Site Visit Report*

- Briefly summarize the events that took place during the visit (a page or two, issue as soon as possible after visit).
- Outline the schedule of events to follow (including any follow-up visits, phone calls, and other action items).
- Let the site know when a detailed report will be first drafted.

3. *Develop an Outline of the Plan*

- Create a table of contents for review by the site (within a couple of weeks of the visit).
- Obtain site approval for the table of contents.

C. Putting Together the Report

1. *Resources and Schedule*

- Determine the resources available to write appropriate sections of the plan (e.g., Do we have the right MES person to write that part?).
- Agree on a realistic schedule and communicate this to the site.

2. *Communication with the Site*

- Set up appropriate communication with the site to obtain follow-up information from survey.
- Determine any outside vendors or resources that will be needed.

3. *Preparation of the First Draft*

- Ensure each section is written by the responsible person in the time allotted.
- Review each section for completeness and overlap with other sections.
- Have a neutral person review the report prior to issuing the first draft.
- First draft preparation of a comprehensive report for a medium-sized pharmaceutical manufacturing facility should take about a month.

4. *First Draft: Issuance and Follow-up*

- Allow two to three weeks for site to review first draft of document.
- Arrange brief meeting with site to discuss first draft. (One site representative may be enough.)

  Has the draft met expectations so far?
  Does it address the priority areas in the right way?

Is it specific enough? Too general?
Does it take full account of the current plant business environment?

5. *Subsequent and Final Drafts*

- As in the first draft, commit to a specific completion schedule for each draft.
- Try to make as few drafts as possible.
- Issue the final plan report, keeping the budget cycle in mind.

D. Plan Upkeep and Change Control

- Ensure that the plan has a version number so that changes to the plan can be recorded and old versions archived.
- Give ownership of the plan to a facility representative and ensure that any changes in philosophy are recorded.

E. Next Steps

It is important to remember that the ten-year plan is a living document. It must be modified from time to time to reflect the rapidly changing face of the facility's business environment. That is why plant ownership of the document and good change control are essential.

Bear in mind that this is a ten-year plan. Consideration must be given, therefore, to what plans should be made in the three-year and one-year time frames in order to meet the ten-year goals.

1. *The "Three-Year" Plan*

To draw up a three-year (or medium-term) plan for systems integration, much the same methodology will be adopted as has been described above; however, the three-year plan will be much more specific. It will describe what level of automation will have been achieved after three years. For this type of plan, budget planning could begin almost immediately. The following should be given consideration.

a. Who Should Write the Three-Year Plan? Consideration should be given to having either a systems vendor or a knowledgeable, experienced consultant prepare the three-year systems plan. The vendor or consultant should be conversant with current hardware, software, and systems issues in the facility environment. This will be especially true if the vendor or consultant has previous experience of systems integration at that site.

The involvement of site personnel is of vital importance at this stage. No longer are "Star Trek" requirements being mooted; concrete proposals are being generated that will soon affect the capital budget profile of the facility, and hard justifications will be sought by plant management for such spends.

b. How Detailed Should the Three-Year Plan Be? The facility should be very clear about its requirements from a three-year systems integration study. Questions that should be asked in advance of starting such a study could include the following:

- What level of detail is required by management?
- How much money will have to be spent in order to satisfactorily reach this level of detail?
- Should the study be throughout the plant, or just a small process section?
- Should the study ask hard questions about perceived problems with facility ''legacy'' systems? (If yes, don't ''expose'' your vendor or consultant. Back them up!)
- What should the eventual output of the three-year plan be? Enough detail to go for a project proposal to management?

2. The One-Year Plan

As its name suggests, the purpose of this plan is to ensure that systems integration projects that are already in the budget fit with the three- and ten-year plans. It is really a check of the existing plant IS plan.

VII. EXAMPLES OF EXISTING INFORMATION SYSTEMS PLANS AT SB

Two examples of IS plans will be described here. One was created for a new biotech manufacturing facility that broke ground in April 1995, and the other was created for a penicillin formulation facility which celebrated its twenty-fifth anniversary in 1993.

Each plan will be described briefly, and the issues surrounding the preparation of each plan will be outlined. Some comparisons and contrasts will be drawn between the two plans.

A. New Biotech Manufacturing Facility: Ten-Year Automation Philosophy

This plan was based on the anticipated automation needs of a multipurpose ''market entry'' biotech manufacturing facility. Design of the facility began in early 1994, and construction began in April 1995. The following issues and concerns drove the creation of the document:

- This is a ''green field'' site. There were opportunities to ''do things properly'' on this project that were not available at existing sites.

- In the hiring process for site personnel, people with systems experience were brought on board early. No ''retraining'' was required.
- While there was the chance to avoid the integration problems that plague other sites, there was still a budget to be adhered to. The design philosophy of the building was very much ''Buick'' rather than ''Cadillac.'' This was reflected in the automation philosophy.
- Early on in the design it was decided that the process would be controlled using a DCS. This was because similar pilot plant processes had been successfully automated using a DCS in the past.
- Around the time the design began, SB signed a preferred vendor agreement with a DCS vendor. This permitted the automation philosophy (and hence the design) to be done around that system.
- The facility will be a multipurpose, market entry manufacturing plant for a suite of biotech products in SB's R&D pipeline at time of writing.
- The automation philosophy delineated a phased plan for automation as follows:
  1. The initial phase (to be executed as an integral part of the construction and startup of the building) addresses implementation of DCS, PLC, LIMS, a warehouse management system (WMS) with bar code readers, and a building automation system (BAS). There will be very limited integration between these systems, because the priority is to get them up and running so that product can be made as soon as possible. However the DCS and LIMS have been specified on the same hardware platform (open VMS), allowing relative ease of future integration. The WMS was specified to communicate with SB's corporate MRP2 solution. (See Tables 2–4 for a matrix defining what level of integration would take place during this and subsequent phases.)
  2. Phase two of systems integration had two goals: complete the automation of the manufacturing process and plan for the integration of man-

Table 2 Systems Integration during Phase 1

	DCS	PLC	BAS	LIMS	WMS	MES	MRP2
DCS	—	Yes	No	Yes	Yes	Yes	Yes
PLC	Yes	—	No	No	No	Yes	No
BAS	No	No	—	No	No	Yes	No
LIMS	Yes	No	No	—	Yes	Yes	Yes
WMS	Yes	No	No	Yes	—	Yes	Yes
MES	Yes	Yes	Yes	Yes	Yes	—	Yes
MRP2	Yes	No	No	Yes	Yes	Yes	—

Table 3 Systems Integration during Phase 2

	DCS	PLC	BAS	LIMS	WMS	MES	MRP2
DCS	—	Yes	No	No	No	No	No
PLC	Yes	—	No	No	No	No	No
BAS	No	No	—	No	No	No	No
LIMS	No	No	No	—	Yes	No	No
WMS	No	No	No	Yes	—	No	Yes
MES	No	No	No	No	No	—	No

Table 4 Systems Integration during Phase 3

	DCS	PLC	BAS	LIMS	WMS	MES	MRP2
DCS	—	Yes	Yes	Yes*	Yes*	Yes*	Yes
PLC	Yes	—	No	No	No	No	No
BAS	Yes	No	—	No	No	No	No
LIMS	Yes*	No	No	—	Yes	Yes*	Yes
WMS	Yes*	No	No	Yes	—	Yes*	Yes
MES	Yes*	No	No	Yes*	Yes*	—	Yes

*Asterisk indicates further integration that will be in place as a result of phase 2.

ufacturing execution systems. Both of these goals will be accomplished after the facility has been started up. Some process areas were deliberately omitted from the scope of automation during phase 1. These would be handled after start-up under a separate justification. MES will require justification also, along with a careful analysis of SB's needs in this complex area.

3. The goal of the third phase of automation is to have a high level of systems integration in order to deliver the final product with maximum efficiency. Ultimately, a single, common facility database will exist for the process, labs, utilities, warehouse, and production. Batches will be scheduled, monitored, and analyzed automatically.

Table 2 is a matrix that defines the level of systems integration that will be in place for the biopharmaceutical manufacturing facility by the year 2005 (ten-year plan).

Table 3 describes what level of systems integration will have been achieved upon completion of the first phase of the automation of the new biopharm facility.

Table 4 describes the level of systems integration that is planned to be in place upon completion of the second phase of the automation of the new biopharm facility.

B. Existing Penicillin Manufacturing Facility: Ten-Year Computer Integrated Manufacturing Vision

This plan was prepared for an existing single-product penicillin manufacturing and formulation facility that has undergone significant changes in its twenty-five-year history. The facility uses an intermediate from another SB facility as a raw material, and processes it into a final product that is packaged on site. At the time the plan was issued, some of the overriding facility issues were as follows:

- Some equipment and instrumentation in the facility is antiquated. In some areas there is no instrumentation at all.
- There are pieces of equipment (e.g., centrifuges) and areas of the facility (e.g., utilities) that have standalone control systems (PLCs, controllers). There is no integration between these systems.
- A small DCS was installed to control a sterile spray drying operation in the plant. It is planned to expand this to a larger DCS application covering other manufacturing areas on the same platform.
- It is planned to implement a pilot MES application at this facility over the next two years.

The ten-year plan for the automation of the facility appears diagramatically in Fig. 1, which demonstrates how a systems architecture was developed following discussions with plant management and operations. In addition it shows how systems integration helps drive the delivery of the product to the customer.

Fig. 2 graphically demonstrates what is planned for plant floor automation in the ten-year plan.

C. How Do These Two Plans Compare and Contrast?

At first sight both these facilities appear to have very different automation philosophies. One is a green field site where upfront systems planning will have very predictable results. As yet, there is no "installed base" of systems to reckon with, nor is retraining of personnel a big issue. In addition, attaining synergy between different systems (e.g., having the DCS and the LIMS on the same hardware platform) in a green field site can be a relatively straightforward matter.

In addition, people in a new facility tend to have open minds about what IS can do for them, budget constraints notwithstanding.

However, it can be difficult to plan for systems in a green field site if key area managers have not yet been appointed. Production, QA, and engineering management play a key role in systems planning, and it is of vital importance to have their early buy-in.

In the existing facility, the key question that must be dealt with when plan-

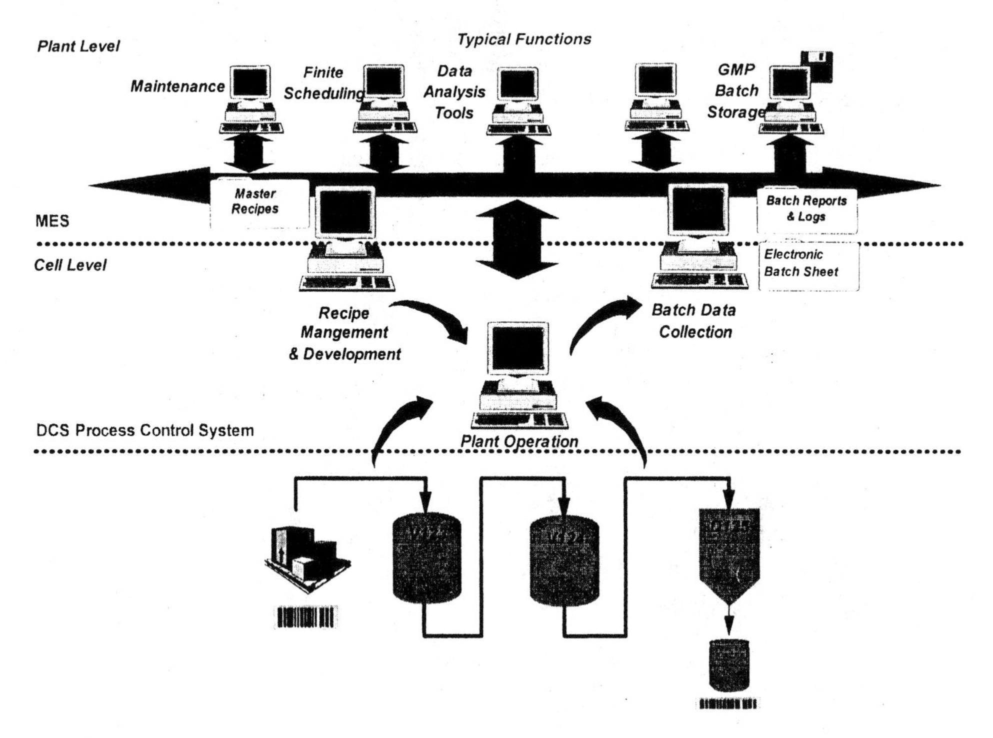

Fig. 2 Systems architecture for bulk processing area—penicillin plant.

ning IS is, "Where does the facility want to go, based on what is in place already?" This can cause IS planning to become quite complicated.

Also, in an existing facility it can be difficult to explain to people the benefits of automation if they feel their jobs are potentially at risk. That is one of the reasons "plant ownership" of the plan is of key importance.

Existing facilities, however, have a management structure in place that has the power to make timely decisions about the future of systems at the plant. Management has ownership of the 10 > 3/1 plans that the IS plan must blend with in order to meet the business goals of the facility.

The methodology for creating an IS plan should not vary that much between a new and an existing facility. Some areas that work in one plan may not be necessary in another, but if the steps outlined in Section VI are addressed, a thorough analysis of IS needs at any facility can be produced.

VIII. CONCLUSIONS

- In a manufacturing environment of increasing complexity and automation, IS planning is becoming a high priority.

- Information systems planning can help avoid one of manufacturing's bigger problems today, the "hodgepodge" of legacy and standalone systems found in plants. Many of these "point solutions" create bigger problems than they solve in the long run.
- Systems integration (resulting from good IS planning) can yield significant payback for a manufacturing facility in the areas of increased efficiency and productivity, operating cost savings, and better adherence to regulatory controls.
- An IS plan for a manufacturing facility should take account of areas such as the long-term business plan of the facility, the current situation (if any), site regulatory needs, the goals and scope of the systems plan, and budget/resource issues.
- For any facility, it should be possible to follow a relatively straightforward methodology to develop the IS plan.

BIBLIOGRAPHY

Cubberly, W. H. *Comprehensive Dictionary of Measurement and Control*, 2nd ed., Instrument Society of America (ISA) Publications, 1991.

Adler, D. J., J. A. Herkamp, J. R. Wiesler, and S. B. Williams, "Life Cycle Cost and Benefits of Process Automation in Bulk Pharmaceuticals," Advances in Instrumentation and Control, presented at Instrument Society of America (ISA) show, Anaheim, California, Oct. 23–28, 1994.

Considine, D. M. *Process/Industrial Instruments & Controls Handbook*, 4th ed., McGraw-Hill, 1993.

Micklovic, D. T. *Real-Time Control Networks*, ISA Resources for Measurement and Control Series, 1993.

3

Information Technology Planning for Electronic Batch Record Operations

Joseph F. deSpautz

INCODE Corp., Herndon, Virginia

I. PHARMACEUTICAL INDUSTRY CHALLENGES

Historically, manufacturers of health care products have focused their investments on research and development (R&D) for competitive advantage. Changes in the worldwide market for health care products are forcing manufacturers to focus on the supply chain to lower costs, reduce order and manufacturing cycle times, and enhance customer service while maintaining or improving quality and regulatory compliance.

Market pressures, increased quality, profitability, and enhanced regulatory compliance are the primary manufacturing challenges that support supply chain strategies. Business strategies are being coupled to create complex manufacturing objectives. Business issues are placing demands on existing information technology infrastructures and people, considered by many to be the most important asset in these times (1).

A number of research studies and surveys conclude or confirm that the key investment drivers in manufacturing across all health care product segments are (2–4) the following:

- Validation
- Document management
- Production management
- Production optimization
- Manufacturing costs

The manufacturing issues are linked to validation and document management on the plant floor as batch record operations, manufacturing unit operation verification, data recording, and quality test results are all required to meet U.S. Food and Drug Administration (FDA) current good manufacturing practices (cGMP) compliance and product quality standards. Automation is one of the keys to improving productivity and efficiency, and maintaining quality, providing such benefits as the following (2,5–10):

- Improved batch record accuracy
- Reduced labor costs
- Improved record keeping
- Improved speed of batch release records
- Facilitating FDA approvals

Considering that automation projects can be multiyear efforts, and integrated pharmaceutical information technology strategy is essential. These manufacturing automation projects have to be successful and yield the return on investments that are anticipated by management. Proliferation of these systems will continue to grow in the coming years.

II. INCREASING PRESSURES ACROSS THE SUPPLY CHAIN

Customers are demanding access to the greatest variety of products and packaging delivered to them in the fastest possible time at minimum cost. Reductions in worldwide cost of sales is occurring while organizations are developing methods to integrate common and sometimes redundant facilities. Integration of complementary organizations to make an efficient supply chain organization are occurring as a result of mergers and acquisitions. Rationalization and divestiture strategies are happening simultaneously.

A number of global process manufacturers have active information systems (IS) plans to implement critical enterprise resource planning (ERP) business functions to support supply chain initiatives. One component of the IS strategy is integrating the ERP business applications to the plants' manufacturing systems, manufacturing execution systems (MES), distributed control systems (DCS), scheduling, and so forth for real-time information sharing and decision support.

Competitive pressures are requiring more efficient use of manufacturing capacities by extending and improving existing process lines and facilities, eliminating bottlenecks, and efficiently using people. Introduction of DCS, supervisory control, bar code devices, programmable logic controllers (PLC), and preventive rather than corrective equipment maintenance systems are some of the application areas being addressed. Paperless environments or electronic batch record operations are being considered as a necessity for competitive manufacturing. Pharmaceutical companies are striving to support shorter order times or ''time to market'' to increase customer service and satisfaction.

Quality initiatives to provide higher yields and more consistent products are part of the strategy to maintain profitability. Stated goals of some companies include the achievement of a twenty-four-hour cycle time metric. With a national average for all manufacturing of eighty hours of queue and delay time for each hour of value added labor, there are many areas for improvement. Information integration allowing quicker access of necessary documentation, increasing manufacturing flexibility, eliminating redundant data entries, and automating manufacturing positions are operational areas that are being investigated to support these manufacturing objectives.

III. MAINTENANCE OF QUALITY

Obviously, product quality and consistency are the most important critical success factors in pharmaceutical operations. Statistical process control (SPC) and statistical quality control (SQC) are programs that are being implemented to support multiple business issues. Reducing the cost of nonconformance is being addressed by coupling process control and quality assurance (QA). Through real-time scheduling of the process with the quality laboratory, visibility of the process is improved by making information available to operators in ''near real time.'' This enables the development of analytical and in-line process control and optimization efforts to improve yields and process conformance.

Getting it right the first time by developing the appropriate documentation needed during pilot operations can be achieved by bringing together production engineering, process engineering, and research with manufacturing. Integrated information with access by all is required for this type of concurrent development.

IV. cGMP CONFORMANCE FOR NEW SYSTEMS

Compliance with cGMPs is a constant obligation. As operations initiates new programs, adherence to standards and quality procedures is required. As an example, cGMPs require that more than 100 different kinds of approved written procedures exist and be followed. Additionally there are eleven references in section 211 of 21CFR that would potentially influence electronic records and electronic signatures. Associations and manufacturing groups have and still have a keen interest in electronic records, identification, and signatures. There was a large response to the advanced notice of proposed rulemaking (ANPRM) for proposed rule changes for electronic records; electronic signatures. On March 20, 1997, the FDA issued its final ruling resulting in the present guidelines for electronic records and electronic signatures. MES process control, testing, and quality systems are introduced, they may require system-extensive validation protocols and efforts, especially to support electronic batch record operations (11).

V. ALIGNED MANUFACTURING OBJECTIVES FOR PROFITABILITY

Manufacturing objectives are being aligned to support corporate business strategies. Reduced manufacturing costs and increased profitability are being achieved by applying manufacturing resource planning (MRP-II) through corporate, divisional, and plantwide planning systems. Just in time (JIT) techniques are being applied to reduce work in process (WIP) inventories and increase shelf life. Shrinking manufacturing cycle times by eliminating scheduling queues and data transfer delays are being planned through real-time scheduling of quality testing with production.

The use of electronic batch record (EBR) systems throughout the life cycle of documentation is an important objective in the industry today. With the continued recognition that an empowered workforce is an essential part of the change, improved visibility and control of the entire manufacturing process is being required through the electronic access of information and documentation.

VI. ORGANIZATIONAL DYNAMICS

There is a top-down push to have more information available to more workers to support manufacturing objectives through better decision making, process optimization, and responsiveness to customer queries. Plant operations are creating a ''bottoms-up'' demand to have systems support manufacturing operations rather than corporate management information systems (MIS) functions. MIS budgets are remaining relatively flat according to the latest market research studies. Budgetary constraints and ''right-sized'' MIS staffs have resulted in less support for existing corporate systems, an emphasis on ''packaged'' solutions to manufacturing issues, and a greater empowerment of end user communities.

Information technology (I/T) is becoming the framework for manufacturing automation strategies because timely, accurate, and auditable information is essential in this highly regulated industry. This I/T framework has to support business objectives by being flexible, capable of growing to meet increasing demands for information and reporting, and permitting the sensible inclusion of new information technology that may be required by manufacturing. Because there are equipment, process lines, automation, I/T solutions, documentation, and operators on the plant floor, a convenient term for discussing these generators and users of information is process control system.

VII. OPERATIONAL INTEGRATION

For operational integration to achieve world-class performance, it must include consideration of the company's business issues, organizations of direct and indirect people, and existing I/T infrastructure. Information availability and accessibility are the basic requirements needed to support business issues. Manufacturing, logistics, sales, marketing, and customer service must have demand access to the information that they need. To support global operations, the information distribution services must be networked throughout the organization. The services must support the variety of devices on each user's desktop: Microsoft NT, MS-DOS, OS/2, UNIX, workstation, radio frequency terminal, and so forth.

People are the critical element of the success of this integration schema. Technology must support users by providing efficient and understandable interfaces for the plethora of applications that people will have to use in their expanded roles. The I/T framework will have to support the inquiry-based information needs of today knowing that these needs will change. Operational integration requires education and training at all levels in the organization. This will ensure that the common corporate vision is understood by all levels of the organization and that the applications will truly be used to run the business.

VIII. MAKING INFORMATION TECHNOLOGY WORK FOR OPERATIONS

An I/T strategy will need to integrate information from quality, manufacturing, management, and corporate systems for everyone to use. Specific information will have to be integrated in a disciplined, auditable way that supports cGMP compliance. Capabilities that are key to a successful strategy and resulting implementation framework include the following:

- Recognizing that "it's the application that matters"
- Allowing distributed multivendor systems
- Opening system network and platform architecture
- Supporting client/server and other computing styles
- Being compliant and supporting industry standards
- Allowing protection of investments
- Being flexible to accommodate growth and change
- Making computer validation an integral part of the application life cycle

The framework must support the I/T elements of three domains—enterprise, plant or execution, and control. (See Fig. 1.) The enterprise includes the interfacing and interoperability of business applications, such as ERP and MRPII; functional manufacturing logic for operations, manual and semiautomatic work instructions, and batch record creation on the plant floor and MES; and

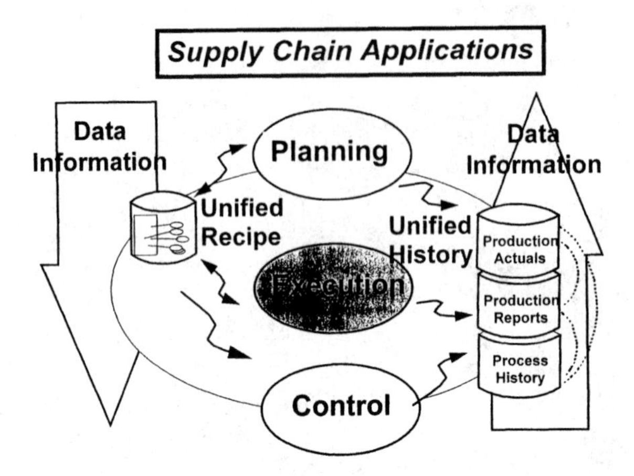

Fig. 1 Pharmaceutical information technology domains.

synchronized process operations of automated and semiautomatic processes residing in the control domain. Traditionally, I/T planning has ignored the MES and control domains.

Compliance to industry standards will promote efficient system design practices for in-house developments. Conformance or future migration to standards can be used to influence software application vendors. Facilitation of integration through the use of common data management technologies will allow a ''remove and replace'' environment once the overall system is validated. Investment protection in existing systems can be achieved while taking advantage of emerging technology as new systems are developed using the same standards.

IX. VALIDATED SYSTEMS ARE REQUIRED FOR REGULATORY COMPLIANCE

All compliance documentation must be maintained according to cGMP throughout their life cycles; therefore, the computer systems that produce the documentation must meet the system validation criteria throughout operations as defined by validation manuals and plans. This commitment to validation being an essential component of the I/T strategy, it is then built into application; it cannot be added after installation. Using this integration platform, enterprise-level systems can be effectively implemented within regulatory compliance environments—and the cost, time, and resources requirements are kept to a minimum. Configuration

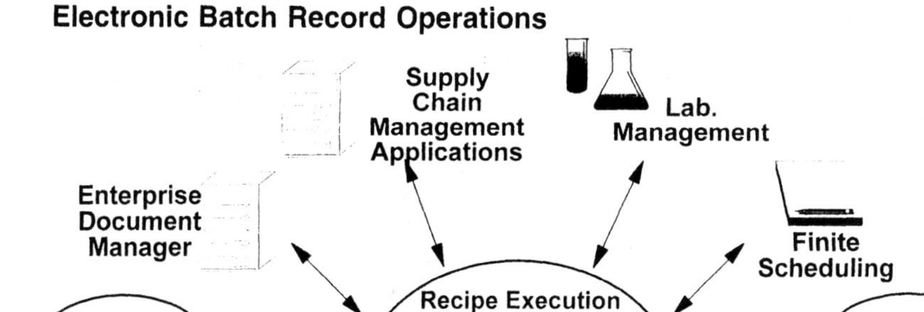

Fig. 2 Pharmaceutical data model.

management, documented standards, quality assurance procedures and standards for software maintenance and development, and testing tools are elements of the life cycle methodology.

X. PHARMACEUTICAL MANUFACTURING DATA MODEL

From a functional perspective, the I/T framework translates to a data model to support the operational strategies developed to comply with the company's business directives. This data modeling strategy supports operations as well as interoperability to the other business functions. (See Fig. 2.)

A manufacturing data model for all shared manufacturing and production information facilitates information access across the organization. This data model can be an amalgam of models for manufacturing resource planning, enterprise planning, laboratory management, and document management from different application providers.

At the center of the strategy is the data warehouse of the company's shared information needed for manufacturing, quality, and business functions. Applications will still maintain its own data structures, while 10 to 20 percent of the

Table 1 Production Documentation

Information types	Responsible department	Document sources
Formulation material usage	Process development	Standard formula
Batch record	Quality	Product formulation
Master device record	Technical services	SOPs
Equipment maintenance profiles	Process engineering	Equipment logs
Operating parameters	Process engineering	Validation profiles
Quality standards	Quality assurance	Product monographs
Cost data	Accounting Production	MES collection systems
Setup instructions	Production	Set up SOPs
Labeling specifications	QA Labeling development	Approved text Artwork
Quality test procedures	Quality control	Laboratory records
Policies/procedures	Administration	Company documents Personnel information
Completed batch record device history record	Production	Plant operations Process monitoring MES equipment
Safety/hazard	Safety Health Environment	MSDSs Safety/hazard SOPs

data to be shared will be maintained in the data warehouse. There can be many information sources distributed throughout the organization. This information will be defined by a common data dictionary. Relational database technology is the basis of the data warehouse.

XI. PRODUCTION RECORD KEEPING FOR REGULATED INDUSTRIES

Compliance with cGMPs is a constant obligation in all regulated industries, including ethicals, OTC, biologics, diagnostics, veterinary, medical devices, and consumer packaged goods. Table 1 shows the responsible departments and document sources to control documentation throughout its life cycle—from design to creation, activation, revision, and archiving. These control activities include access security, revision and change control, review and approval cycles, maintenance of product approval lists, signatures, second person verification and approvals, and maintaining secure audit trails of activities to support cGMPs.

Schuber (12) outlines an implementation to support document requirements at a high-volume manufacturing facility, noting the extensive paper documentation that must be addressed. (See Table 1.)

XII. PROCESS GENERATES DOCUMENTATION FOR LOT RELEASE

Many of these documents are developed as a result of the actual process from assays analysis, laboratory testing, actual variances in materials, process and results, and exception reporting from manual operations. A typical completed batch record or device history record contains two to four times more information (and is therefore two to four times larger) than the original master batch or device record. These records must be captured in a validated computer environment to support cGMP. Some of the information must be passed back to the business systems for analysis, archiving, and control. The complete record must be maintained for lot or batch tracking and release of product to the manufacturer's customers. As international health, North American Free Trade Agreement (NAFTA), and FDA issues and regulations change in such areas as product performance and distribution documentation, a complete production record must be maintained to ensure accuracy of information. Many products have multiyear product lot releases that must maintain document continuity.

XIII. PHARMACEUTICAL INDUSTRY DICTIONARY: DATA DEFINITIONS AND STRUCTURES

During development, pilot phase, document development, and the production process, a wealth of data is accumulated on procedures, materials, machines, people, costs, quality control (QC), quality assurance (QA), operating environment, and so forth. Unfortunately, most of these vital data are stored in paper documents and are not readily available for development, decision support, or in-process analysis.

The shared data warehouse would form a ''holding area'' for operational information to support real-time and ad hoc needs. For example, the data extracted from corporate systems, as well as process or work position data (from the batch record), would be instantly available for use in quality analysis, process optimization, finite scheduling, customer service, and so on.

Use of a data warehouse model does not require the conversion of existing applications' data structures to any specific data product set. Standard database access protocols will be used to transfer data to and from the data warehouse. It is the integration of the applications or functions that occurs through the shared data.

XIV. I/T SERVICES TO SUPPORT THE STRATEGY

Repository services that are networked throughout the organization to allow storage, translation, data conversion, and presentation services to users and applications

An electronic batch record system (EBRS) capable of supporting current and future document requirements

A document management system for all production-related documentation (including complete document control capabilities) that supports regulatory requirements

Support for existing applications and future applications that are needed for world-class manufacturing and performance

XV. REPOSITORY SERVICES PROVIDE THE LINKAGE

Access to information should be independent of an application, a user's desktop device, or the operating system. Information should be accessible anywhere on the network.

Multiple applications on separate systems can deposit, extract, and exchange data using the data dictionary and the repository services. Applications can act as either "creators" or "consumers" of shared information. They can easily exchange vital information, yet perform their primary functions completely independently of each other. For example, a laboratory information management system (LIMS) can exchange sample testing status with an MES workstation for in-line operator control and processing in order to maintain the real-time status of a batch.

Functional integration is achieved in the data warehouse using standard repository services. Desktop users having any type of presentation device may access information stored in any information source. The repository services will locate the information, transmit it to the appropriate device, and translate it into the proper device format for display or use by the requester.

Functional manufacturing requirements to support a company's specific business objectives include applications for the following:

- ERP
- Manufacturing resource planning (MRP)
- Quality
- Process control (supervisory and distributed control systems)
- Factory data collection
- Maintenance and calibration

Typically, these applications will be commercially available or developed in-house to run on a variety of platforms such as Microsoft NT, VMS, Ultrix, UNIX,

MV, MVS, MS-DOS, OS/2, and Macintosh. The I/T framework will be required to support a heterogeneous computing environment to allow a ''plug and play'' environment through well-defined interfaces and protocols (i.e., standards).

XVI. BUSINESS SYSTEM INFORMATION DRIVES MANUFACTURING EXECUTION

Between the business planning activities and the plant floor, various functions translate business objectives into production plans, schedules, and documentation, as well as the actual data from completing production to closing the manufacturing loop. Activities include

- Resource management
- Formula and process management
- Batch management
- Extensive document management and creation
- Production costing, evaluation, and accounting

The information to define the dispatch order lists for plant operations on what to make, how to make it, and what materials to use on what process equipment, need to be defined before product can be produced. Also, to support health, environmental, safety, cGMP, and other regulatory compliance issues, an enormous amount of accurate auditable documentation must be generated and made available to the plant floor before product manufacture is initiated.

XVII. DATA OWNERSHIP ISSUES

A portion of this information may reside in plant-level databases. Some information must be supplied by the business system, while other information is available through plant and corporatewide document repositories. This leads to ownership issues that can virtually stop projects. Any effective I/T strategy must deal with these conflicts.

- Who maintains the formulations or recipes with bills of materials and work instructions?
- Forecasting needs bills that are at the family level.
- Production planning needs the recipes with available materials.
- Regulatory assurance requires that the recipes be maintained to agree with regulatory submissions or documents on file.
- Operators need detailed material allocations and work instructions in the proper recipe sequence (section, stage, phase, etc.).
- The master batch record (MBR) has to be consistent with the documentation on the plant floor

- All of the various forms should be under versions control with cogent routing and approval lists for sign-off.
- Control elements such as ladder logic, setpoint control, and other equipment-specific parameters must be maintained and selected based upon the specific version of the recipe to be run
- Which systems will be validated?

Any effective I/T strategy must deal with these data ownership conflicts. The concerns usually reduce to the ERP practitioners and the manufacturing personnel who need the detail and exact manufacturing recipe. Different systems can have different recipe structures as long as the data model(s) will support the common shared information. Shared databases, translation tables, and transaction processing are some of the ways in which this information can be shared. Cool heads and effective mediation are sometimes required.

Another form of conflict that needs to be addressed in the strategy is how to interpret the business-processing rules. Different applications for different domains need to support how warehousing, local stores management, and manufacturing do business. The business model should be known and supported by each of the different applications in the different domains. Some of the typical areas for discussion are the following:

- Who maintains the inventory item names? They must be consistent across all compliance documentation.
- How will lots be allocated for production? Does the company have soft or hard lot allocations for consumption?
- What is the level of container tracking within the warehouse? Can containers for the same lot numbers have different release statuses? One business process rule could allow the release of the portion of the received lot that is required for production. Another rule could require that the entire receiving lot be released when approved by QC.
- Will electronic status be used for release of materials? Will raw and intermediate blends have release status on the paper label (e.g., quarantine, released, on hold)?
- What is the practice on segregating raw materials in the warehouse?
- Many facilities have only sufficient space for storage of all of the materials for one or two days of production. What will be the strategy to replenish these stores? Will it be order-driven or defined by historical consumption?
- Which system will provide lot traceability and genealogy?

XVIII. PLANT AND MES PROCESS EXECUTION

Information flows continually between the enterprise-level systems and the plant-level MES systems. During operations, real-time queries from business systems

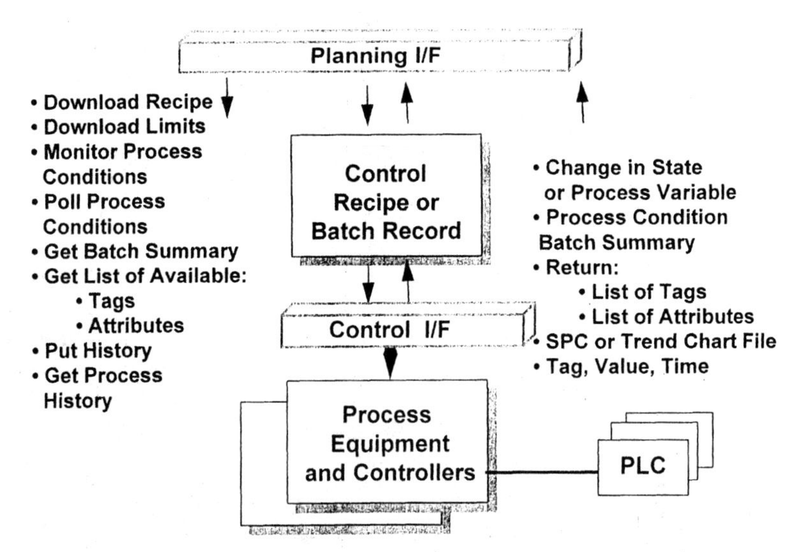

Fig. 3 Information flow between ERP and MES domains.

are occurring to support customer requirements and requests, and internal demands for product status, issues, and costs. (See Fig. 3.)

Information from the actual processes, operator actions, materials consumed, and product made must be passed back to the business system modules to close the loop on open dispatch orders. Actual values from production are passed back to be compared with standards and specifications to analyze the batch processes as well as to record completed product and consumed product records. These close-the-loop information requirements are passed to enterprise systems according to requests and other parameters.

XIX. PROCESS TO MES TO BUSINESS SYSTEMS YIELDS BENEFITS

The source of customer service information is found in the plant and control domains as product is being made and resources are being consumed. Real-time availability of this information is a powerful tool for meeting business and manufacturing strategies. Grayson and O'Dell (1) reported how a paper mill implemented a shared production and business information system with employees that included process and business data. Within six months, eight production records were broken with no change in personnel and equipment. Baxter (2) is aggressively bringing together vendors to integrate the MES environment to the business system environment. Downline-loaded recipes and work schedules and uploaded production results bridge the gap between business and plant floor or process control systems.

XX. KEEP THE INFORMATION WHERE IT IS REQUIRED

The ERP domain has to support the business and process models of the organization, wherever they may reside—whether corporate, division, or plant. Business applications can be the originator of all activities. The plant-level MES application model can supply unique local requirements and maintains a complete production control record for cGMP environments. In a multiplant environment, there may be different models, depending on the products, equipment, and organizations involved. In all cases, to support an EBR environment, this record has to be available to the business system. This flexible schema of using the process model to augment the business model can support business system document management requirements as well as maintain an auditable, validatable, plant-level document vault to support QA practices for local regulatory compliance.

XXI. PROCESS CONTROL MUST BE LINKED TO MANUFACTURING EXECUTION

The Computer Integrated Manufacturing (CIM) implementation at Baxter's North Cove plant, which uses an MES integration platform for a considerable amount of data collection equipment, has yielded many gains (3). In the sterilization area, the automated systems verify setups, monitor temperatures and other parameters, and provide event monitoring and alarm processing.

Of major importance (3) is collecting information from the process equipment and operators to automatically generate the detailed batch records required by the FDA. The completed batch record contains the information that verifies to a high degree of assurance that the process has consistently produced a product meeting its predetermined specifications and quality attributes. One significant benefit is that the MES solution minimizes the human error involved in record keeping and speeds up the processes of record verification and keeping. Scale recordings, online SPC, and monitoring and control of process lines all yield benefits as this integration of MES to process control equipment continues within the plants. References 1, 2, 8, 9, 10, 12, 13, and 15 present experiences and perspectives on the costs and benefits of equipment integration, paperless environments, and enterprisewide integration.

Increased productivity can be achieved through the information integration of external devices to automate manufacturing functions and process monitoring systems to the operator's workstation (14,16). Electronic signature will be an important component of this information integration. Verifications and checks that can be performed by MES applications relieve the verifiers to perform more value-added tasks.

XXII. SEPARATE REGULATORY DOCUMENTS FROM MANUFACTURING INFORMATION

The framework can offer a dynamic aid to all phases of a document's life cycle. The data warehouse (multiple sources, distributed, if required) would provide the repository for documents. Separate data warehouse sources would be the repository for shared manufacturing and production information not required for cGMP practices. This separation of data would allow specific I/T to be used to optimize system performance in a cost-effective manner.

XXIII. ELECTRONIC BATCH RECORD SYSTEM STRATEGY

A paperless environment is defined as the transfer of batch records and other documents and data using computer systems. Paperless operations or EBRS can provide a higher level of productivity as well as QA to support such business issues as "shorter time to market" and reduced cycle time. Some companies believe that the future competitiveness of the industry depends upon the implementation of EBRS. Another current belief is that the technologies and framework underlying these paperless environments will become the platform for automation and integration. The development of world-class manufacturing principles within the workforce are keyed to these automation and integration strategies.

In defining the strategy to support EBRS, one has to consider the entire life cycle of a document from document design, creation, control, delivery and use, through retention and archiving. An additional function, information management, is required to address the control of data that have been collected from EBRS and other devices. Documents in the context of an EBRS can be any type of informational forms, such as MBRs, Standard Operating Procedures (SOPs), process instructions, master production schedules, and logs (i.e., any type of information that is maintained for reference, review, use, etc). (See Fig. 4.)

XXIV. DOCUMENT DESIGN AND CREATION

The creation function includes designing, creating, and revising documents by users working throughout the organization having access to information anywhere in the organization. Features needed for this function include the following:

- Text, graphics, and image capabilities
- The ability to both import information from existing information structures and use existing tools (Commercial Computer-Aided Design and Word Processing applications)
- Copy, same as, global commands, word processing

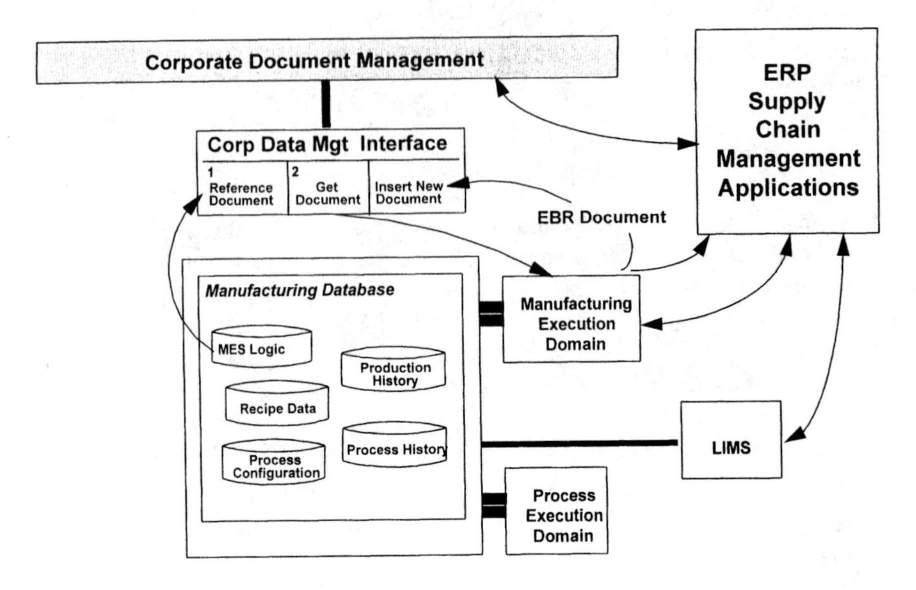

Fig. 4 Document management integration strategy.

- Access to repositories of company documents
- Index and keyword searches
- Audit and control of user access
- Compound document support

The I/T framework must provide a compound document architecture to completely support the pharmaceutical manufacturing environment. Electronic exchange of batch records and other production documents require the transfer of text, graphics, and images.

A compound document environment will allow the interchange of information between authoring and other creation-related systems. An author using import tools can gain access and use label drawings from a computer-aided design file or the package insert text from a word processing file for use in his or her document. Maintenance and management of appropriate authors and their activities with audit logs is a requirement.

XXV. DOCUMENT CHANGE CONTROL FOR cGMP COMPLIANCE

All of the production-related documentation, including batch sheets, packaging specifications, material safety data sheets, equipment instructions, safety information, and labeling, require methods to control their life cycle from design through archiving. This ''control activity'' is supported by the following features:

- Hierarchical data structures
- Version control
- Access control
- Review and approval cycle generation
- Change notification
- Activation of the document for actual production
- Query and database access
- Ability to manage heterogeneous data
- Secure audit trails of all activities

The I/T framework must provide a document management system by which electronic documents can be created, accessed, and so forth while providing the required pharmaceutical organizational controls and procedures to satisfy cGMPs. Security can be provided at the user access and document levels. Access control can be assigned to the document and specifies whether a user can read, make changes on, or delete a portion of the document. When a change is made, the system prevents other users from updating the same document; however the document can still be viewed. The privilege level assigned to each user determines whether the user is allowed to view, create, change, or delete information on the document. Users should be able to define and track hierarchical relationships between documents. Creation of dependencies for the purpose of notification is another feature required for effective document development. The document management system would provide tracking, access control, change notification, and archiving of documents across the network. The review and release mechanisms should be configurable for expedient approval processes.

The system should manage nonelectronic data such as historical files, logbooks, completed batch records, and drawings on hard copy or microfilm. This would allow users to monitor documentation projects electronically and manage hard copy data. If documents are archived to other storage devices, their history can still be retained online.

An active revision control system must be in place to maintain tracking of documents in creation, documents in review, and released documents. The document management system frees users from concerns over the existence of multiple originals, latest revisions, and change notification issues. Standardized database/query functions for customized reports and access to multiple databases for greater user accessibility should be provided by the document management system.

XXVI. ON-DEMAND DELIVERY AND USE

The document delivery and use function includes the distribution of EBRs to users as needed. The users work at workstations or positions within work centers throughout the plant. Once in place, the documents are used by operators to perform the designated steps of instructions, log data, perform calculations, and so on. To enable operators to manipulate documents, the system must:

- Provide simple-to-use user interface
- Zoom in and out on detail
- Present work instructions
- Support simple and multiple checkoff lists
- Display mixed text, graphics, and images
- Receive keyboard and/or barcode input
- Receive direct output from manufacturing devices
- Receive secure operator ''signature'' data to support existing and emerging guidelines
- Function in a secure operating environment

Electronic signature is a term signifying approval, authorization, or verification of specific critical data entries, as in the pending new guidelines. Electronic signatures are at the crux of the paperless environment. Devices and systems to determine and verify the actual person performing specific acts or being allowed entry to specific areas are readily available based upon industrial and governmental security requirements. A central issue is cost. Costs may be separated into procurement costs and the recurring costs to maintain and use the devices. The latter costs, being composed of expenses for inspection and testing, lost productivity, lost efficiencies, and potential reduction in job enjoyment, can be significantly more than the procurement costs.

XXVII. DEVICE DATA COLLECTION FOR HIGHER LEVEL OF QUALITY ASSURANCE

Increased productivity and operator efficiencies can be achieved through the use of external devices and integration of process control systems to the EBRS. Data collection vendors have developed and provided support for a wide range of automatic ID and input/output (I/O) level devices (pulse counter, parallel printers, electronic scales, radio frequency tag scanners, etc.); peripherals (wands, slots, lasers, magnetic strips); and economic, multifunctional, and modular data entry terminals and displays. These devices can reduce input errors, inhibit actions until data entry, make accurate calculations, put information online quicker, and automatically time and date stamp data. The online information can be used to support manufacturing strategies and is at an increased level of QA over manual systems. Provisions for verification of system and device input and output data will become a part of the ''operating environment'' and will have to support the various cGMP requirements already in place.

XXVIII. INFORMATION MANAGEMENT

Information management is the task of storing station information in a database in which it is available for batch records, area, room and machine logs, or user-defined reports. Information management features include the following:

- Linkage to other manufacturing applications
- Exception reporting
- Decision support systems
- Standards-based query and database access
- Interfaces to support users and applications

Interfaces are needed to run Windows environments on workstations and menu interfaces on character cell terminals. Callable interfaces that adhere to standards will allow information access to applications across the network.

Linkage to MRP, QA/QC analyses, and process optimization functions will allow data to be transferred to these applications. Exception reporting and decision support functions can increase operational effectiveness through easy-to-use procedures.

The information available in these systems is transported into the data warehouse to be used by operations through the EBRS and separate collection systems. All levels of the organization are interconnected through information. The data dictionary would define the information required for supporting the distributed operational applications that are in the system.

XXIX. DOCUMENT RETENTION AND ARCHIVING

The document retention strategy has to support regulatory compliance guidelines for time limits on retention. The system has to archive the batch record documents and provide these document to future requesters. The security of the records and the ease and rapidity of access and retrieval, each in accordance with cGMP procedures and practices, will be requirements.

Benefits can accrue by archiving other manufacturing information such as event history, machine data, exception data, and batch record data-type data in usable formats. These data may be retrieved for statistical and trend analyses by process engineers for process optimization and costing analyses to support such objectives as cost reductions and increased yields.

XXX. SUMMARY

If paperless environments are to be a major component of U.S. pharmaceutical competitiveness, then the EBRS must be built on an I/T strategy that will support operational needs. The system must provide a set of features that allow efficient and productive use of people while providing as high or a higher level of QA as in existing manual systems.

The key to any successful EBRS is getting the right information to the right people at the right time. This means using computing technology to provide appropriate access to accurate and timely information in an automated fashion—whether or not that information resides in a different application, department, or device.

An effective I/T framework must support information integration while protecting investments in computing equipment and applications. The framework must bring together I/T with world-class applications and a comprehensive set of people-focused programs to support pharmaceutical manufacturers requirements through the end of the 1990s and beyond.

XXXI. OPERATIONAL INTEGRATION CHALLENGE

Successful operational integration must include considerations for the business issues, people in the organization, and levels of technology employed for systems. The people/technology integration provides the human–machine interfaces needed as people must have access to information. Cross-functional programs form the basis of the people/business integration to align the organizations to the common enterprise purpose. The business/technology interface is the identification and planned use of the company information sources distributed throughout the organization that are needed to run the business. This information must be available to all users, regardless of where they are located in the organization. To succeed in this operational integration will allow a pharmaceutical company to achieve world-class performance and competitiveness. The challenge to achieve this integration can be expressed by three questions. How can I make the best use of technology in ensuring the success of my business? How can I ensure that the technology helps the work of my people? How can I get my organization to team together to improve the performance of my business?

REFERENCES

1. J. Grayson and C. O'Dell, *American Business: A Two Minute Warning*, Chap. 17, Free Press, A Division of Macmillan, Inc., New York, NY, 1988.
2. "The Benefits of MES: A Report from the Field," white paper #1, MESA International, Pittsburgh, PA, 1994.
3. Advanced manufacturing research survey commissioned by Digital Equipment Corporation, Marlboro, MA, 1993.
4. AUTOMATION: Your Prescription for Survival in the 90's, *Pharm. Proc.*: P 1 (1993).

5. Putting information technology to work, *Chem. Week*: Vol. 151, No. 16, Riverton, NJ, 22–25 (Oct. 23, 1991).
6. Integrated manufacturing: Barriers and opportunities in the Fortune 500, *Adv. Mfg. Res. Rep.* Boston, MA (April 1990).
7. D. H. Sinason, A dynamic model for present value capital expenditure analysis, *J. Cost Mgt.*, *5* (1991).
8. T. J. Williams, ed., *A Reference Model for Computer Integrated Manufacturing (CIM),* Instrument Society of America, Research Triangle Park, NC, 1989, pp. 163–176.
9. T. J. Williams, *The Purdue Enterprise Reference Architecture*, Instrument Society of America, Research Triangle Park, NC, 1992, pp. 313–333.
10. D. Davis, Profit found in MRP II execution integration, Mfg. Syst. (July 1994).
11. B. Meserve and J. deSpautz, Use of electronic identification and signatures for integrated operations, *ISA Trans. 32*: 215–224 (1993).
12. S. Schuber, Product, not paper: A manufacturing execution system installation at SmithKline Beecham, Pharm. Tech.: 34–39 (Nov. 1993).
13. J. deSpautz, Quantifying the benefits of automation, *ISA Trans. 33*: 107–112 (1994).
14. J. S. Cardarelli, Identifying and reducing the hidden factory costs in cGMP regulated manufacturing, *ISA '94 Adv. Instr. Control,* (October, 1994).
15. D. J. Adler et al., Life cycle cost and benefits of process automation in bulk chemicals, *Adv. Instr. Control* (October, 1994).
16. T. R. Sweet, Pharmaceutical manufacturing competiveness: The role of manufacturing execution systems, *Proceedings of the Industrial Computing Conference,* October, 1993, pp. 305–312.

4

Human Factors and Information Systems

James L. Vesper

LearningPlus, Rochester, New York

I. INTRODUCTION

Implementing a new information system in a manufacturing, laboratory, office, or support area is a sizable investment. Beyond the financial outlays, time, energy, reputations, and opportunities are invested in the project. In addition, the system and information produced from it will be long-term reminders of how successful—or unsuccessful—the solution turns out to be.

Simply having a technically sound solution doesn't ensure success. The people who will be using it must also be considered, as well as the organizational, work, and performance environment in which the technology will be used.

"People issues" extend beyond simply training people in the new system, although it certainly includes that. The system must be usable in the environment in which it is intended to be used. People must be motivated to use it. Figure 1 identifies some of the broader people issues and shows the relationship of the technical solution, people issues, and training to the success of the project.

Human factors (also known as ergonomics) is an applied field of study that examines the person–machine interface. In our discussion of human factors we will broadly apply the definition so that it overlaps with other disciplines such as organizational psychology and organizational behavior.

This chapter will discuss some human factors issues that can affect information systems projects. The goal is to show the importance of taking a broad, integrated approach to development and implementation of an information sys-

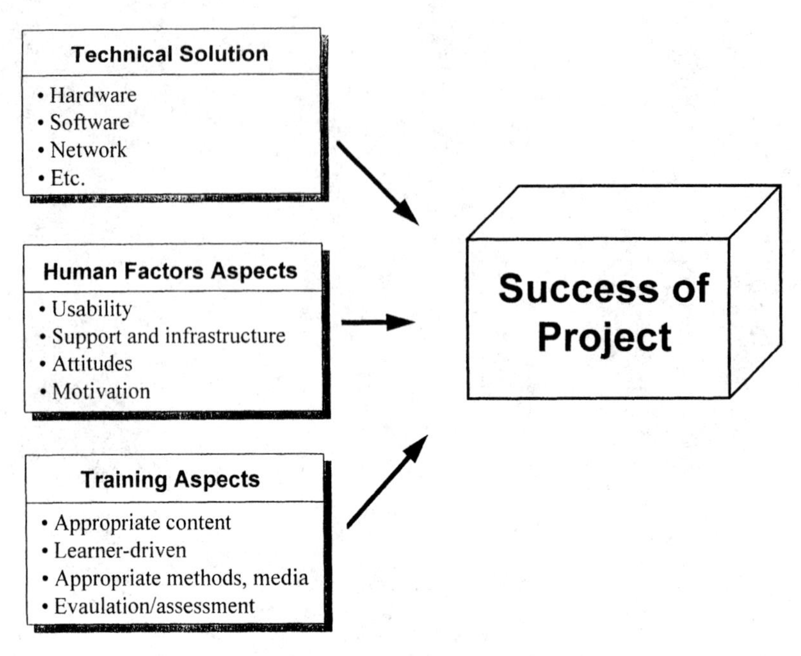

Fig. 1 Relationship between training issue and project success.

tem, including human factors, as one element in the system can affect another. Suggestions are given about specific things that need to be considered, along with some approaches for collecting information.

An example of emphasizing the technical elements of the solution at the expense of the other parts is described by James Fallows (1) in his book, *National Defenses*. Extremely complex technology was used by the U.S. Department of Defense in its ''Worldwide Military Command and Control System'' and ''Command–Control–Communications Intelligence'' network (Fig. 2). In his analysis, Fallows shows that the use of costly and overly complicated technology

- Diverts resources from other elements of implementation, such as training
- Makes hands-on training and practice too expensive or too impractical.

In other words, in situations in which training is critically needed, time and money for instruction and opportunities to practice are not available.

II. USABILITY

Usability consists of features designed into the hardware, software, and implementation of the system so they meet the needs of the users. A system that is highly usable makes no special demands on the person using it. This goes beyond what is typically called ''user friendliness''; the physical and organizational environment in which the person uses the device is also taken into account. An example of usability is a computer with a touchscreen interface and input device designed to accommodate the work gloves the user would be wearing.

A. User Needs

No matter if it is a technical manual, a regulatory submission, or a novel, there is one particular characteristic that distinguishes an expert writer from a not-so-skilled one. Expert writers carefully consider—and meet—the needs of their audience.

The same holds true for an information system. A successful system accommodates the needs of its users. This doesn't happen by chance; early in the project, the users and their needs must be identified. In the requirements phase of a project, whether it is simple or complex, developers must talk to the users and discover what their real needs are. Doing this after a magnitude budget has been prepared is too late.

The questions used to gather this information are rather simple; however, frequently in the race to address the technical issues they are asked but not found in the final solution. Some examples of questions are listed below; actual questions vary according to the specific project.

1. *Who Are the Primary and Secondary Users of the Information System?*

- What are their literacy skills? In what written language?
- How comfortable are they with interacting with a computer?
- What experiences have they previously had interfacing with a computer?
- Are the users young or old? How much experience do they have in their jobs?
- Are the users at one site or are they located in different locations? Countries?

2. *How Are People Currently Doing the Task?*

- What difficulties are they facing?
- What will the effect of the new system be on their current duties?

3. *Where Will the System Be Used?*

- Where will the users interact with the system?
- Are there safety issues related to the use of electrical equipment in the area?
- Is the area one that is cleaned, sanitized, or fumigated frequently?

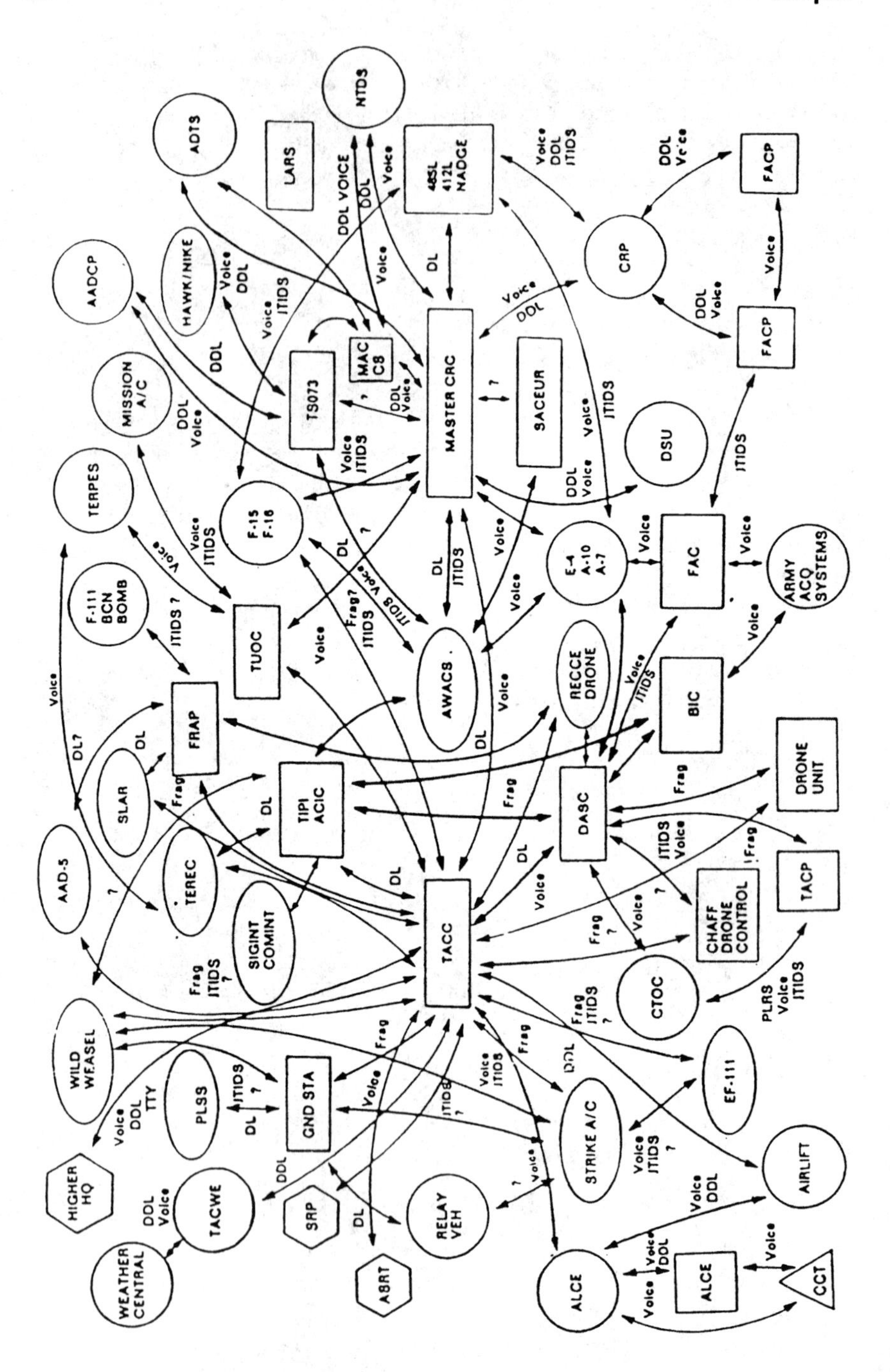
NTDS
ADTS
LARS
485L
412L
NADGE
FACP
CRP
FACP
AADCP
HAWK/NIKE
MAC
C8
TS073
MASTER CRC
SACEUR
MISSION
A/C
DSU
TERPES
F-15
F-16
E-4
A-10
A-7
FAC
ARMY
ACQ
SYSTEMS
F-111
BCN
BOMB
TUOC
AWACS
RECCE
DRONE
BIC
FRAP
SLAR
TIPI
ACIC
DASC
DRONE
UNIT
AAD-5
TEREC
SIGINT
COMINT
TACC
CHAFF
DRONE
CONTROL
TACP
CTOC
WILD
WEASEL
PLSS
GND STA
STRIKE A/C
EF-111
AIRLIFT
HIGHER
HQ
TACWE
SRP
RELAY
VEH
WEATHER
CENTRAL
ABRT
ALCE
ALCE
CCT

- Will the user be wearing any special clothing that might make operation of the equipment difficult?
- What is the work environment like? Are there special lighting or noise considerations? If the system signals an error with an audio tone, will the users be able to hear it?

4. *How Will the Users Interface with the System?*

- Does the system automate an existing task or is it a completely new and different task?
- Are users expected to interact constantly and concurrently between the task and the system or interact periodically with the system?
- Will users communicate with the system using a keyboard? Touchscreen? Mouse? Voice?
- Will the interface be adaptable to the particular things the user does or will there be one general, noncustomizable interface that all will use?
- Will there be a systems terminal or interface at the workstation or at other specific locations?

5. *When Will People Use the System?*

- Will all users be trying to get into the system at the same time, say, at the beginning of a workshift?

6. *What If . . .*

- If the system crashes, what should be done? Who should be contacted?
- What does a systems failure mean to the work in process?
- Can activities continue if the system fails?
- Are there backup manual procedures that will go into effect in the event of a systems failure?
- Could a failure potentially affect the health or safety of the worker? The community? The environment?
- What is the probability of a critical failure?
- Are users expected to react to a failure in a specific way?

7. *What Can Be Done to Help People Prepare for the Changes and the New System?*

Fig. 2 Schematic diagram of the command-control-communication-intelligence network (U.S. Defense Contractor's Chart [1]).

8. Approaches in Gathering the Questions and Issues

Questions such as these should be asked in the earliest phases of the project. Potential users should be involved in discussions, as they will be most affected by the systems. Techniques such as group brainstorming, brainwriting, or online discussions can be used.

Another source for information would be from people who have implemented similar systems, such as user groups, other companies, vendors, or consultants. Their ''lessons learned'' may be helpful.

Testing a prototype of the system with naive or new users is also a way to collect information. (This technique is discussed in more detail in Chapter 5.)

9. How the Information Can Be Used

From the data collection process there will be a number of possible solutions to meet the needs. There will undoubtedly be some right and wrong ways of addressing the issues, but many of the answers will depend on the vision that management, the developers, and the users have for the solution. Some approaches used in the solution may require more design and development efforts, and subsequently, less training is needed. In other situations, the decision may be to rely more on well-trained people than trying to automate a complicated decision process. As mentioned earlier, it is important to understand how *all* the elements of the information system (e.g., hardware, the interface, user training needed) are related to each other. Answers to the questions (such as those listed earlier) will be useful in the requirements document. Also, they will be of interest to the potential users and management.

Much of the information will be valuable to those who will be providing training. For example, if people are expected to interact with the system using a keyboard and typing skills, training personnel would need to assess the users to determine if they have the skills that are expected. The information may also affect other aspects of the performance environment. For instance, there may need to be decision trees (i.e., a type of job aide) that can be used manually in the event of a serious system failure.

B. Interface Standards

The success of how well the system and user interact is primarily dependent on the interface standards that are developed and applied. Based on studies of office automation, three issues are particularly important.

- Consistency. Actions and responses should be identical throughout the system. For example, cursor movement and insertion/deletion of characters should be similar in all parts of the application. Carroll and Mack (2) show that if there are differences, users will try and invent their own ''rules'' for interpreting the inconsistent behavior. When possible, there should also be consistency with other applications the users may have used. That way, people can use the foundation of knowledge and skills they already have. An example of this is found in Macintosh standards; virtually every program written for the Macintosh operating system makes use of identical keystrokes for cutting, pasting, copying and so forth. (Standards used by Apple are available in their developer's kits and also on several online services such as America Online.)

- Clarity. User and system responses and visual icons should be easily understood. Error messages are known for being cryptic and extremely frustrating to those trying to figure out what a "type E-847 failure" means, and more specifically, what needs to be done to correct it. Graphical user interfaces (GUIs) that use icons for particular functions provide a more significant challenge to the developing team. Icons need to be simple, readily understandable in the various cultures using the device, and be applied consistently. Such interface designers as Tognazzini (3) can provide suggestions, but it is essential to test the images with a large sampling of the potential users.
- Metaphor. Metaphor is the implicit or explicit image or comparison that is invoked in a user by an electronic system. Most people using word processing systems for the first time make comparisons to typewriters (2). Metaphors come from other experiences people have had. For example, many electronic document systems have the capability of adding electronic Post-It notes that can be examined on the screen, but are not a part of the actual document. The metaphor gets stretched when in some applications the electronic annotations can be verbal (audio) as well as text or image.

Metaphors can be powerful, in both the positive and negative sense. When there is a high correlation between the electronic system and image, users can take what they know from previous experiences and apply it to the electronic system. If there is a difference between the two, or if the metaphor breaks down, it can be very unsettling to the user.

One other aspect of the interface is esthetics—what the interface looks like. Obviously, this has a significant subjective factor to it, but there are still some timeless principles of design that can be applied to the interface. Simplicity, balance, use of "white space," borders, weight, and so on can all help to make a more appealing, inviting interface. Another approach is to provide the users with the opportunity to customize their own interface, changing colors, electronic "wallpaper," and so forth.

III. ATTITUDES AND DYSFUNCTIONAL BEHAVIORS

The success of a system in accomplishing its purpose is certainly affected by how usable it is, but there are additional factors that are related more to the organization, its formal and informal reward systems, and the users' attitudes.

Several authors (4,5) have identified the fears and attitudes that people have when new types of office technology are introduced in their organization. These include the following:

- Fear of being replaced by new equipment
- Anxiety of having to learn how to use new, sophisticated technical equipment
- Fear of the unknown
- Loss of control
- Changes in interpersonal relationships
- Fear of failure
- Lack of understanding

The "fear factors" can be especially high in people who are experiencing an automation project for the first time. In operational or maintenance areas, many employees will have never used a personal computer before. The introduction of computers for many is a major change in how they view their own status in the organization. For example, a bulk chemical pilot plant was being automated so virtually all of the equipment could be controlled by computer monitors and keyboards. Experienced operators who had served decades in the facility and become masters of the valves and gauges suddenly became novices in controlling the rigs by computer. Younger operators, even though they had little computer experience, were much more comfortable using the electronic system.

Attitudinal factors can cause people to resist change. Furthermore, dysfunctional behaviors can arise in people as they react to all phases of information system projects. Some of the behaviors become so destructive that they contribute to or actually cause failure of the project. Dickson and Simmon (6) and Peterson and Peterson (4) identify five such behavior.

- Aggression—The individual attacks (physically or nonphysically) the object causing the "problem"
- Projection—Blaming the system for causing problems that are in fact caused by something else
- Avoidance—People withdrawing from frustrating or stressful situations
- Defensive planing—Planning done with great reluctance has less than efficient and effective results
- Chronic skepticism—Constant doubting, questioning, and disagreeing with the new system

A. Addressing Dysfunctional Behaviors

Peterson and Peterson (4) offer a summary of suggestions for minimizing dysfunctional behaviors. They are

1. Have a supportive climate for acceptance of the new information system that includes top management support and a conduciveness of risk taking.
2. Have clear and open communications from top management regarding the equipment/project and its purpose.
3. Get employees involved early in the process so they feel ownership in the project.
4. Plan the scope of the project so people know what tasks and personnel will be affected.
5. Determine the users' needs and act upon them.
6. Provide education and training to both management and end users regarding the philosophy, benefits, and skills needed to fully implement the system.

IV. SUPPORT AND INFRASTRUCTURE

Another factor that can affect the success of a new system is the amount of support provided with it. This extends beyond training to coaching and the availability of immediate assistance for when things begin to go wrong. Some implementation plans solve this by providing a "key operator" in an area who has undergone more extensive training and is available to answer questions. Other times a "help desk" is established with experts who can solve problems. Sometimes this assistance is provided by the vendor or a third party on a fee or subscription basis.

The attitude of the support personnel toward the users is also a factor that can affect the success of an IS project. Often technical staff will immediately assume that the user is to blame and will resist the idea that there may be a problem with the automated system.

Electronic performance support systems are another way to provide help to the user. These can be relatively simple or very complicated and include not only written instructions or suggestions, but high-quality images and video that can show standards or demonstrate skills. These systems are described more fully by Geary (7).

V. MOTIVATION

People may not use a system because they have no incentive for doing so. In fact, there may be a *disincentive* to use it. An operator doing in-process weight checks may be able to do the calculation, graph the result, and determine how to respond faster than it would take him or her to input the numbers into a computer application he or she is beginning to use. Sometimes the system needs to provide relatively low value-adding features, from an organizational standpoint, that users enjoy as an incentive. When the French government replaced paper telephone directories with electronic terminals (''minitels''), the response was not enthusiastic. After several years, interactive fantasy games prompted people to get their minitels out of storage and into use (8). More recently, some people reluctantly agree to get a personal computer on their desk because it is the only way they can have the flying toasters and swimming fish screen savers.

At some level, all of us want to know ''what's in it for us'' related to a behavior, attitude, or course of action. We internally calculate a cost/benefit ratio, and when we find it in favor of the particular action, we do it.

Sometimes organizations unknowingly reward the wrong behaviors. Engineers may not put through change requests because they know the requests will take too long to process; it is worth the risk to make the small adjustments, get the equipment running and the product made, and hope that someone will not notice the change. In another example, the document control clerk at one firm tracks the time it takes for SOPs to be modified and the number through her area. In order to meet her management's expectation for ''productivity,'' she puts through documents that have very minor changes when it would be better if the changes were held and consolidated into one revision.

Incentives for people don't need to be monetary. Recognition by management and peers, attendance or presentations at team meetings, and so forth, can be motivators for people. Just as people have different value systems, people can be motivated by a variety of factors. An effective incentive program should provide something that is meaningful to the people involved.

VI. CONCLUSION

For a new technology or a new information system to be successful, human factors—specifically related to the users—must be considered at the outset of the project. An active process must be employed to determine how to make the system usable for the users and also to foster positive attitudes and behaviors so people will utilize the system. Getting and keeping users involved, asking, listening, communicating, and being open to their comments is critical.

VII. ACKNOWLEDGMENTS

The author wishes to thank Farrow Beacham, Eric Cohen, Bonnie Meath-Lang, Ph.D., and Jim Wanzenried for their assistance with this chapter.

REFERENCES

1. J. Fallows, *National Defense*, Random House, New York, 1981, pp. 51–54.
2. J. M, Carroll and R. L. Mack, Learning to use a word processor: By doing, by thinking,

and by knowing, *Human Factors in Computer Systems* (J. C., Thomas and M. I. Schneider, eds), Ablex, Norwood, New Jersey, 1984.
3. B. Tognazzini, *Tog on Interface*, Addison-Wesley, Reading,: Massachusetts, 1991.
4. C. M., Peterson and T. O. Peterson, The darkside of office automation, *Fundamentals of Human–Computer Interaction* (A. Monk, ed.), Academic, London, 1984.
5. Z. Quible and J. N. Hammer, Office automation's impact on personnel, *Personnel Admin.* 29:25–32 (1984).
6. G. W. Dickson and J. K. Simmon, The behavior side of MIS, *Bus. Horizons*, 13:39–71 (1970).
7. G. J. Gery, *Electronic Performance Suport Systems*, Weingarten, Boston, 1991.

5

Instrumentation and Process Control System Strategy

David J. Adler

Eli Lilly & Company, Indianapolis, Indiana

I. INTRODUCTION

During the last fifteen years, this author has seen a wide variety of process control systems implemented in the bulk pharmaceutical industry.* The process control systems consist of the field measurement hardware, the field control hardware, the process control computer hardware, and the process control computer software. A typical automated facility consists of batch equipment controlled by a vendor-supplied process control system. This batch unit operation equipment consists of material handling, pumping, scrubbing, waste treatment, columns, utility equipment, filtering, and drying, as well as batch reactors and stills. Field instruments and valves control events in the batch production area through the process control system. Processing steps are monitored under the watchful eye of the production operator seated at a console in the remote control room. The operator is responsible for the many batch unit operations in the production area. The process control system steps the batch through sequenced operations that allow the process unit to produce the desired product. The process control system generates alarms to inform the operator of abnormal activity. Process information is collected in a data historian for later retrieval and analysis by production and technical personnel.

---

*See D. J. Adler, J. A. Herkamp, S. B. Williams, and J. R. Wiesler, "Lifecycle Cost and Benefits of Process Automation in Bulk Pharmaceuticals," ISA Paper, Anaheim, California, 1994.

II. DELIVERY OF PROCESS CONTROL SYSTEMS

Process automation is typically delivered to a major bulk pharmaceutical facility as part of the overall design and construction of a new processing plant. In this industry, however, many existing manually operated plants have also been renovated to incorporate process control systems. The delivery of a process control system requires the design of the instrumentation and process control strategy. The field instruments are purchased and installed in the field while the process control code is developed, written, and tested. The process control system is documented to meet regulatory requirements. Finally, a successful start-up of the process control system occurs that enables the batch unit operation equipment to produce the desired high-quality product. Other measures of a successful start-up are the delivery of the project on schedule and within cost estimates.

The two major factors involved in a process automation project are hardware purchases and personnel expenses (Fig. 1). Personnel delivery costs include the engineers needed to design the field instrumentation and the process control personnel needed to develop and code the automation strategies. Hardware delivery costs include the purchase, construction, and installation of the field instrumentation as well as the purchase of the process control system hardware. On several process control systems delivered in the early 1990s the ratio of hardware and personnel costs were found to be approximately equal (Fig. 1).

In the 1990s, process control system project delivery costs were about $4000 per input/output point. This average does not take into consideration the complexity, the experience level of the personnel, the pace of the project, and the level of automation of a process control system. All of these factors can influence the cost to deliver the process control system. Process control system delivery costs for ten major facilities over the past fifteen years have indicated a sharp increase compared to the consumer price index (Fig. 2).

Project delivery costs for process control systems have increased at more than twice the rate of inflation. This increase in cost compared to inflation can be attributed to a much higher level of functionality and regulatory requirements

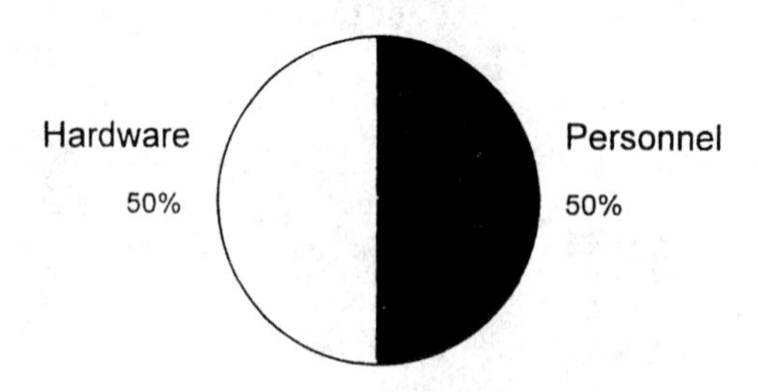

Fig. 1 Delivery cost—several automated facilities.

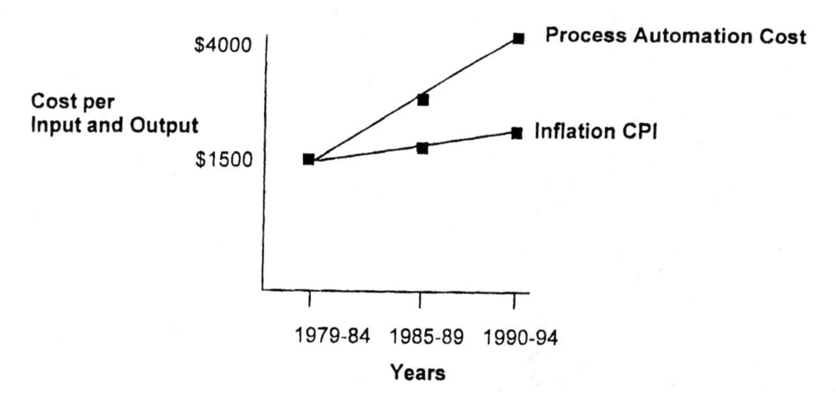

Fig. 2 Delivery cost.

on process control systems in the 1990s compared to the early 1980s. The huge increase in documentation requirements to meet regulatory computer validation regulations has increased project delivery costs significantly. Alarm management, data historians, and sequenced batch unit operation are the functions now delivered as standard features of a process control system. These features have increased project delivery costs significantly, but have also extended the process control system's capabilities.

III. MAINTENANCE OF PROCESS CONTROL SYSTEMS

Significant effort is required to maintain the process control system in a bulk pharmaceutical facility. A dedicated staff of process automation personnel is needed for the maintenance and optimization of the installed process control system. The required personnel make the many changes and repairs to the pharmaceutical process control system. In addition, their efforts result in improvements to the manufacturing batch unit operations and processing equipment.

The cost of process control system maintenance consists of two major factors. These are the hardware purchases and the personnel expenses. Personnel maintenance expenses include instrument engineers, instrument technicians, process control engineers, process control technicians, system managers, and system analysts. Hardware maintenance purchases include service contracts, replacement parts, and technology upgrades. In the maintenance of process control systems, personnel costs were found to be much higher than the hardware costs (Fig. 3).

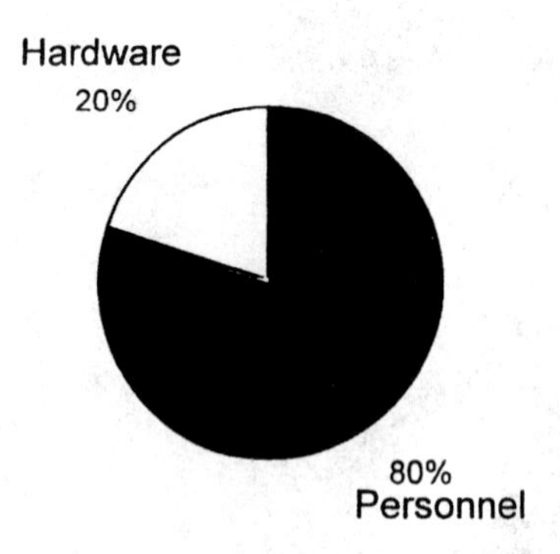

Fig. 3 Maintenance cost—several automated facilities.

The average cost of process control system maintenance varies widely, depending on the size of the facility, the number of process improvement changes needed, and the flexibility of the facility. The largest factor in the maintenance of the installed process automation system is the cost of the process control personnel. Having a process control support staff with a high level of experience can minimize the total number of personnel required. It is more cost-effective to finesse a process control problem with process control system expertise than muscle it with a large number of inexperienced personnel.

The conventional wisdom of the engineering community is that 80 percent of the cost associated with automation of a bulk pharmaceutical plant occurs during the delivery of the new facility. This is not the case. The maintenance cost of a process control system is equal to or greater than the cost to actually deliver the new process control system. The process control system maintenance cost for software and hardware support in bulk pharmaceutical manufacturing is 50 to 60 percent of the total automation cost during the life of the facility (Fig. 4). The reason that process control maintenance costs are so significant is that the automated bulk manufacturing facility is used for a long period of time.

The installed process automation system must be maintained to ensure successful operation. Significant effort must continually be expended to keep the automation operational and to make the necessary enhancements. This is summarized in a pie chart (Fig. 4) for two automated facilities that have been in operation for longer than ten years. It should be noted that both of these facilities are still in operation. Maintenance costs will continue to become a larger percentage of the life cycle cost as long as these facilities continue to be used.

The fact that the maintenance cost makes up a high percentage is not a bad thing. Bulk pharmaceutical facilities are designed to be operational for a long time. It would be expected that the process automation system would need to be

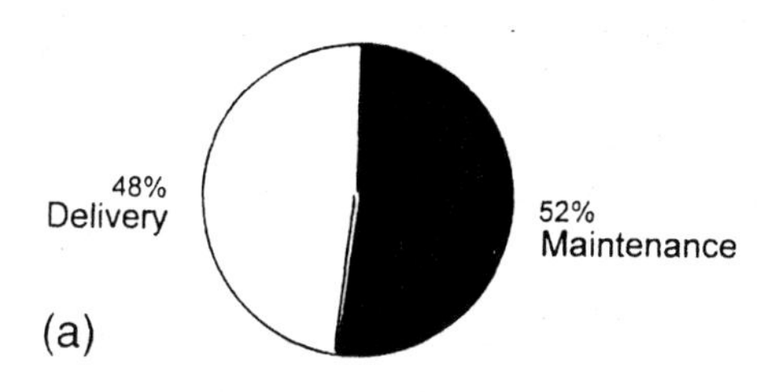

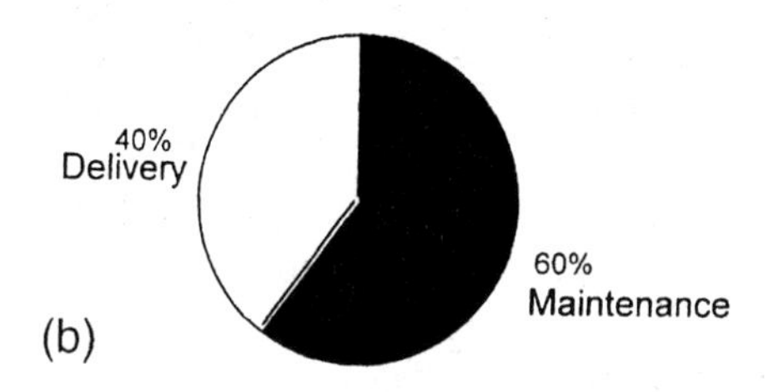

Fig. 4 Process automation cost. (a) 15-year-old facility, (b) 13-year-old facility.

maintained and upgraded to meet the changing requirements of the bulk facility. Many enhancements are needed to the automated plants to meet changing product requirements and customer expectations. The real value of the automated system is its ability to assist production personnel in quickly adapting to these new conditions. In fact, to make project delivery decisions based solely on the capital cost can cause higher life cycle costs for the bulk pharmaceutical facility. It is indeed important to consider the long-term maintainability when making project decisions. These project decisions made during process control system delivery can make a process retrofit possible five or ten years into the future.

IV. BENEFITS OF PROCESS CONTROL SYSTEMS

The tangible benefits from process control systems are the following:

1. Lowered net personnel requirements
2. Yield enhancements
3. Reduced lot variation
4. Increased operational capacity

The intangible benefits include the following:

1. Improved product quality
2. Improved operator morale
3. Regulatory compliance
4. Fewer physical operations

Automated bulk pharmaceutical facilities required significantly fewer production personnel than comparable manually operated facilities. The reduction in production operators has to be balanced with the need for maintenance personnel for the process control system. Typically, a dedicated, automated plant requires 25 percent of the personnel needed in a manual plant. With one product running many lots in a processing plant, the process control and technical personnel can learn much about the process. This allows for continuous incremental improvement.

Figure 5 summarizes the experience of one facility. This facility was manually operative for many years. In the late 1970s, it became fully automated. The many changes to a dedicated processing facility can have significant impact over ten or fifteen years. The biggest personnel reduction is not realized at project completion, but rather after the maintenance staff is able to analyze the operation and improve the process as well as the process control system.

A number of factors can improve the product yield. Two major factors are tighter process control and process information. Yield is the conversion efficiency of starting material into final product. In this industry, it is not uncommon to have yields of initial raw materials into final product that measure less than 50 percent. The ability to systematically improve the overall yield is a significant factor in the ability to deliver cost-effective products for our customers.

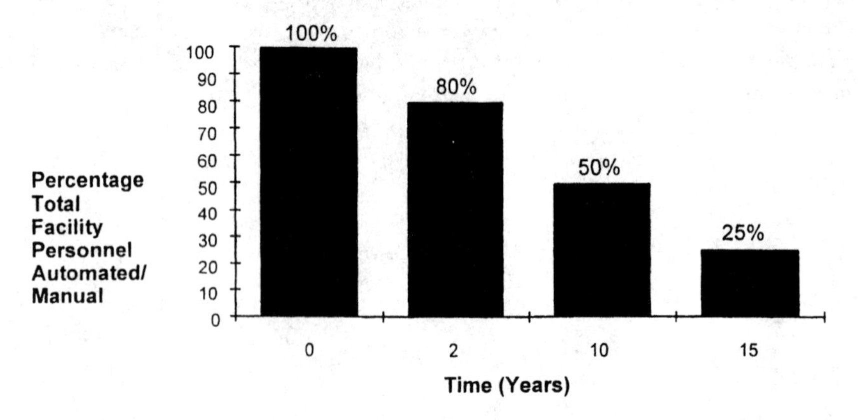

Fig. 5 Personnel reductions—one automated facility.

Process control of time, temperature, and pH, for example, are critical in this industry. Process control systems can improve the control of critical variables. Process information is also available from the use of a process control system. The data historian information is used by the technical support personnel and production operators to analyze and understand the process. The production operators use statistical process control to understand the operations they control. The technical support and production personnel use the data historian information to make many incremental improvements. The result of the efforts to drive the yield learning curve is improved control and process information (Fig. 6).

One measure of quality is reduced variation. Lot-to-lot and shift-to-shift consistency can allow for reduced variation in yield. Batch sequencing is one tool to achieve this consistency. Process sequencing is achieved by linking a series of unit operations together through a series of automated batch steps. This enables the operation to proceed in the same way from lot to lot. The application of sequencing typically reduces yield standard deviations by more than 50 percent. This reduction in variation allows the technical support staff to make smaller process changes without the impact of the change being masked by the normal variation from lot to lot. In general, the largest improvements in yield are seen after sequencing is implemented and the process is continually improved. For one process that was run manually, the unit operation equipment was upgraded to run in automated batch sequencing, which significantly reduced the yield variation (Fig. 7).

The capacity of an automated dedicated bulk pharmaceutical facility can increase by a factor greater than two over its life. The process control system and information management system are significant factors in contributing to this improved capacity. Especially for those products that are successful in the marketplace, these capacity increases can meet the increased demand without

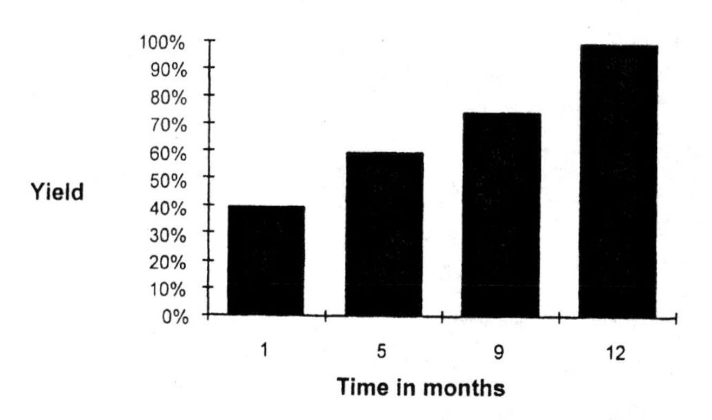

Fig. 6 Yield improvement—one automated process.

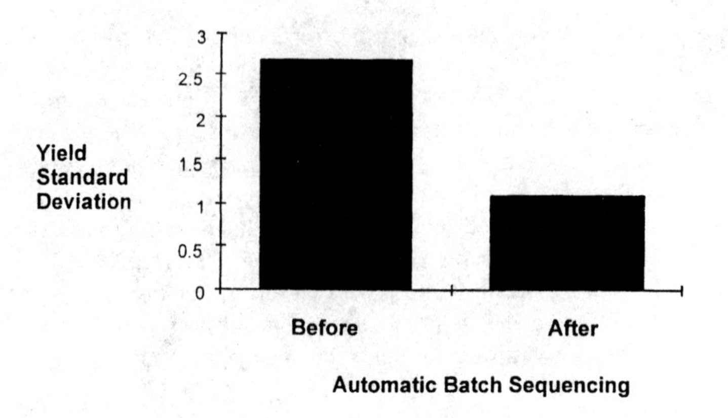

Fig. 7 One automated process.

significant capital investment. This can reduce the need for additional capital investment in new facilities. In addition, the unit cost is reduced if the fixed cost can be spread over a larger number of units. The higher capacity of the plant can allow the needed inventory levels to be reduced. A lower level of inventory is needed to react to changing market conditions for a plant with a higher capacity. This is especially true if the capacity gains were realized by process control and process improvements rather than additional capital projects.

Figure 8 concerns one plant that has been operational for several years. It should be noted that management was willing to invest the incremental dollars for process control and technical personnel to achieve these improvements.

Life cycle information has been obtained for several automated bulk pharma-

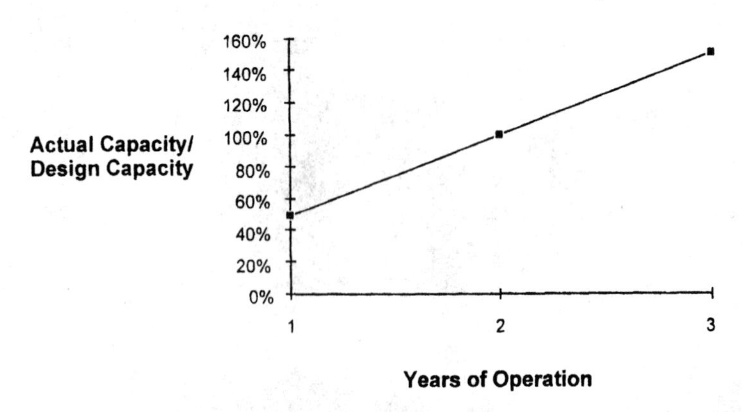

Fig. 8 Improved capacity—one automated plant.

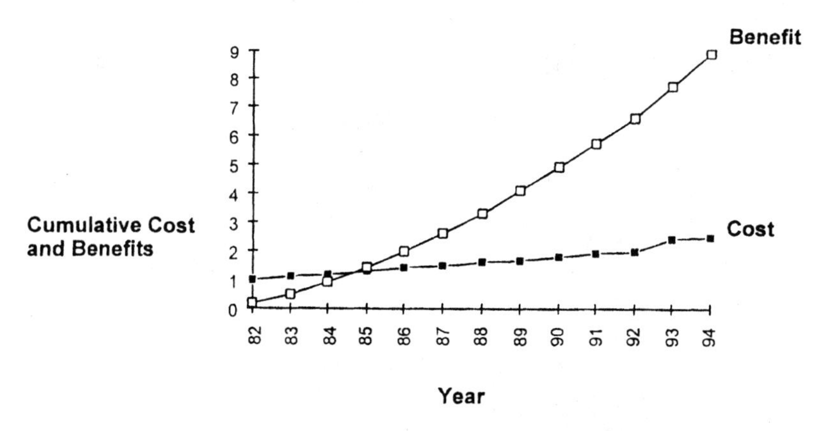

Fig. 9 Life cycle analysis—one typical automated facility.

ceutical facilities. Figure 9 summarizes the typical costs and benefits for one large automated facility. In 1982, a large initial outlay of capital was required to design, purchase, and install the process control system. By 1983, the process control system was successfully started up and the new facility was operational. This operating facility required ongoing process control maintenance. The annual expense for process control hardware and personnel is approximately 10 percent of the initial investment in 1982. This annual maintenance expense was relatively flat until 1992, when the ten-year-old process control system needed a major upgrade due to its obsolescence. This upgrade is approximately 40 percent of the initial investment.

The tangible benefits of a process control system are yield improvements, inventory reduction, personnel reduction, and capacity improvements. There are benefits in the first year of operation after the process control system is implemented. The incremental changes by the maintenance personnel have a larger benefit, however, because of the cumulative effect of these many improvements. In the tenth year, when the process control system is upgraded, a boost in benefits occurred with the increased power of the upgraded process control system. It should be noted that the costs associated with the delivery of the project are less than the long-term maintenance costs, and the life cycle tangible benefits are significantly larger than the life cycle costs. In addition, a trained, dedicated staff is needed after start-up is completed to realize the desired process improvement that will give these tangible benefits.

V. SUMMARY

Process control systems have gained significant financial benefits for the pharmaceutical industry by the industry's investment in capital and personnel in automation technology in batch bulk manufacturing. Experienced process control personnel are needed to achieve the benefits of improved yield, increased capacity, reduced personnel, and reduced variability. With the ideal combination of process control system and personnel, a company will easily experience the benefits of an automated process. Ultimately, the benefits derived from an automated process far outweigh the costs of delivery and maintenance.

6

Automation Life Cycle Is More Than Looking at Cost: It's a New Tool for Competitiveness

Steven B. Williams and David J. Adler

Eli Lilly & Company, Indianapolis, Indiana

Competitiveness is the issue. It's producing more of what the market demands faster and at less cost than the competition. Competitiveness is about quality and responsiveness. It's also about meeting government regulations as well as the business issues of ever-higher rates of return on funds invested. In the pharmaceutical business, competitiveness goes hand in hand with earning a reputation for leadership and integrity. Until recently, many of these issues seemed to reside outside the bulk manufacturing arena. No longer!

Advanced automated manufacturing provides the consistency, the repeatability, and the continuous improvements required to keep firms in business. With the deepening need for automation in the pharmaceutical industry has come new responsibilities. Engineers must think in terms of the manufacturing process as a business. They must prove to management that for every dollar invested in the "business" process, the larger organization will be paid back at least two, three, and four times. Engineers have to do everything they've always done and more.

This chapter describes the automation life cycle model and how it can be used to meet the twin needs of bulk product manufacturing and cost competitiveness. The conclusions and insights are based on data collected by the authors over the past fifteen years at Eli Lilly.

Section I develops a model for understanding automation system life cycle costs. It's through a firm understanding of what costs are involved and what the anticipated "economic value added" of the system will be that a firm justification for investment can be made to management. It describes spreadsheet-based tools that are helping engineers at Eli Lilly and Company better understand the cost and payback implications of systems over the life cycle.

Section II explores ''function points,'' a new concept in the manufacturing arena. Function points offer a different way to measure the size of process control applications from which effort can be predicted and against which productivity can be measured. By knowing what effort is required, project managers will be better able to manage the critically important software development process. The decision to focus heavily on software technology is a conscious one. Developing custom application software for each new system is one of the most difficult and costly aspects of the pharmaceutical manufacturing process. It's also an area that offers the most potential for higher levels of operational efficiency and product quality. Understanding the software development process and being able to compare that process project by project over time is essential to maximizing the return from an automation investment over its life cycle.

Section III offers several examples of ways to help automate the process of software development during the apply and install stages of the life cycle.

Section IV arrives at the important conclusion that 75 percent of the benefits of automation can only be obtained through continuous improvement and an ongoing commitment of engineering and technical resources over the life cycle.

I. JUSTIFYING THE INVESTMENT IN AUTOMATION: A LIFE CYCLE COST MODEL

The automation systems described and used as examples control a variety of unit batch processing operations common in the bulk pharmaceutical industry—for example, fermentation and organic synthesis. Control systems include both distributed control system-(DCS) and programmable logic controller-(PLC) based architectures. In rough numbers, 33 percent of the input/output (I/O) for these systems are analog, with the remainder discrete. It's a belief that the general principles in the following discussion can be applied to most, if not all, control solutions in the bulk pharmaceutical industry.

The definition of automation life cycle cost is the total cost of implementing and maintaining a system over its life; it is therefore more than the cost of acquisition and installation. The life cycle cost model proposed here takes into account, for example, the inflation/time value of money and the tax implications on long-term investments. That is the cost side. On the benefits side, the model provides a way to calculate the value of the investment in automation—the economic value added of the investment—or the lifetime payback.

This model presents to management the full justification of the investment—from costs to anticipated benefits. Eli Lilly and Company financial services and corporate engineering have developed computer-based tools to make justification a life cycle endeavor. It's presented here to help describe what areas are essential to consider in a life cycle cost model.

The life cycle cost model is in a spreadsheet format. It allows project personnel to, first of all, load in cost assumptions. Initial one-time costs include the following:

- Design and specification
- Acquisition/purchase
- Engineering
- Installation
- Process control application software

Ongoing costs are calculated on a per-year basis over the expected life of the system and include the following:

- Training classes
- Support personnel
- Maintenance and optimization
- Repair
- Spare parts

On the plus side, the model allows personnel to put in the savings and payback that are anticipated, including the following:

- Increasing product yield
- Lowering unit cost
- Increasing production capacity
- Achieving net reductions in production head count over time

Also included in the life cycle cost model are the following:

- Anticipated life of the system
- Expected system upgrades and replacement during the life cycle
- Corporate tax rate
- Hurdle rate—the cost of capital

These are the key elements in the life cycle cost model. It's not simply an ROI statement; it's looking at every cost and benefit over the life of the system that can potentially be in operation for ten, fifteen, or twenty years.

Justification is based on the reality of the situation. That reality looks at the system over a span of years—far beyond acquisition and installation—to calculate the anticipated total economic value added to the organization of the investment over the entire life of the system. It must be above the hurdle rate of the proposed automation system to be a viable candidate for management endorsement.

Incidentally, the new computer-based tool allows engineers to perform

Table 1

Year	Average project cost per I/O device
1979–1984	$1,500
1985–1989	$2,500
1990–1995	$4,000

''what if'' scenarios. An engineer can ask, ''What if I'm wrong by a factor of two—what would happen?'' The tool lends itself to sensitivity analyses. It's right on the desktop helping make the justification process become not only faster and more interactive, but more specific to the needs of the application solution.

II. A NEW WAY FOR ENGINEERS TO MEASURE SOFTWARE DEVELOPMENT AND ITS IMPACT

One point is to investigate the automation life cycle from a cost and benefit viewpoint. As stated above, it will focus primarily on software. Why? In a typical automation project at Eli Lilly in 1978, for example, approximately 75 percent of the costs of automation were associated with hardware; however, if one looks at the numbers today over the life cycle, software is replacing hardware as the more significant cost. Software is an extremely important contributor of continuous improvements in a highly automated system.

During the application engineering stage of the life cycle, project managers must estimate the effort and associated cost of writing application software. It's also extremely important to have some measure of the value of that code—''What is it giving us toward the bottom line?''

To determine a rough estimate of the cost of a project from a control system point of view in the past, project management counted I/O and stopped there. The concept was sound—there was a rough equivalency project to project based on the number of I/O. In a hardware-dominated environment, the I/O method alone was a good rule of thumb. Table 1 shows how those costs have varied over time.

In a hardware-dominated system, I/O counting makes sense. Today, however, there is a problem with only counting I/O, because it does not take into account many software-related factors such as functionality level and how much repeatability there is in the system.

To illustrate, consider a fermentation area of 2,000 I/O with ten identical fermenters. Software for that area may involve basically developing code for one fermenter and then repeating the same program ten times. Consider a second system that has the same number of I/O but no repetition in programming. The effort to develop the software could be almost ten times higher. From a software point of view, the systems are really not equivalent at all.

Consider the relative amount of effort required to program a tank farm system versus a chromatography column system of the same I/O count. More functionality will be programmed into the chromatography system, and it will take more effort. Counting I/O doesn't present the total picture in a software-intensive environment.

In this environment, then, how do project managers not only estimate hardware costs by counting I/O but also estimate software costs? How do they effectively allocate engineering resources so that projects are completed on time, within budget, and with the required functionality?

This suggests taking a page from computer science. The concept of ''function points'' offers a promising tool to allow engineers to be able to talk about the costs associated in a way that would make project-to-project comparisons more meaningful. In the future it should be possible to use function point measurement to better predict the number of resources required to deliver the project, the number of resources required to maintain the project, and the cost associated with it so that better judgments on the investment can be made.

A. What Are Function Points?

Function points are a quantitative measure of software functionality. A project manager looks at each required function and awards so many function points. The function point concept considers whether one is putting in a simple message display or a highly proceduralized operation. There is a different rating, depending on the class of the function and its complexity. For example, an analog input point would be assigned four function points. A flow totalizer, which utilizes an analog signal and includes flow control logic, would be assigned thirty-one function points. Function points aren't independent of I/O, but instead attempt to understand the I/O point and its relationship to the functionality of the system.

How would one use this to better manage a project and add value during the life cycle? Knowing the number of function points for a system and building a database of knowledge, engineers will be able to predict with growing confidence how many function points can be completed in a work month. If, in midstream, engineering calls for new capabilities from the system—a large number of new function points being added—project management will have a gauge as to what resources will be required to meet milestone dates.

Function point analysis is a relative measure that helps project managers understand and compare the size and productivity of software projects. The concept provides a way to better manage and understand resources. With this

Table 2 Results of Function Point Counting

Project	Characteristics	I/O count	Total FPs	FP/ (man month)	FP/ (I/O point)
A	Flexible Procedural control Interlocks Extremely high repetition	1,200	19,000	430	16
B	Dedicated Procedural control Interlocks Very low repetition	1,900	27,000	110	14
C	Flexible Procedural count No interlocks Extremely high repetition	6,800	103,000	280	15
D	Dedicated Automatic functions Interlocks Low repetition	11,500	71,000	130	7

concept/tool, management of software throughout the life cycle of the system will be greatly enhanced.

B. Function Point Project Data

Work on counting function points for automation systems is in its early stages. Function points were developed for use in the computer science area. The method needs modification to make it suitable for use with automation systems. Work has been done by Steven Williams and Tammi Shoemaker at Eli Lilly and Company to make those adaptations and count four different automation systems. Data considered include the apply and install stages of the life cycle. Results of function point count appear in Table 2.

FP/man month is a productivity measure. Projects A and C are based on one complex unit that is repeated many times. Projects B and D have multiple unit operations, which widely vary. The data show that the level of repetition is likely to be a major factor in determining productivity and thus in being able to predict the time and staff needed to complete the apply and install phase.

FP/I/O point illustrates that the level of functionality specified for the automation systems for the four projects varied by over a factor of two; some areas delivered more functionality from their I/O.

Flexible and dedicated facilities can have the same level of functionality.

Project D had a restricted time frame and thus the functionality was intentionally limited. Functionality has been added to project D during the operate and maintain phases of the life cycle.

Procedural control adds significant functionality to the system. The level of staff support depends on the number of requirement changes for the system. Based on the results presented, 100 FP/man month is a starting point for determining required levels. Additional work remains to be done for more accurate numbers.

Adding and changing functionality as we learn more about the process is important to obtaining the maximum life cycle benefit.

III. ILLUSTRATIONS OF WAYS TO AUTOMATE THE SOFTWARE DEVELOPMENT PROCESS

Function points in themselves, however, do not produce software at less cost. Computer-aided software engineering (CASE) tools do. CASE tools are a major evolving technology for maximizing the investment in automation over the life cycle.

A few years ago, after beginning to work steadily with CASE tools, a team of automation engineers found that some requirements in a unit batch processing system, say control of flow, needed several different ''pieces'' of software in order to meet the requirement.

Likewise, one piece of software often was found to fulfill several different requirements. The same kind of many to many relationships that one sees in a relational database is found to exist between functional requirements and software design.

With this insight, they set up ''system requirements'' in one table and then ''design objects'' in another. A relational database was used to tie the two tables together. With software standards for design objects in place, they were able to put their efforts into coming up with a relatively small set of objects that can be combined into a relatively large set of requirements. The quality, consistency, and repeatability of this approach makes the software development effort extremely productive; there is far less duplication of effort. The point is that many of the effort and cost issues involved with application software development can now be better addressed with the maturing CASE and database tools widely available.

Automatic I/O configuration provides a strong example of what this means. When an input or output is set up, it requires that a number of parameters be entered. For example, should the input be inverted? What is the description of the input? What's the tag name of the input? All these things lend themselves well to a relational database. To create a productivity-enhancing tool, a database was loaded with an exhaustive compilation of information about inputs and outputs. The team created a program that takes information and turns it into code that can be read directly into the automation system. When it's done, the system is configured—all inputs and outputs are defined.

That same database could also be used for setting up a data historian. It's amazing how often the same database information can be used over and over again. If one looks ahead, it's possible to get six or seven tasks done that traditionally would have been typed one line of code at a time.

The point of describing these examples is that strategies and technologies such as the ones listed above recognize the impact of software engineering on the automation life cycle and attempt to measure, control, and make it more productive. It is only through such efforts that the costs are controlled and the value maximized at each stage of the life cycle—justify, apply, install, operate, maintain, and improve.

A. Installing the System Is More than Gantt Charts and Wires and Screwdrivers

Something that is very significant at the installation stage and start-up is how well the software works as it's delivered to the users. The authors have experiences ranging from rolling out software for the first time in the field to testing it thoroughly before it is placed in production use. Ideally, one wants to have it tested thoroughly before it gets to the field.

When a DCS system is being tested with software, one needs to throw at it all the possible failures that one can think of to make sure the system reacts correctly. Trying to do that in the field is an impossibility. Recently the authors were dealing with a highly toxic reactant. The system had to take special action if a rupture disk blew. Actually blowing the rupture disk in the field was out of the question. On a simulator running Allen–Bradley Company PLC-controlled I/O into a Measurex DCS system, the authors energized a signal that said ''rupture disk blown now.'' The test results showed what corrections had to be made to the control software.

If the failure rate in the field is 1 or 2 percent after having gone through lab simulation, it's more than 5 percent without it. The bottom line in life cycle thinking is that if a mistake can be found during specification, it's really cheap to fix. If a mistake is found during design, it's more expensive. If it's found after code is written, it's even more expensive. If one finds it in the field, it's real expensive. This is not a lineal relationship but an exponential one. Offline software testing is a valuable life cycle tool.

During the installation stage of the life cycle it's a good idea to benchmark control loops. Early on, while tuning a control loop, an engineer can intentionally change set points or introduce a process disturbance, and then capture the trend data. The data are filed away as the benchmark for the performance of the loop. Future trends can then be compared to the initial ones. In effect, one can say

"This is what it looked like to begin with, and this is what it looks like now." With the benchmark process, one can be assured of having the "key" parameters stored away.

These examples definitely are not exhaustive of all the issues related to software and maximizing the value of the life cycle. The authors present these examples as thought starters.

IV. BREAKING NEW GROUND IN OPERATION, MAINTENANCE, AND IMPROVEMENT

The life cycle model forces those in charge of automation to look at both the front half of the life cycle—justify, apply, and install—as well as the back half—operate, maintain, and improve. With this model, it's no longer enough for design engineering to deliver a system. It's incumbent on design engineering to improve the system over its life. The old "handoff" from design engineering to operations just won't cut it anymore.

Here is why! Data from ten major facilities at Eli Lilly indicate that less than 50 percent of the life cycle dollars deliver a project. That's where 25 percent of the benefits of automation come from. An important aspect of automation is that one needs to make another 50 or 60 percent investment over the life cycle to get 75 percent of the benefits of automation.

If a project team installs a system and then takes all the support people away after six months or a year, the company will be missing 70 to 80 percent of the potential benefit of that system. To understand this, let's begin with a fundamental question—"Why does a pharmaceutical company automate?"

Fundamentally, automation aims at reducing manufacturing costs through decreasing process variability. One of the primary differences between a manual process and an automated process is the ability of the automation system to deliver repeatable operations and continuous incremental improvements. One way automation does this is through programmable systems. One can change the performance of a system without having to add expensive hard components. Another significant contributor to continuous improvement is electronic data gathering. Using data to determine what is going on in a process is a fundamental feature of automation systems. Putting that information—those data—in the hands of the scientists, engineers, operators, and technicians allows these various professionals to make better decisions.

How does this translate? It translates into the fact that one makes many, many more improvements because the data are there to drive those decisions. That's one significant piece of the puzzle.

It's amazing that over ten or fifteen years one can make many small changes that don't seem very significant at the time, but one can look back after ten years to say, "Wow! We cut unit cost down by more than 90 percent."

Table 3 Life Cycle Model Existing Process Automation Investments

Plant number	Age of facility (years)	Benefit/cost ratio
1	17	3.75
2	14	2.50
3	11	11.25
4	6	3.50

The cost per kilogram decrease is much more significant in those facilities that are automated *and* have the technical support/maintenance personnel to drive those costs down. Facilities with long-term dedicated process control talent drive the learning curve and reduce the cost of production over time.

The gist of this is that the same people and tools that help apply and install the system can bring significant value to the operation, maintenance, and continuous improvement of that system.

Does this mean that operators will be replaced by control engineers? No! It means greater partnership and teamwork between the two groups and other groups than ever before. To reap the 75 percent of the benefits of an automation system, there had better be that sense of shared responsibility. These systems blur the whole concept of who works for whom. The team's effort is all directed toward the never-ending improvement of the process.

The definition of maintenance includes far more than preventive care and repair. The maintenance person is the one who makes things better, who drives the learning curve. This definition of system maintenance personnel would include process automation engineers, technicians, computer scientists, systems analysts, and instrument technicians.

At this juncture, someone must be asking, ''With all this overhead in highly trained personnel, how can any payback be made?'' First of all, let's look at the costs and then the payback.

Based on data collected for more than fifteen years, over the automation system life cycle the costs during the operate, maintain, and improve stages will be greater than 50 to 60 percent of the total life cycle cost. This includes both overhead and development tools. That's the cost side.

Now let's look at the actual net present value—the payback—experiences of four existing bulk manufacturing facilities at Eli Lilly using the life cycle model for the process automation efforts. Table 3 summarizes these results.

These facilities all had significant process automation costs throughout the whole life cycle. However, the benefits were even greater. This is the reason to continue to make these investments in the future. The process improvements facilitated by process automation have had a significant payback.

The bottom line to this is that one needs experienced people making decisions on process improvement. There is often a mindset that these people are overhead and the company is better off reducing overhead. This view ignores the big picture implication that by cutting out $100,000, the company may lose $200,000 in productivity gains.

That's not a good decision, but engineering personnel may not always do a good job of explaining to management why it's not a good decision. This is one of the reasons the life cycle model is so important. It shows the real situation, the pluses and minuses, and the impact of automation on the profitability and longevity of the enterprise.

For every dollar engineers ask management to spend, there must be two or more dollars paid back during the life cycle. One must make promises of what can and cannot be delivered. With an investment of ten staff years, the company had better be paid back at least $2 million. The authors' data support the assertion that this is what a company can expect if operation and maintenance of automation is truly seen as long-term optimization and improvement.

It comes back to being data-driven. If one manages by data, one can predict future performance based on an understanding of past performance. If one understands the automation investments made in the past, one can be more successful in predicting what investments should be made in the future. That is what the life cycle model is all about.

7

Managing the Manufacturing Control Domain

Sean M. Megley*

PerSeptive Biosystems, Cambridge, Massachusetts

I. PROCESS MONITORING

The environment of process monitoring in the pharmaceutical industry is process-parametric, largely batch-operational, and dependent upon validation integrity. The parametric aspect compares the actual physical measurements at certain moments in the process to the specification under which the product was licensed to manufacture. A regulated industry is required to produce its product within those specifications, but this observation is only to establish a context, since the reader is probably most aware of those operating constraints. The batch-operational segment of process monitoring is a temporal measurement that regulates the genealogy, time, and transition that a material undergoes from state to state. In biologics, with live cells, the expression of proteins occurs within such a distinct time period and is optimal when this expression peak is not overshadowed by cell mortality, debris, and by-products. Validation integrity in the context of process monitoring has several important factors to consider. *The integrity of any batch is dependent as much on the physical resources as it is on the knowledge resources that contribute to the capture, analysis, and interpretation of process data.* Validation integrity is a concept that focuses on the initiation and conservation of system validation. This section of the chapter will focus on this triangle relationship (Fig. 1).

* *Current affiliation:* Vanstar, Jamestown, Rhode Island.

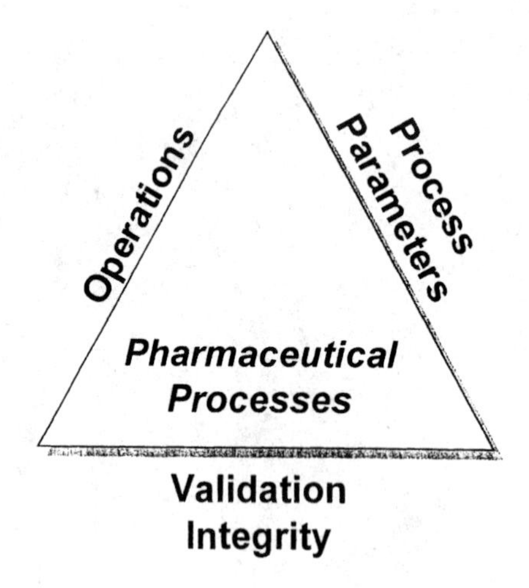

Fig. 1 Triangle relationship of validation integrity.

The material is presented in an applied and additive manner. For someone investigating these technologies, some baseline start-up topics are presented. For the person interested in improving his or her present system, this material will address some ongoing operating issues that may be of help. In all phases (starting, ongoing, retirement), strategic assessments are necessary to ensure the success of the process and ultimately the entire enterprise.

To my mind, it is paradoxical that many process automation environments are isolated and distinct from the information environments. In facilities that are relatively enabled with desktop and central computing resources, automation assets lie untapped and underutilized. This inscrutable paradox can be understood better by an exploration of the five major components of a process automation environment. Organizations that only address components do not get the economical benefits that can be realized by focusing on automation as a whole system. In the systems approach we can reveal some of the process tenets that, if applied, can help increase your project's success forecast. Then, rather than trying to change the way the process works to fit your way of doing business (1980s computerization), maybe we can find ways to use every attribute of the process to improve the way we do business (1990s process centered).

The pharmaceutical process has a primary context, the chemical or biotechnology process, and secondarily the business processes of design, start-up, and operation. The primary context has a huge influence on the nature of the business processes, while the business processes have a relatively minor impact on the nature of the pharmaceutical process. There is a great advantage to *understand this and then exploit it.* Next decide how rapid the deployment of the business

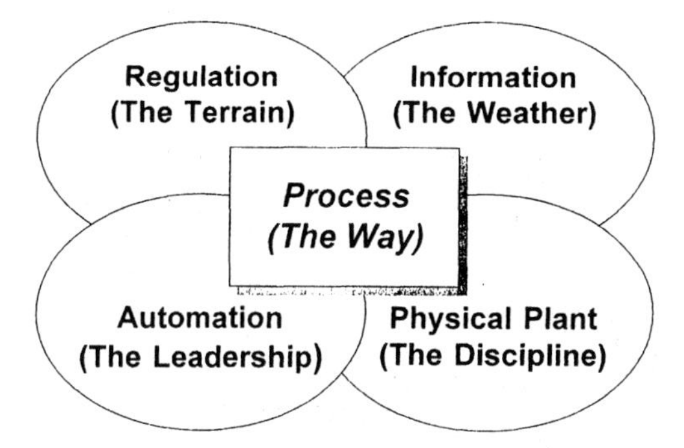

Fig. 2 Five areas to assess before resources are committed.

activity will proceed based upon your resources. This means to define the way you are going to do business and clearly communicate this to everyone, show them the way: ''*The Way means inducing the people to have the same aim as the leadership.*''* By taking steps to understand and communicate your aim, you will have increased your project's primary value.

Figure 2 depicts areas that should be assessed before committing resources. These five areas are the focus of *The Art of War*, but also apply to the resource wars that automation systems incite. The regulatory terrain of the pharmaceutical industry has a significant impact upon all attributes of information. Generation, analysis, and storage of the data is as important as the actual product; without that information a batch of product is useless. The timespan of information for a new drug begins with discovery and product development. At the time of submission, clinical data are the key factor. During the life of the product, manufacturing data and ongoing adverse reaction data management are the primary issue. Factors to consider at the initiation of a new suite or product focus on clearly noting those information items that indicate compliance with the regulatory agencies and those needed to consistently produce the product. When the regulatory information is a subset of the information needed for production, the perception is that this extended information becomes a legitimate regulatory requirement. This ''wrapping yourself in the flag'' is expensive. Although start-up information requirements are different from ongoing requirements, most companies don't differentiate, and when people change jobs or move on, the basis for that original information requirement becomes obscure and inherits legitimacy. The downside of this is that the information requirement is never questioned. Information gathered for regulation would be identified and regularly reviewed. Strategy is required to be successful with a validation and production project. Risk can increase

*Sun Tzu, *The Art of War*, 6th century B.C.

by not measuring the scope of the information/validation requirement. In all cases, computer-based information requires validation and ongoing validation integrity support, so to consider the information requirement while ignoring the initial and ongoing validation requirement is pointless. A parallel strategy should thus be considered to address a concurrent validation integrity program. In this mode, the information systems are designed with the validation planned. Safety and chemical use information are consonant components of the regulatory terrain. By assessing these components in the early phases of the project, they can be engineered into the environment without any additional information-gathering costs. Genealogy and lot tracking should be considered elemental regulatory requirements.

Information is much like the weather, because it is always changing. In biotechnology the seasons actually are a consideration, since some contaminants are common in the summer and others are promiscuous in the colder months. Information in a pharmaceutical process is a *temporal attribute* of the product. At what time and for what duration did the product experience this transformation as indicated by the interpreted data? Since both an entire product line and each batch are dependent upon the information reliability, the value of the information and product are the same. Success in the information domain can be achieved by adequate planning and infrastructure depth. From initiation to termination (Fig. 3), reliability and integrity issues are forces acting on the infrastructure. The infrastructure strength will allow expanding data requirements to be absorbed while transformation to the infrastructure occurs. In the 1980s, computer systems were focused on capacity planning as the critical success factor. In the 1990s that

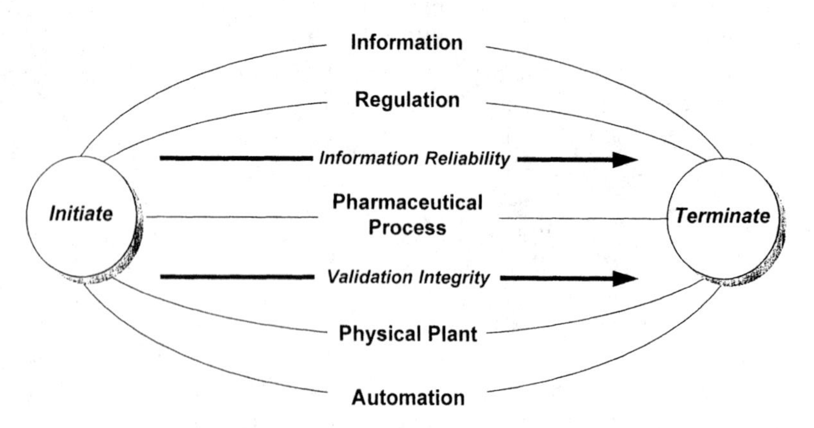

Fig. 3 Reliability and integrity issues from initiation to termination.

focus has shifted to communication and capability—communication that enables peer-to-peer data transfers, command, and control; capability that is based upon flexible data structure, real-time graphics, and client/server paths that can address all levels of information sharing. Timing is an important factor for information/automation projects. The following list of factors can make the difference between a successful project and costly derailment:

- Are all the software products you are planning on using released? How many sites?
- Will (assume) this be a validated system and can the module you are building be validated?
- Are all computers that are needed ready and available? What is the life of the platform?
- Can you bring the right staff together for the right length of time and keep them pointed in the right direction? Extended projects weaken the staff.
- Are the consultants you are using stable financially? Do they have and use standards for development and implementation? Is their interim project style compatible with your management reporting requirements?
- Are the stakeholders in the project committed and do they understand the way you are planning to proceed?
- Are there opposing camps and do you completely understand their positions?

The physical plant of a pharmaceutical facility has an impact on the discipline and operations with respect to information and automation utilization. Rooms are isolated by design, therefore a widespread network is necessary. Adequate network access and systems are essential to avoid ''pocket systems'' in which local inventory is tracked on a clipboard or material status is inherent by material location. *You should never have to enter a process area to gather information.* The discipline to use information and automation systems correctly minimizes human intervention for non-value-added events, which in turn minimizes *contamination*. The working organization has an impact on the information that is required to run the facility efficiently. In a fully integrated environment these information needs are in harmony with the regulatory requirements and do not swell to facilitate organizational boundary issues. Boundary issues arise when information is generated outside the production event to status the production event. For example, a documentation group maintains a batch genealogy, which is produced by production. However, the quality group needing to have the genealogy at its disposal for regulatory issues may duplicate this information, leading to swollen information, which adds no value. Logistics of material transfer are the most important aspect of designing an information environment with validation integrity. This integrity is based upon the accuracy of the material transfer from the following possible attributes:

1. Lot
2. Type
3. Status
4. Quality
5. Quantity
6. Method of transfer
7. Completeness of the information transaction.

Automation can only be successful if all of the preceding attributes have been addressed and integrated into the process. Automation is essentially the lieutenant making the decisions of the commander. In some facilities, automation is the commander, where all decisions have been entrusted and encoded into the knowledge form that is used to make decisions on a serial, distributed, or synaptic basis. The degree of automation is widely varied, and can range from instrumented to articulated. In an instrumented environment the process would be observed and data captured for batch information. On the other end, the articulated environment would be able to monitor, request material, process intermediates, and discharge products. It is inherent in the degree of automation what quality of results are going to be achieved. When the process is fully defined and nonvariant, full automation will produce high-quality products. When the process is transient, the incidence of intervention will increase the potential for error and variable product quality. As much effort should be given to elimination of process variation as possible. During the production phase of the product, any overrides or exceptions should be immediately run down or they become a ''way'' of doing business. Human factors in automation environments should focus on effective communication. Communication deals with how the information is perceived. Studies indicate that 51 percent of the population is graphic, 26 percent is linguistic, and 23 percent uses kinesthetics for their most effective communication modality.* This means that at least half of the automation interface should be graphic, and the balance should utilize characters or speech communication. Kinesthetics relate to things in a way that they ''feel'' them, and essentially a predominantly feeling person would not be the best-suited for automation operations.

A. Plantwide View

Pharmaceutical plants are heterogeneous environments in which mainstream processes are facilitated by branch support processes. It is not likely that all the branch processes are automated in the same manner as the mainstream. *In a strategic formation the most capable system should be deployed on the most cost-impacting process.* This usually implies the most expensive system as well. Fig-

*M. Brooks, *Developing Business Rapport*, HarperCollins, New York.

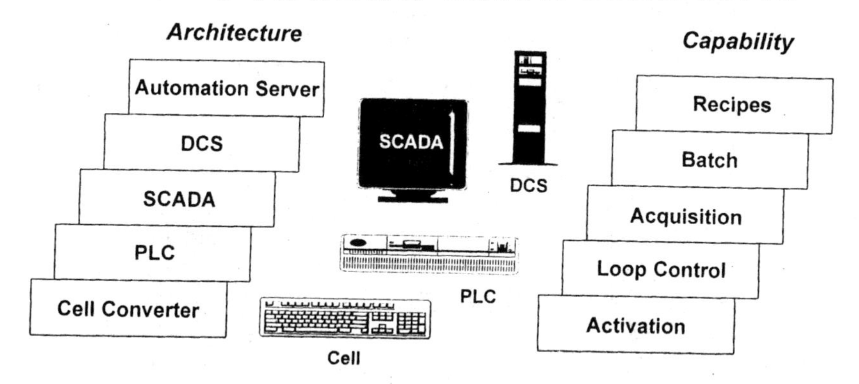

Fig. 4 Ladder of increasing capability, architecture complexity, and cost.

ure 4 depicts the ladder of increasing capability, architectural complexity, and cost. An automation environment is a continuously changing milieu. It is possible for some periods of time to "freeze" an environment. However, the daily use of the environment itself will often cause changes that must be planned for and managed. Figure 5 relates to the changes that may come indirectly from issues unrelated to the information and automation systems. Production plans, process changes, material quality, and environmental variation could cause your strategy to become compromised. It is most likely to prevail if there is as much consideration of capability of the architecture as there is capacity (Fig. 5).

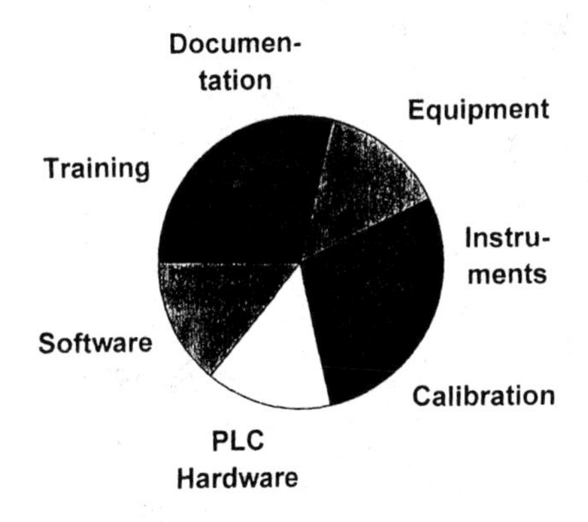

Fig. 5 Changes that may come indirectly from issues unrelated to the information and automation systems.

B. Cell Controllers

The first level of automation, cell controllers, are generally task-specific machines that are used for production and laboratory processes. In the biotech industry, backup cell culture (BUC) labs use ''biocontrollers,'' which control fermentation. Laboratories across the board have a great number of analytical devices with embedded computers. Computers are more general than biocontrollers, but have highly specialized software that communicates with the robotic lab devices. Both types of systems perform similar functions for the pharmaceutical process, perform repeatable process steps on material, gather the data, and perform analytical or process decisions. The other attribute that is important at this level is the degree of integration that the cell controller has with respect to the manufacturing execution system (MES) or laboratory information management system (LIMS). In small single-product facilities the tendency is standalone. In the long view, this has numerous problems with data collection, product quality, and communication. The integrated cell controller can have a wide degree of connectivity functions. Data gathering, analytical decision making, and upstream instruments can be accessed if the controls are on the network. Recipes can be used if the controller is capable of participating in a client/server conversation.

1. *Automation Capability*

Opportunities at the cell controller level exist for creating a uniform facility look and feel with heterogeneous equipment. Process recipes can be used at all levels. The recipe for a fermentation batch is relatively the same for 10 liters as it is for 7,000 liters. Relative is the key word. Material charges are related to the ultimate product goal, but pH, temperature, pressure, and other control factors are only related to the unit measurement, so a recipe can be scaled up relative to batch size. This is very important, because the scientist, process developer, and technician all can review and understand the recipe no matter what level of production is involved.

2. *Information Capacity*

The information capacity is going to be dependent upon the number of products or variations that the cell controller has to control. That is also dependent upon the configuration of the controller as a task-specific device or a general process client. The trade-off is that a specific task configuration will take X amount of manpower hours every time a new product is introduced. Configuring the controller as a process client may take 5 * X for the first configuration, but all subsequent configurations, using recipes, might only take 0.1 * X, so the flexibility factor is important to consider. This relates back to capacity, because the controller has several limits—the number of process recipes it can store and the number of process batches it can record. A network-integrated controller may have no recipes locally until execution and may upload data continuously or upon batch completion.

3. Start-up Considerations

a. Hardware In order to develop a stable facility and ensure support on a highly reliable basis, part of the start-up review should include consideration of equipment failure, repair, and support. Critical spares are needed to ensure batches in progress do not get lost due to a $5.00 fuse. What about spare computers? If your project can sustain the additional cost for spares at the outset, purchase them. Technology moves so fast that perfectly working equipment that is current today can obsolesce in months. Computer chips burned especially for your control task should also have spares. They should be purchased and vaulted to ensure that if your controller breaks down, you can replace it with ''in-kind'' parts. Disk drives also wear out. The duty cycle of a commercial computer is much higher than a civilian model. Don't expect an office computer to pull 365 * 24 hours of service without some problems. Power is also a never-ending source of excitement. *Assume the power will fail.* You can use local battery devices for hours of protection. Even if your facility has a standby generator, get the battery; those systems are not invincible. If your power protection is thin, what happens on a power down? Can your process recover and be reset to continue? Do you want to consider integration into the building alarm system?

b. Software At this level the software considerations are related to the chip set on the controller and the data collection software used to chart the collected parameters. The chip set functions should be verified and documented. A family of controllers approach can be taken if you can establish that they are all the same version. So once you examine in detail the process control algorithms in one controller, you could presume that all other controllers perform in the same way. However, this is an assumption that must itself be documented. You must still check out all instruments to assure that they are connected and adequately operating. The software for the data collection must be accounted for in three ways; what computer and operating system it is running on, what functions the program is specified to provide, and what data are gathered and how they are stored. One way to document the computer itself is to use a program that examines all the pertinent parameters and writes a report. You can write this yourself using batch procedures, or purchase a utility. You want record capability, memory, OS version, start-up files, program versions, sizes, and dates. If you are in an open lab and the computer may be used for other tasks when off-line, a virus protection scheme may need to be considered. Strategy for the validation of the software should be commensurate with the size and complexity of the system. The more modular and decomposable the system, the easier it will be to validate and maintain. Like may quality issues, validation cannot be put into the system after it is built. Validation of software starts with design, testing, and deployment. The data generated during a batch is going to consume space. A simple calculation of the typical size of a file multiplied by the number of batches will predict how often the data must be removed. Consider whether the process can be stopped to remove the data and if the size of the files can be moved with portable media. Networking a device at this point now has a major advantage.

c. Training Successful projects consider training a critical part of the path. Training is a formal transfer of skill and knowledge. On-the-job training after start-up tends to be a watered-down, just-punch-the-buttons training in which rote behavior is transferred. Serious errors are usually attributed to human errors, which is always related to training. Training is beneficial to everyone. Technicians can provide valuable insight to process engineers. Process engineers can explain why the programmed systems react to the process conditions. This complete understanding is essential to a smooth operation. Good training, clear documentation, or online support will make the technicians confident in the operation of the facility.

d. Procedures and Documentation In addition to the batch procedures, the procedures for start-up and initiation are critical to long-term facility operation. When there is an equipment failure, the start-up method used several years ago is a distant blur. The cost of documenting every step of the installation may seem unnecessary, so you need to consider how long you expect the process to be in operation. Any time the answer is years, any replaced item should be completely documented so that replacement, even ''in kind,'' can be accomplished with the same results.

e. Validation Since validation has been mentioned in every section so far, a separate section on this topic seems to be redundant. But what is often missing in validation strategies is the evaluation of the validation itself. You can overdo it without adding to the confidence level that you achieve during the examination. Your goal is to ensure that your system does what you specified it is going to do. To that end, the validation must be thorough and effective. The regulatory requirements are interpretive, and on the day of an audit the light is different from that during the start-up period in which the validation was executed. It takes top-down management discipline to do the right level of validation. At this point capable leadership is highly valuable.

4. Operations

Immediate resolution of exceptions and regular review of operation status are ideal disciplines. Human nature has a sensitivity to the *new and changing* while *the old and repeating* dulls the senses. Status quo is only a human perception. The equipment is wearing out, the computers are getting older, and the plant is changing every day. System maintenance is as important as paint and grease. Rather than address this in a checklist fashion, the focus will be on two major thrusts that were diagrammed earlier; information reliability and validation integrity.

a. Information Reliability As operations continue, information residue should be managed. The review of a raw data and the decision to store it or the "interpreted" form should be made. I have heard "Save it all, we don't know what questions we may need to ask!" The truth of the matter was that no one ever came back and asked for the raw data again. In research the requirements are broader than in production. Whatever the decision, be consistent with the procedure and follow the procedure. Work files or files created by reports often create large amounts of residue. Versions of files created during development are often unnecessary checkpoints that will not be returned to. In this matter, it is best to take a full backup, vault it, and purge all but the operation versions.

Security is a topic worthy of mention. Training and discipline are required to have an effectively secure environment. In the regulated industries, operator identification is required on any critical step in the process. That means that passwords and rotation of passwords on a regular basis are required to secure the data entry of operators. Leaving "the password" on the computer so everyone can use is a severe breach in policy, procedure, and discipline. Security is a foundation discipline; it must be conveyed to the personnel, and the policy for failure to follow this discipline must be clear.

b. Validation Integrity The concept of validation integrity should be ubiquitous in the pharmaceutical industry. The *integrity* of the state of the equipment and computer system is a dynamic, which in any moment must remain intact. This means that the equipment must be operated in an approved manner by a trained operator with certified software on approved material. If any of these factors is compromised, then the validation integrity is compromised. This also means that it is deeper than software testing; it is a management practice. Systems personnel have been scapegoats, and seen as the last point where quality is stuffed into the system. Their role is to ensure that the system section stands certified, but the operation and production use of the system still bears the brunt of the proper usage.

C. Programmable Logic Controllers

The programmable logic controller (PLC) is today's building block in heterogeneous environments. The cost, speed, and density of the devices have made them very popular for continuous and some batch duty. The downside of the deployment is the ladder–logic programming, which is obscure to all but technical groups.

1. Automation Capability

PLCs can be deployed in active, process decisions are made, or passive, data I/O multiplexing, modes. In the active mode parameters would be sent to the PLC and a process cycle would be engaged to meet the criterion. This introduction of the PLC as part of a pharmaceutical environment is going to assume a fully networked implementation of the equipment. A passive implementation would use the PLC to concentrate and transform field instrument signals to a digital format. The data are then polled by a supervisory or automation server. In the active mode configuration the PLC logic must be decoupled from the product parameters so that the equipment remains independent of the process. This allows rapid validation and redeployment. Since the equipment is divided into equipment functions and recipe processes it can be decomposed into simpler tasks to certify.

2. *Information Capacity*

PLC capacity is register- or memory-based. An attendant supervisory or automation server must actively scan the PLC to collect data that the PLC has updated at its programmed scanning speed. When the PLC is parametrically configured, it can process as many different recipes as the parameters represent. Static programming should be avoided unless the PLC will never be used for more than one or two variations. The savings of parametric configuration should be realized on the second task. At that time the programming is already complete and the changes are implemented as a change in data, not logic. It is important to understand that the PLC is not best suited for a widely varying, potentially strategy-changing problem. A DCS or automation server would be better suited for that task. PLCs are also best suited for number processing, multimode character and number tasks; likewise, material identification or operator conversation are better suited for an automation server.

3. *Startup Considerations*

a. Hardware PLCs typically are deployed with higher I/O counts and wider physical assets. A database of all I/O should be developed in design and maintained throughout the life of the implementation. During start-up this database is used to I/O checkout and instrument calibration.

Critical spares should be considered for high-risk implementations. In high safety and environmentally sensitive implementations, redundant processing may be considered. The whole philosophy of redundancy can be extrapolated from the instruments through communications to data collection systems. The safety, equipment, and cost factors should be carefully reviewed in the design phase of any project.

b. Software PLCs are configured. The logic is represented in an electrical circuit or ladder logic. Important factors that must be documented are PLC version and size, PLC configuration tool, and the revision of the PLC configuration source code. Since the PLC is configured "live," the program must be offloaded and stored. Discipline must be exercised to ensure that any "tweaking" is accounted for and revision control is in place.

When a PLC is deployed in a DCS/PLC scenario, the DCS/PLC mapping is also considered part of the PLC software. This map provides the DCS with the highway address and starting register of the PLC at which data registers will commence. These registers may represent instrument values or process parameters, depending upon the configuration. PLC I/O is considered DCS I/O, and can reduce the physical footprint of current DCS termination cards. Depending upon project talent, functions may be stashed at various levels in the architecture. To have and maintain the highest validation integrity, the functions should be implemented at the highest level to avoid concealment. It is also key to avoid any "fixed" algorithms that are product-dependent. It is sometimes unavoidable, but minimizing and localizing these functions is then the next best approach.

Automation server polling of a PLC can be accomplished over an Ethernet network. The PLC presents a RS232/RS244 interface that is polled by the server in a handshake protocol. This conversation could send parameters to the PLC and recover data. This allows the PLC to be minimally configured and have the automation server determine strategy via a recipe. This topography can be used for laboratory, HVAC, and near-time process equipment. Since the network does not guarantee a time schedule, real-time control is not possible. The critical strategies must be handled by the PLC. However, in most monitoring situations in which one-to-two-minute sample cycles are used, this network uncertainty is not relevant. Network delays would be in a matter of seconds. More of the automation server role is discussed further in this chapter.

c. Training Validation requirements should be the first training program that is considered. It is the fundamental discipline that all other training programs will rely on, as well as the weakest link in the training programs. Why do chemical/pharmaceutical operators need to understand validation? Because they are part of a regulated industry, part of a regulated process, and the persons most likely to compromise a million dollar batch if they don't. Validation is a fundamental requirement that when properly approached can yield substantial benefits to the production organization.

Operation of a PLC system is based upon equipment and operator interface input and output. It makes sense to divide the training to focus on these areas. It is the system engineer's job and project manager's responsibility to see that thorough training information is placed into a permanent record for the facility. Such fundamental topics as "What does it look like when it's OK?" should be addressed during start-up because there "will never be time later."

A power-up sequence should include the power engagement from the circuit breakers to the equipment and any communications equipment needed to complete the PLC network. Some processes may have dead-stop start-up sequences different from warm starts, which have different ramping strategies. These distinctions should be clear in the documentation. Data for the PLC is usually downloaded upon system start-up. If anything must be manually done from a full power-up sequence, you need to rethink the risk of skipping that step. PLC downloads may also have to occur after the battery period has been exceeded. Here is where the discipline of the organization comes to play. Do you have the laptop ready, the cable in hand, the knowledge of the PLC software, and the correct revision of the program to go and correctly complete the restart? If you answered maybe to any of these parameters, create a detailed procedure to clear the question.

Planned power-down events should begin with the monitoring software being disabled. The operating technician should be trained in the complete method to conclude normal operations and the sequence to ''down'' any software processes. Batches should be concluded and notes in the operating logs should reflect the planned event.

Emergency shutdown procedures should be simple and clear. Training on these methods can mean the prevention of dangerous and expensive midstream halts. The training should focus on problems that could require an emergency shutdown and on what information reveals the true state of the equipment. The difference may be the use of a calculated point versus a raw value that is presented on a meter. Verifying the fault is as important as responding to the alarm. All alarms should be reviewed by production, quality, and systems engineers. If the alarm is real, correct the condition. Do not leave alarms that can be ignored, because then real alarms can be missed.

Normal restart requires that the operator establish that the process equipment is in a state ready to proceed and that the software is likewise in agreement. Determine if you plan to allow resumption or intend to start new batch recording as a matter of operations. It may be inconsequential to the material, but irrevocable from a regulatory position. Any halt/restart should be documented, explained, and evaluated. Training of the operators to be forthright will aid in long-term success of the facility.

Operation training is relative to the manner in which the PLC is deployed. If the operator is in-line and required to make decisions, the boundary conditions for the acceptable and unacceptable must be documented. If the operator is ''monitoring'' the time sequence of checking the process, the critical parameters should be part of the process training. Scheduling the operator may be required in some process, and alerting the operator may also be part of the operating plan. In a regulated process the identity of the operator will come into play. Security training must be included in operations training. Policy must address this issue to ensure that it is implemented on the plant floor.

d. Procedures and Documentation A database of instrument calibration records must be maintained to ensure that all instruments are properly maintained. Depending on the facility, any plan to schedule or base calibration on usage will impact the calibration agenda. This requirement is related directly to the use of PLCs, but when looking at the total plant information strategy, all systems and instruments that deal with critical process functions have to be managed in this manner.

4. Operations

Information reliability is related to the confidence that the information you are using to operate your process is consistent and reflects the process accurately. The reliability of the information can be compromised if instrumentation, data manipulation, or communication is inhibited. To reliably operate your process, the data should be directly reported by the PLC or automation server. No secondary "spreadsheet" setup should be permitted to be used as a deciding factor. If that is actually needed it should be incorporated into the baseline system. If not, ancillary calculation systems with inherent human error can predict incorrect results.

Validation integrity is an ongoing process of review, operation, data gathering, and consideration. *Kaizen* is the Japanese word for continuous improvement. While improvement of processes is not considered continuous, validation monitoring is important. Prior to going online with a process, those areas most susceptible to change with operation should be identified and programs established to manage their state of readiness. *If the "price of freedom is constant vigilance" the "cost of validation can be reduced by constant vigilance."* This cost may be the closing of a plant or process if an ongoing validation breach is not detected. A cycle should be planned in the areas shown in the Fig. 5.

D. Distributed Control Systems

The DCS brings a complete solution to the pharmaceutical environment: field I/O, data highway, real-time control, data integration, and batch operations. However, depending upon the integration level of the DCS into the overall information infrastructure, some of the standard components may not be suitable. This happens from the DCS vendors trying to be all things to all users. It requires generic to point of limited usefulness.

1. Automation Capability

At the beginning of DCS projects a "style" evolves that impacts the system for the life of the installation. You can put all process and equipment logic into DCS coding, making it the repository of all production knowledge. Alternatively, you could put equipment logic into the DCS and put the process knowledge into a "recipe." This has an impact on personnel requirements, validation, revalidation, and transferability of the DCS environment.

2. Information Capacity

DCS information exists in several temporal forms. In the controller, data exist in a real-time format and live through the end of a batch. In a standard DCS offering, a batch data manager can be used to collect data as needed on behalf of the active batch. This activity occurs on the attendant configuration computer. It is worth mentioning that the shift of a DCS into a client/server architecture changes the personnel requirement from a straight DCS programmer to a vertical DCS/client programmer. These are more commercially available skills and they make staff recruiting more attainable.

The use of a data warehouse concept dramatically leverages the information capacity of the DCS. A data warehouse is conceptually a database in which all data collected with a batch are stored. All batches end up in the warehouse and retrieval may be against one or many batches. This capability is usually in the site custom level.

3. Startup Considerations

A DCS is best suited for a wide area or field deployment. A database of all I/O and processor equipment should be developed in design and maintained throughout the life of the implementation. During start-up this database is used for data highway testing, I/O checkout, and instrument calibration.

Critical spares should be considered for controller, critical devices, and single point of failure. In high safety and environmentally sensitive implementations, redundant processing may be considered. DCS systems have built-in redundancy which is only a factor of financial investment not additional engineering effort. Since a portion of the DCS may be exposed to a ''public'' network, consideration for validation of the network hardware may be necessary.

a. Software DCS languages at this time are somewhere between the second and third generation. Due to the ''register'' mentality, this manipulation is the primary object in the language. The handling of character information in a straight DCS is messy and contrived. Again, the client/server plan rings many more capabilities to the table. Using the server to process character information and the client to process local numeric data gives the greatest capability.

Automation server integration into the DCS divides the configuration job into two sections: DCS drivers and recipe server. The job of the driver is to provide access to equipment and provide strategy for controlling that equipment on behalf of the recipe. The job of the recipe server is to communicate with the DCS unit, sending down parameters and scanning DCS data registers for batch data. During the start-up this driver testing can be done with recipes. A family of recipes can be developed to use the driver in boundary, nominal, and excessive limits to test driver resiliency. Any changes in the equipment isolates software changes to the driver only, not a recipe change.

4. Operations

The *batch operations* themselves execute in a controller. At this point we need to have a basis of understanding the DCS hardware architecture. The configuration computer, which programs the DCS, is connected to the plant Ethernet. This computer is used to configure and download the controllers and console. The console is connected to the DCS highway and the plant Ethernet. The controllers live on the DCS highway and communicate with subordinate termination cards that are directly connected to process equipment. The project I helped to formulate used a Fisher/Rosemount DCS system. Most DCS systems have similar configuration tools, controller, and control loop capability, although the standards employed by each system vary. The batch operations are typically the sequences of states the equipment transitions through to achieve the desired effect on the batch material. *Process and equipment information are intermingled.*

The *control loops* described by the configuration tool relate to the instruments and equipment reactions by source code programming. A control system engineer performs this task. The process engineer usually does not work at this level. While some control loops are product-specific, others are configured in a more generic manner. The standard control loop is independent of the batch operations that call it when control is needed. Control loops combine into groups for programming efficiency; however, the modularity and validation impact of this division can be significant. *The worst-case scenario is that a small change in a DCS operation spreads throughout the configuration so that instead of a minor revalidation test, a major recertification effort is the result.*

Where are the data logged and stored? In a DCS environment, data exist in many places and temporal conditions. Field instruments sensing physical conditions reflect a current into the termination card that converts the information to a digital format. The digital values polled by the unit operations controller (UOC) are stored into the data registers. Batch operations and control loops review the information at different intervals for sequence decisions and control loop reactions. Data can be targeted onto a graphic console or into a data collection database. The database is running on the network-connected computer and the communication between this computer and the controller is facilitated by the network interface. Batch reports can be generated by the controller or the database.

5. *Validation Integrity*

Specification and development of DCS applications vary by company. The transformation of process knowledge into automation actions follows this scenario; the process developer writes a specification that is process-oriented, material-based, and time- and condition-oriented. The automation engineer takes this specification and *translates* the specification into automation jargon, at which point the process engineer no longer can recognize the original requirements. As the process is developed and tested, the process engineer and operator are molded into the automation view of the process. *Associating units, operations, and control loops as devised by the control engineer is artificially reorganizing the process knowledge because of the limitations of the DCS language.*

Validation of a standard DCS goes down to the source code level. Each point is checked, then each control loop is tested and each operation is verified. Failure, recovery, and alarms are examined to ensure that every action and reaction of the DCS can be proven to act according to the *automation specification.* Then the material validation must occur that ensures that the process transforms the material as planned according to the *process specification.* Often this effort can become redundant and time-consuming because it is perceived that it is better to err by overexamination than omission. *Consider that it is better to decompose the problem into separate equipment and process components and do the job once, with 100 percent coverage.*

Transportability is important to consider when research groups are developing processes that are going to move into manufacturing and scale-up. Ideally the research DCS configuration is copied and moved to the manufacturing DCS. The ideal is difficult to achieve with a standard approach because the research DCS must exactly match the manufacturing DCS point for point or the operation will not work. Conversion is almost always required. It is better than writing the process from scratch and some efficiencies are present, but it is a low-level problem once again.

Upgrades and changes to the process, equipment, and DCS environment are continuous. Software revisions, equipment enhancements, and process optimization are some of the driving factors that cause changes. In order to support these changes and keep the validated DCS in operation great consideration must be made. Is the change isolated? Can it be verified easily and are any peripheral impacts possible?

E. Automation Server/Automation Client

The following concepts are a summary of an implementation of a client/server DCS (CSDCS) project where I helped formulate the information architecture. The most essential principle in adapting a DCS into a CSDCS is to segregate process and equipment functions. This is key to defining equipment *drivers* and the development of process *recipes.* In software engineering terms, the decoupling of the recipes and drivers is the focus. An equipment driver is a software program that provides access to and control of a particular control module, much as a printer driver in Windows allows access and control of various printers. The driver functionally will be examined in more detail later. For now it is important to understand that a driver provides the connection to use the equipment without the need to know the internal operation of the equipment.

A recipe is made up of the operations, phases, and process steps that transform the batch materials from raw material to final product. In addition, the recipe expresses the data collection, process parameters, quality samples, and operator instructions. Follow the following rules for driver/recipe module decisions:

1. If it is related to the equipment and independent of any recipe running on the equipment, the knowledge belongs in the driver.

2. If it is related to the recipe and independent of any equipment that it runs on, the knowledge belongs in the recipe.

For example, the need for temperature control is basic to a recipe, but the use of an HV01 valve to provide steam is dependent on the local equipment. If the recipe calls for temperature control, then the driver is responsible for knowing how. *Therefore the recipe is independent of the equipment that it runs on and may be run anywhere that the equipment driver can provide temperature control within the range needed. Now you come to having CSDCSs that are* functionally equivalent, *versus DCSs that must be* identical *in order for recipes to be transportable.*

In a full CSDCS environment the *recipe server* fulfills the mission of providing requested recipes to *unit servers* and accepting completed batch information into the *data warehouse*. In addition to this primary role, the server also has revision, validation status, and resource unit information about every recipe in the database. A recipe server can support multiple suites, while a unit server is a dedicated suite resource. A trained person is assigned the responsibility to insert recipes into the recipe server. The guard the database to ensure that the revision of the recipe is correct and that the recipe has been certified by quality, production, and engineering as suitable to the task.

The unit server sends recipe steps to the CSDCS or user interface. The server also logs security, data points, and recipe step completion. The unit server is in contact with every executing unit in the suite, so for management, the scope of the server is limited to a single suite. The computing and performance capability of the server is much greater than this assignment. Risk and failure management play a factor in the resource allocation. The products that make up the unit server layers will be discussed in the section on application interfaces.

A data warehouse in concept is a single database in which all product, equipment, and material information is stored. In application, the data warehouse is a collection of databases and access methods that have utility in all phases of the manufacturing processes. Recipes are managed, and served to requesting unit servers. Completed batches, an separate database of a single recipe execution, are logged into the warehouse. A critical tenet in the use of the data warehouse with batch information is *read-only access*. Information may be added to the batch database but never modified.

Validation of a CSDCS has advantages over a DCS due to the modularity and segregation of process from equipment. The equipment drivers are compact and focused on task, and easily identify the actions and reactions they need to perform. Clearly, using the CSDCS, recipes can be written as validation recipes that test the driver functions with different challenges and record the results of those challenges. Likewise, the process portion of the CSDCS is simpler to validate because you are only focused on the transitions called for by the recipe. The equipment drivers have already been validated and the recipes work within those driver limits. The recipes can also be enriched with additional data collection to support process validation. Following certification the data collection can be commented out of the recipe or removed. *The greatest benefit from the CSDCS validation profile comes at the introduction of the second product; the equipment validation remains intact and the recipe validation now is significantly less than a complete DCS validation effort*!

Transportability is intrinsic to the CSDCS. Driver standards applied throughout a company cause the drivers to share common communication. Recipe servers are connected to common DCS interface programs. When recipes call for heat, pressure, or material, they are not concerned with *how* it is provided. The driver takes care of any local customization.

F. User Interfaces

X Windows plays a key role in delivering the CSDCS information and automation windows. Following the drivers and recipes, the information and automation windows provide access to the layer of the CSDCS that is relevant. The X technology is a tremendous step forward in the delivery of automation throughout a facility. Within a single X Windows terminal, multiple process and information computers can be sponsoring sessions that the operator can move from window to window as needed. In the CSDCS scenario the operator relies on two primary windows. One window has all the automation in focus and the other window has batch recipe information. The unit server has a session running for each recipe that is in progress. The CSDCS has a session through which the operator can access any unit that is in operation.

The automation server, or CSDCS, has several essential functions: graphics, data access, driver communication, and alarms. The graphics are typical DCS graphics with set points, color-enhanced equipment diagrams, and trends. In the CSDCS they are provided by a software option called the network operations server (NOS). This provides control functionality from a remote terminal. This is direct CSDCS communications in which the operator can view the status of equipment and answer alarms. The data access is provided by a program called the computer highway interface program (CHIP). CHIP is configured to have points that are evaluated by the process controllers and stored in CHIP for access by data-logging programs. CHIP is bidirectional and provides the driver communication points between the unit server and CSDCS. Alarms are always handled directly by the CSDCS. Equipment limits, failures, and process limits are detected by the drivers, and the alarms are posted. The operator acknowledges the alarm, reviews the condition that caused it, and initiates a corrective response. For example, if a temperature alarm is set to post when the vessel rises 5 degrees above the set point, an alarm will sound. The operator would determine what action would resolve this (perhaps a heater circulation outlet has been restricted), and implement the correction. Recipes do not implement equipment alarms. Recipes, however, can change alarm levels, which is a key distinction. For safety and speed, the CSDCS is the best level to deal with these evaluations.

The unit server provides functions that deal with recipe processing, unit status, and data evaluation. When the recipe is selected in the data warehouse it exists as a model, which becomes a specific recipe when batch, quantity, and equipment assignments are made. The operator accesses the unit server, and selects the equipment unit where a recipe has been sent. The operator initiates the recipe and begins to monitor the recipe step execution, interacting with the unit server whenever operator input is required. The unit server role in information gathering is distinctive to the CSDCS environment. Prior to this, system engineers contrived awkward methods of soliciting information from operators within a framework that was designed to do automation tasks. The problem was that the DCS had very limited ways to deal with character information, which is the core of batch reports in a regulated environment.

The unit server also maintains a unit view so that supervisors and operators can review the unit status at any point, and this view can be used to place equipment in and out of service. In order for any unit to accept a recipe for processing it must be "available." This is very helpful in a multiproduct facility in which such common resources as waste and buffer solutions can be viewed as units. With a single unit status change these common resources can be isolated for repair and maintenance. The data evaluation segment of the unit server has two media, trend graphics and recipe input. The unit server can dynamically trend data as it is logged from the CSDCS and it can also background prior "best batches" to see if the current batch is following a successful profile. A recipe can also use CSDCS data for calculations and recipe branching decisions. For example, a material charge might be based upon the present level of material in a reactor. When the recipe started this may or may not be known. In the case of a branching decision, the recipe may determine from instruments measuring material by-products that the batch may be contaminated, and prevent further processing and wasted material.

The control panel is a unit server function, which allows an operator to control recipes. The recipes may be run in automatic, or manually. This allows testing and stepping through recipes in a validation exercise. The recipes may be suspended and terminated through this interface. Every function point in the control panel is security checked to determine that the person attempting the function is authorized to do so.

Recipe tracing allows the executing recipe steps to scroll backward and forward so that the operator can see the history and future requirements. The steps are time stamped or time estimated, which is helpful so that human intervention can be planned.

Parameter tracing shows the values that the unit server is sending to CSDCS for a recipe step. A process developer may want to monitor these values during the initial runs of the recipe and turn them off at a future point. In recipes in which feedback calculations are made, the parameter trace is used to view those results.

System-to-system linkage is another synergy that a CSDCS can provide. Since the recipe has access to information of events that have recurred and will occur, a LINK recipe statement can be used to issue a parametric transaction. For example, a material charge may call for a reactor charge, which has an exact value following execution. The LINK will create a transaction that can be sent to the material management, batch records, and lab systems to record and log the event. *The important point of this interface is that it is parametric, not programmatic.* Changes in the recipe or equipment drivers will not change the LINK function. The data you select may change, but the basic socket remains intact.

G. Application Interfaces

The recipe server receives complete recipe databases from the recipe notebook. The ''notebook'' is any application that allows the process developer to select recipe verbs and select parameters. The recipe definition language is detailed in Section. The server manages all the recipes in a relational database format. Access to the recipe management functions are limited to ensure the criterion is met on all categories. The interface is facilitated by the open architecture system (OASYS) from Process Control Industries (PCI). OASYS is a multitalented system that features X Windows interfaces, database access routines, and real-time and event data acquisition. In the recipe server role, OASYS is utilized for consistency, while the application that really takes advantage of the capabilities is in the unit server.

Unit server processes are the core of the CSDCS. It is also the layer at which the specific DCS manner of data presentation becomes a critical issue. In the concept of the CSDCS, it was envisioned that any DCS, PLC, PC, or controller could be used as an endpoint, using the same recipes. The recipe does not know about the endpoint, since it is process-dependent. The unit server, however, must have access to the tags (control points) that the endpoint system is using for control. The parameters are written to the communication tags, and the endpoint system initiates control. This is an important layer distinction, because the recipe server does not directly control any equipment. It has a client that requests parameters that are used to implement control limits. Table 1 has a stack of the layers as they are used in the CSDCS.

TAG is a program by PCI that facilitates communication between different sources and destinations. As part of the OASYS, TAG is the interface that scans data from the CSDCS and forwards it to the unit server. Using this configurable

Table 1

Layer	Information
Recipe server	Process knowledge
Unit server	Recipe status
EVD	Event monitor
TAG	Point communication
CHIP	DCS points
Executive	Process status
Driver	Equipment status

interface has tremendous power and flexibility. Systems can be coupled together without programmatic links. When systems change the configuration can be adapted. Source code links would have to be changed, tested, and recompiled. Another PCI component in the CSDCS is the event director (EVD). The EVD is a conditional mechanism that waits and monitors data conditions. When, for example, a level or temperature target is achieved, EVD will act and send a signal to the program that requested EVD to monitor the condition.

CHIP is the computer highway interface program provided by Fisher/Rosemount Controls. CHIP can ''see'' control points in the CSDCS. This allows server-level access to the control points, which is how the CSDCS communicates with the controllers. When the CSDCS is configured, all the instruments and equipment that are active have their *points* set into specific file/card/channel positions. This is the lowest level of configuration. At the next higher level, *units* that are collections of points used to indicate the status and control of the complete equipment module are configured. A common unit in the CSDCS is a fermentor, used in mammalian cell culture. The unit represents several hundred points of instruments, control loops, and valves.

H. CSDCS Drivers

Drivers are the result of applying such software engineering practices as modularity and coupling into the DCS context. The top driver is the *executive driver*. The executive's job is to regulate communication with the unit server and tell all the other drivers what to do. The diagram in Error! Reference source not found shows the executive controls when it is ready for the next command to be sent from the unit server.

A *control driver* ideally has one and only one function—control. For instance, a temperature loop should take a set point then initiate control and set alarm limits. However, in the case of material drivers, the drivers have sections dedicated to the delivery of a particular material. All of the material functions are kept together for programmer convenience. For most cases a driver should only be tasked with one function in order to keep the unit complexity and validation content reduced. When an executive directs a control driver to engage, the executive waits until the control driver has successfully engaged and signals completion. If the executive does not receive the complete signal within a configured time, an alarm would result.

Interunit communication is needed to operate a process train made up of separate units. As one unit is reaching a point of discharging the completed intermediate product, a downstream unit will be reaching a charge state, enabling the unit to receive the material. In order to synchronize this discharge/charge synapse, the control drivers for the respective units check with each other to see if they are ready to go into the material transfer. Control is actually biased to the receiving unit (charge), which signals the sending unit (discharge) that the required amount has been received. Depending on the instruments available, either unit could control the transfer. If during the transfer either unit senses problems, it can abandon the transfer, signal the other unit of an abnormal termination, and inform the unit executive of an incomplete step. The executive then calls the unit alarm driver, which takes appropriate action.

Alarms are used to indicate abnormal conditions, incomplete steps, and equipment failures. Each driver has alarm processing associated with it. If the control function the driver is supposed to implement cannot be achieved in either magnitude or the expected time, then recovery, retry, or alarm can be processed. In the discharge/charge scenario, if the transfer did not occur in a typical twenty-minute time period, then that may indicate a clogged filter or closed valve. The Driver then initiates control and detects this time out, which now is an alarm condition. *Alarms are only detected at the controller level because no server communication delay is desired. This standard is required for safety.*

Since the CSDCS is made up of a number of cooperative modules, the concept of self-announcement is used to examine the version of driver that is loaded. It's like pressing a Windows HELP button and asking ''about'' the program. In the CSDCS, a graphic screen is the billboard on which every unit executive and control driver writes its name and version. This makes the CSDCS a self-documenting system.

At an enterprise level, validation and development of a library of drivers can be extremely cost-efficient. Think about the effort that would be saved if once a driver was developed, tested, and validated it was stored in a library. Then other control enginners could retrieve it and instantiate it in their unit! *The art form that was once DCS programming has now yielded to applied software engineering of a CSDCS driver.*

I. Recipe Definition Language

The recipe definition language (RDL) is used to construct process recipes. The RDL is focused on making the specification clear and easy to read. For example, calling for a material charge uses the verb CHARGE. A discussion of the verbs follows. By using this standard way of expressing the process knowledge, any person can examine the recipe and understand the operation sequence. *RDL will become to the batch process industry what SQL has become in the database world.*

Verbs have different functions, some interacting with the operator, some directing equipment. The first sets are known as *information verbs*, the latter as *automation verbs*. Information verbs, such as operator information request (OIR), MANUAL, and SAMPLE, are used to gather batch information that may either be used later in the recipe for calculation or used to log information. The automation verbs send parameters to the CSDCS and log information. No operator interaction occurs on the automation verbs. There are several other classes of verbs that can be introduced now—the *navigation verbs* and the *language verbs*. Navigation verbs, such as WHEN, GOTO, WAIT, and LABEL are used for conditional branching and looping. Language verbs such as OPERATION, PHASE, PRINT, and LINK provide recipe segmentation and system output functionality. PRINT can be used to generate bar code labels for product identification. LINK is used to create transactions that will be picked up by other systems, such as material, laboratory, and maintenance information systems. LINK provides a parametric interface to the CSDCS, which standardizes information transactions throughout the organization.

Parameters are the leaves in the knowledge tree that the recipe represents. As OPERATION and PHASE break sections of the process apart into functional branches, each step verb has parameters that detail the way in which the step is applied. In an automation verb the setpoint, alarms, and rate information are sent. In the information verbs the parameters represent the questions and answers the operator will be presented with and select.

Inherent to the process definition are calculations based upon material properties and process stages. In order to support this the recipe server and RDL must support *tag calculation*. This powerful feature allows the process developer to handle this example scenario: charge the reactor with enough material to reach a cell density of 3.4 × 10**6. The volume and cell density are needed to make this calculation. The volume would be read from an instrument and the present cell density would be manually calculated and entered into the batch using an OIR.

The RDL and CSDCS system have been developed based upon the framework proposed by the ISA SP88 batch controls standard. In that regard the RDL is an open industry and language that is nonproprietary. The project team developed a *recipe notebook* to allow rapid development of recipes. This tool is portable, flexible, and as easy to use as a spreadsheet. The recipe notebook permits modeling recipes so that once a basic framework has been worked out, variations on the initial recipe are easy to construct. Once the recipe has been developed it can be printed out for detailed verification. When ready, the recipe is moved to the recipe server with a single press of a button.

Recipe simulation can be performed since the verbs and parameters are stored in a normal database format. The simulator has methods for each verb in the language, and as each verb is presented the parameters are highlighted and displayed. This dry-run capability is highly effective for multidiscipline reviews. To approve a recipe, representatives from quality, operations, and engineering could sit down and simulate the recipe. This would verify step by step that the recipe follows facility standards and that the eventual material produced meets the product specification.

The recipe notebook is bound to an industry (biotechnology, pharmaceutical, chemical, batch process) by the dialect of RDL that is selected. Multiple RDLs may be used at a given facility without collisions as long as the verbs are registered and uniquely defined. For transfer from site to site identical RDLs must be used.

J. Conclusions

Depending upon the level of automation that the process requires and the level of information that the regulation requires, a successful project can be executed if all of these consideration are examined prior to committing resources. The thrust has been to reveal the automation from a building block manner—primary cell controllers through to a fully integrated CSDCS.

The CSDCS, recipe notebook, and RDL will evolve and hopefully be used as models for a biotech application of the SP88 batch control standard. In developing this application environment, the CSDCS has reduced system development, increased system vision, and improved the architecture of the CSDCS so that validation is inherent to the system.

In the future, CSDCS vendors will be able to offer various products that customers can insert into their CSDCS architecture to provide standard functionality. Libraries of validated drivers, database functions, and analytical add-ons will extend CSDCS automation. Equipment vendors could provide equipment and a canned set of drivers, which would mean the customer only needs to develop recipes.

CSDCS vendors should also be able to take advantage of the CSDCS features, reducing the batch programming on controllers and configuring the controllers with menus of drivers. Cost should be driven down by reducing the complexity of the software on the controllers.

In the broadest possible acceptance of the CSDCS, it may be seen by regulatory agencies as a superior manner in which to process biopharmaceuticals and ensure that the systems are validated. The future of the CSDCS will depend on the perception of the inherent value that this elegantly simple architecture provides.

8

Distributed Client/Server-Based Batch Control System Applied as Part of the Enterprise Solution Suite Using Technology

Baha Korkmaz*

The Foxboro Company, Foxboro, Massachusetts

I. INTRODUCTION

The accelerated introduction of new technologies and new tools to apply these technologies provides opportunities for the creation of new enterprise solutions. It was not possible until recently to use the Internet/intranet on your desktop to view batch process, on-demand batch reports or trends, or even to control the plant in some cases. Other technologies that are playing a significant role in applied solutions are object-oriented databases for real-time distributed control systems, CORBA-ORB communication methods for platform and station independence, Microsoft Windows NT 4.0 within a client/server architecture, and most recently, JAVA. We are rapidly moving away from costly point solutions and making a revolutionary leap toward integrated enterprise solutions. This technological revolution will enable users, vendors, and system integrators in this industry to design and implement complex batch applications easily and plug them into the right spot within the enterprise structure. This chapter will focus on the impact of new technologies on batch plant automation. It will also describe the increased role of batch control systems for integration of control with the enterprise.

In the 1980s and early 1990s, the manufacturing industry focused on downsizing and reengineering. Corporations mainly redefined the way they ran the

**Current affiliation:* Automation Vision, Inc., Wrentham, Massachusetts.

business and eliminated outdated, rigid organizational structures. Enterprise resource planning (ERP) systems were introduced. Most of these business systems were still using mainframe computers with central databases and programs. This architecture did not allow them to have the agility required to have comprehensive and error-free planning and scheduling systems. This observation applies to batch control systems as well. Even now almost all batch management and control software packages are monolithic and do not take advantage of object technology. In the coming years this outlook will change drastically as all major players adapt to new technologies in an effort to remain competitive.

The industry standards (S88.01 and emerging part 2, SP95, STEP, etc.) help to define the next generation enterprise and control models. Batch control systems and application solutions for processing industry became more affordable and maintainable with the introduction of the S88 part 1 batch control standard. Applying object technology, distributed networking, and such other enablers as JAVA, ActiveX, CORBA-ORB, and object-oriented databases increased the processing and storage power of networked computers. The introduction of the Internet/intranet is creating an open-ended and a very exciting avenue for total manufacturing automation and business solutions, and the effects will be felt for many years to come.

II. EXPECTATIONS FROM THE NEXT GENERATION BUSINESS AND CONTROL MODEL

As the competition increases and the need for decreased response time to customers demands becomes a major necessity, ERP solutions are becoming more and more functionally comprehensive. The utilization of object technology is the key to the next generation of enterprise and control systems. Currently, business systems, including resource planning, advanced planning, and scheduling systems, are implemented without real integration to the shop floor or process lines. Not having real-time feedback, or historical or predictive information from the control systems inhibits the business systems' ability to perform planning and execution with accuracy. Most of the planning and scheduling coefficients are entered manually as constants or estimates. Linking ERP systems to control systems and integrating the information as appropriate can eliminate critical errors in inventory, delivery, and other long-term business planning.

The following solutions are expected from enterprise and control system models:

- Extreme agility in manufacturing and planning to further shorten the response time to customer demands
- Enterprise to control integration (nonproprietary interfaces and data transfers)

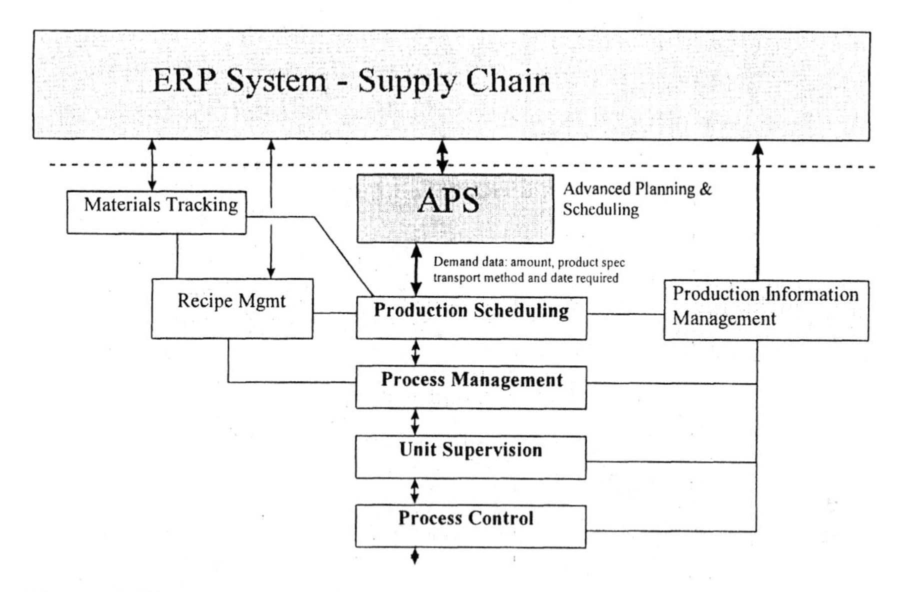

Fig. 1 ERP systems–control systems link.

- Enterprisewide integration and communications (distributed networking, Internet/intranet)
- Modularity, scalability, ease of engineering and use, platform independence
- Manufacturing automation life-cycle support
- Multivendor integration from sensors to the ERP systems

III. ENTERPRISE TO CONTROL INTEGRATION

ERP linkage to the batch control activity model is shown in Fig. 1. There is an established control model for batch-processing plants; ERP systems have their own self-contained model as well. What is still missing is integration between these two independent models. There is a lot to be gained by introducing a comprehensive model that integrates business systems with control.

A. Top-Down View

Enterprise systems handle supply chain planning, dealing with such external issues as demand, supplier capacity, and alternate transportation methods. The enterprise planning step deals with optimized business plans, production capacity, and materials to meet customer or market demands. To come up with an accurate and dynamic planning system ERP systems must be integrated with the rapidly growing segment called advanced planning and scheduling (APS). So far, none of these top-down layers contains real-time data or an online link to control systems. Without this connection, even APS systems will not have total accuracy. Constraint management or plant capacity management problems can be solved with technology enablers. It would be unrealistic to ask APS systems to perform micromanagement by monitoring highly complex real-time plant data. Control systems under the direction of APS systems must have short-term scheduling performed to provide the necessary data for APS.

Other modules of the batch control system that communicate with business systems are material tracking, lot tracking, recipe management (master recipes), and production information management.

B. Bottom-Up View

From the control system point of view, integration plays a role in short-term planning and scheduling, in control recipe updates based on the demand changes (amount, product spec, transport date and method), and in material-tracking database updates.

Manufacturing plants consist of multiple process cells. Each process cell normally has an independent control system (DCS). Short-term planning and scheduling, dispatching, and resource management activities are connected to the real-time control system and dynamically get adjusted based on process cell history, current state, and projected status.

IV. PHYSICAL MODEL CONTAINING ENTERPRISE, AREA, AND SITE

S88 defines a physical model in several hierarchical levels. They are from the top down: enterprise, site, area, process cell, unit, equipment module, and control module. Lower-level groupings are combined to form higher levels in the hierarchy. In some cases, such as equipment module and control module, one level may be incorporated into another grouping at the same level.

Newer batch control systems incorporate process cell and lower-level components of the physical model comprehensively. Applying new technologies for object-oriented and distributed client/server design allows the batch control system to be very scalable and manageable. Figure 2 shows the physical model from a business model point of view. The layers that are under the domain of the process cell are not covered. Batch control system responsibilities are process cell-centric. Each process cell has an independent management and control system. The business systems, including APS, could utilize the physical modeling of S88 as well. It would then deal with the enterprise, site, area, and process cell

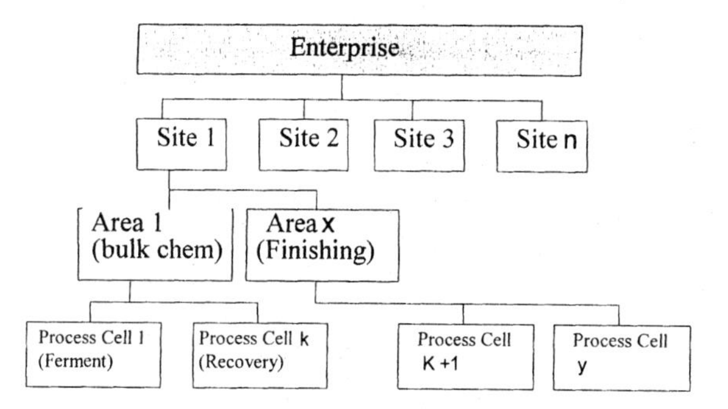

Fig. 2 Physical model of the enterprise.

layers. The process cell is the only layer overlapping between the business and control system models. Physical modeling defines all physical entities, their attributes, their characteristics, their constraints, their capabilities, and the relationship of each to the procedural model. Procedural to physical model mapping enables the process model. (See S88 document page 31.) Each physical entity is an object with attributes, data, and methods. Object-oriented modeling allows abstraction to be represented in the model. Abstraction of the physical entities (class-specific) allows batch control systems to define product-specific master recipes and to perform dynamic short-term planning and scheduling. The same method would apply to business problems as well. Another advantage of modeling and abstraction by utilizing object technology is simulations. To further optimize planning and scheduling systems (long-term or short-term), simulation runs are necessary.

V. PLANNING AND SCHEDULING

Utilizing the physical model concept of S88 allows us to modularize the entire enterprise (Fig. 3). While ERP systems perform their business-related planning and scheduling by dealing with the business constraints, batch control systems deal with process cell-centric short-term planning and scheduling. Short-term scheduling is directly linked to process management and control and is dynamically adjusted based on plant and other production status. ERP systems send demand requests such as amount, product specification, date needed, transportation method, and packaging type to the area/site-specific management system. The site manager then coordinates the activities between process cells (similar to resource management in batch control, which manages units within the process cell) and sends commands based on the long-term plant production plan and schedule. Short-term scheduling systems are responsible for optimizing actual batch scheduling and resource management at run time.

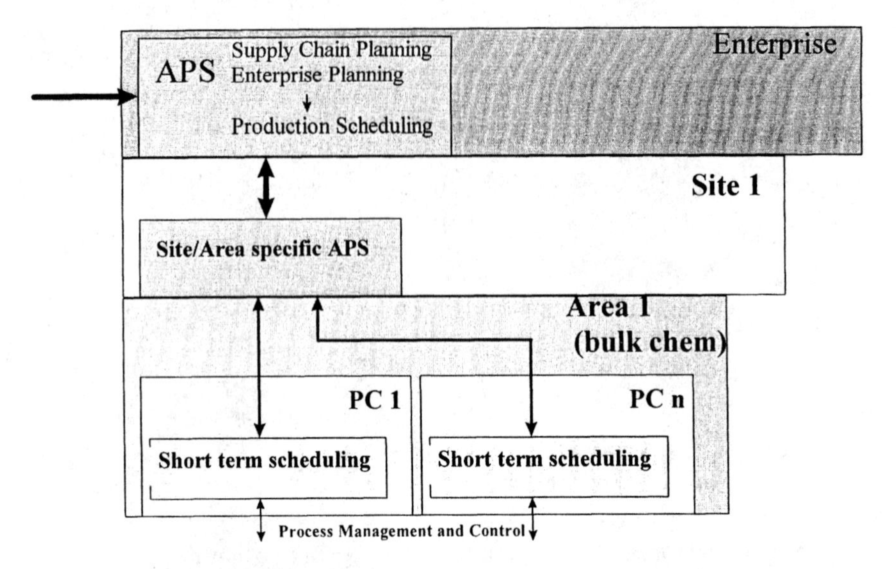

Fig. 3 Planning and scheduling model.

VI. TECHNOLOGY ENABLERS

Appropriate application of technology enablers can produce the following benefits:

- High performance in a worldwide network
- Vendor transparency–ease of integration
- Database independence
- Platform independence
- Flexibility and scalability
- High availability of information–data integrity
- Control system security and robustness
- Modularity and reusability

A. Object Technology

Object-oriented methodologies have existed since the 1970s. It took almost twenty years for technology companies to enhance hardware and software platforms and to develop adequate tools to allow object technology to be applied to its full capabilities. The most popular tools are methods such as OMT Rumbaugh and Unified Modeling Language from Rational. The programming languages adapted to object-oriented software engineering are Visual C++, SmallTalk, and

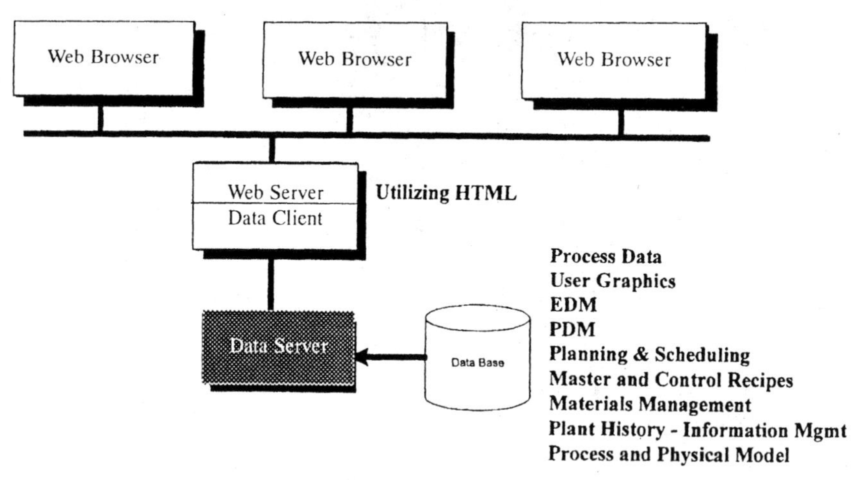

Fig. 4 Internet/intranet.

JAVA. Newly introduced Visual Basic version 5.0 is supporting object-oriented software engineering as well.

Object technology enables scaling up of client/server applications for distributed control and business. It allows modeling and enables software that can cope with the required agility of business and manufacturing plants. Ideally, object-oriented analysis and design tools should provide a model for the application architecture. However, tools for object-oriented software engineering are not yet mature enough for mass utilization. Applying object technology to any business and/or control problem enables reusability, maintenance, and upgrade of the objects. The interfaces to the objects are not affected if the internals of the objects get modified. This means no impact to the object's surroundings.

B. Internet/Intranet

The introduction of Web technology with the Internet (and recently intranet) accelerated the enterprise integration process. These new technologies make integration and automation over the network more affordable and possible. JAVA applications with HTML bring shop-floor information to executive offices. Any information can be accessed from anywhere, providing the necessary securities and fire walls are in place. Control systems need to stay robust and secure while providing online information to the business systems. Figure 4 shows possible connections. Via the Web browser it is possible to access data as well as any user interface, including the process cell, unit, and process control displays. This

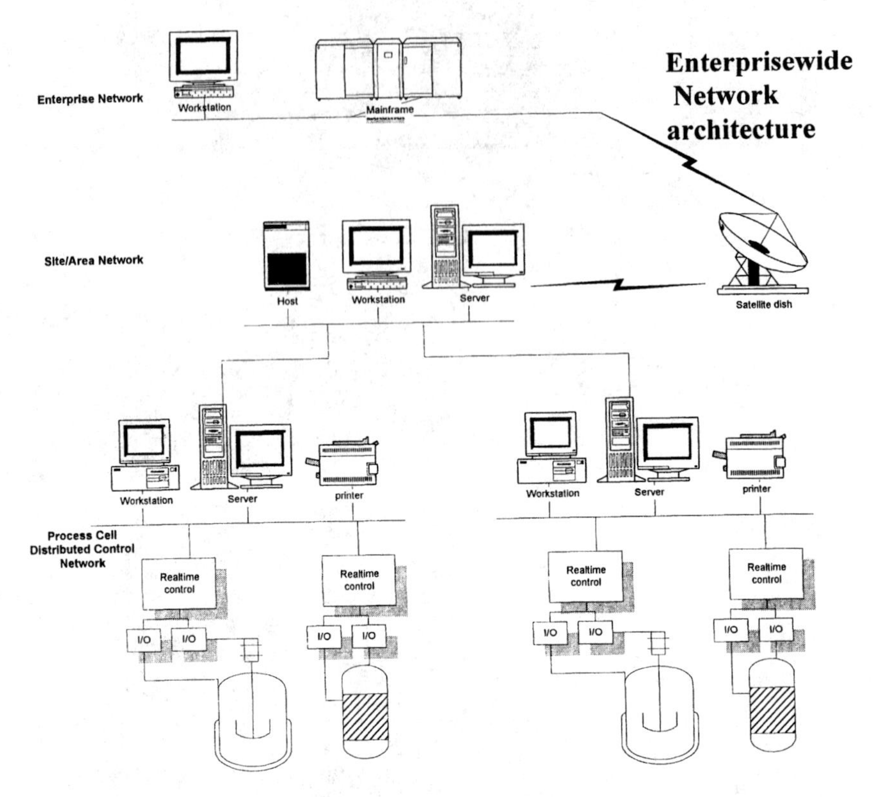

Fig. 5 Enterprisewide network architecture.

technology is making electronic document management, change management, and linkage between hierarchical levels easily applicable. (See Fig. 5.)

C. CORBA-ORB

Application of distributed object technologies became possible with introduction of object request brokers (ORB). CORBA stands for the common object request broker architecture, which is defined by the OMG (object management group). ORB technology is used to build multitier applications, update legacy code, and create Web-based information systems. ORB is a middleware module used in distributed computing environments to provide interoperability between different object-oriented software (Fig. 6).

CORBA-ORB technology allowed the development of station-independent and platform-independent distributed batch management packages. This technology further allows modules to communicate without knowing their residence

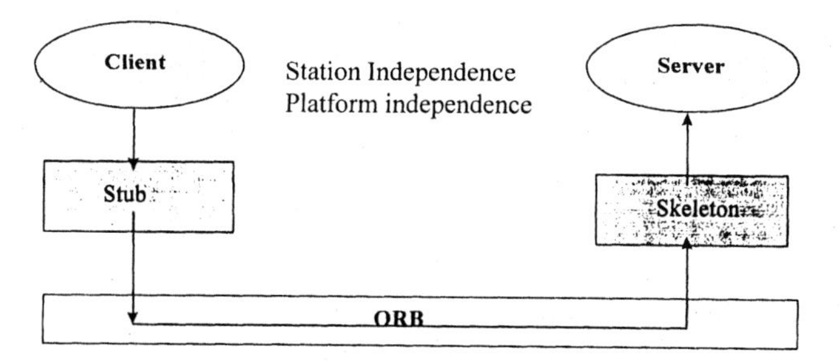

Fig. 6 CORBA-ORB.

location or the platform (UNIX or Windows NT, etc.). Microsoft has also introduced distributed object technologies called ActiveX and Distributed Component Object Model (DCOM; see Ref. 4).

D. Object-Oriented Databases

Object-oriented database management systems (ODBMS) represent another emerging technology. Object-oriented databases should not be seen as a direct replacement for RDBMS systems. RDBMS systems serve well for online transaction processing of textual and numerical data. They will remain as major database systems for such functions as data warehousing. Manufacturing automation systems, however, require more real-time data handling and complexity in the database. Increased agility requirements in automation systems and the distributed nature of control activities make ODBMS systems suitable for these applications. Object-oriented databases handle the distributed nature of data and scalability. They offer clustering in a distributed network and fault tolerance of the data as well. All configuration and run-time databases can exist modularly in a distributed environment. It enables modularization of elements for vendor independence and interoperability between systems. ODBMS systems provide database independence with both ODBC and SQL interface (Fig. 7).

VII. CONCLUSION

The application of the advanced technologies summarized in this chapter will drastically change the way businesses are run in coming years. Both users and

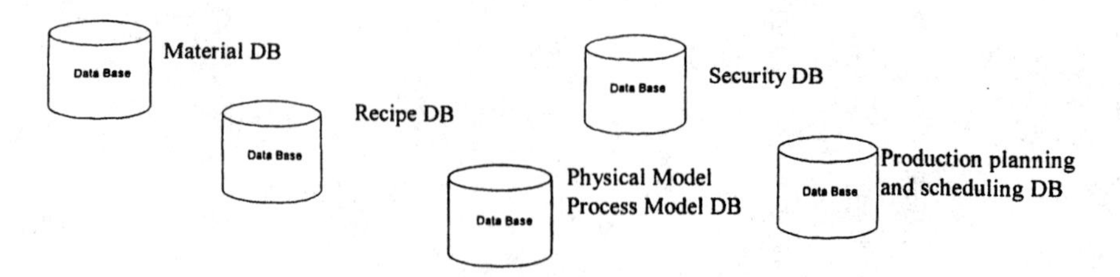

Fig. 7 Object-oriented databases. Distributed object database management system (ODBMS) is ideal for applications that require complex data models. RDBMS served well for online transaction processing of textual and numerical. The new class of applications covers more complicated domains such as process control, manufacturing, telecommunications, multimedia, and authoring. Object-oriented databases handle distributed nature of the data. It is ideal for the modular nature of the batch management and control. ODBMS provides the database independence by providing ODBC and SQL.

the vendor community in manufacturing automation are working on these next generation models. The tight integration of control with business systems, online linkage of shop floor information with advanced planning and scheduling systems, and utilization of distributed object technologies for software development will continue to improve production and optimization of the manufacturing process.

REFERENCES

1. ISA S88.01 batch control standard.
2. AMR MAS report for Dec. 1996.
3. Mastering objects, *Inform. Wk.* (Oct. 21, 1996).
4. Race between CORBA and ActiveX/DCOM, *Inform. Wk.* (Jan. 20, 1997).

9

A CIM Architecture for Validated Manufacturing Systems

Joseph F. deSpautz

INCODE Corp., Herndon Virginia

Today, many automation projects are introducing commercially available enterprise resource planning (ERP), manufacturing execution systems (MES), distributed control systems (DCS), and programmable logic controllers (PLC) applications into pharmaceutical manufacturing. Existing mission-critical systems must be included in the new system projects. Regulatory compliance adds the complexity and effort of validation to the project. System planning for these systems must include how to support these validated systems that may reside on different hardware platforms with different operating systems. System development life cycle (SDLC) methodologies provide an excellent framework for these computer-based projects. System architecture is a more encompassing term for an SDLC. In the literature (1) there are references to different architectural types or models, such as the following:

Type 1: Physical components or collections of principles, models, standards, and guidelines

Type 2: Life cycle identification for integrated systems. Type 1 architectures are typically referenced as components.

Information systems (IS) uses the term *information architecture* to define the physical model of the computer system, hardware platforms, application software, and the collection of principles, models, standards, and guidelines used throughout the enterprise for computer-related activities. An information architecture is an example of a type 1 architecture and often is used to identify the application and technical layers of installed systems. It defines such elements as those in Table 1.

Table 1 Typical Layers of a Type 1 Information Architecture

Application architecture layer	
Logical data model	Graphical user interfaces
Applications	Relational databases
Security model	System management policies
Information exchange standards	System development standards
Technical architecture layer	
Client–server operations	Communication protocols
Network topology	Coding standards
Database access standards	Hardware characteristics
Graphic display standards	Software tools
Operating systems	Hardware platform

I. INTEGRATING INFORMATION, ORGANIZATIONS, AND MANUFACTURING

Some years ago, Digital Equipment Corporation, IBM, and other companies realized they needed to deploy architectural disciplines to ensure that internal systems met the enterprise's business needs. The adding of the business component or business architecture as an independent view of the enterprise information architecture added a level of accountability to the implemented system. The Purdue Laboratory for Applied Industrial Control has spent many years working with industry in developing reference models and reference architectures that include information, business, and technology components. The Purdue enterprise reference architecture (PERA) and methodology (2,3) is well known as an integration methodology for computer integrated manufacturing (CIM) and enterprise integration. Fluor Daniels Company, a major consulting and construction firm, is applying PERA to project work across different industrial areas (4). PERA is a framework for presenting its work practices on system integration projects.

Purdue has extended this work into a specification document (1) for a generalized enterprise reference architecture and methodology (GERAM). The specification uses many examples of architectures and SDLCs for enterprise integration and CIM programs. The specification shows how these architectures fit within the GERAM guiding principles outlined in Table 2 and are all acceptable methodologies for integration projects.

Figure 1 presents the PERA Life Cycle defining three architectural components—information systems, human and organizational, and manufacturing equipment. Tasks are executed and information derived for each of the architectural components throughout the SDLC.

Table 2 GERAM Requirements

- The architecture must cover all the details of the life cycle of the system.
- It should be capable of handling the description and development of any conceivable system, CIM, information system, validation, enterprise.
- It should provide the information, guidelines, and management techniques for the entire life cycle.
- It should be capable of including any and all type 2 architectures.
- It should show the place of humans in all aspects of their involvement in the mission fulfillment components and interaction with information systems in terms of skills and requirements for task execution (1).

II. INTEGRATING VALIDATION WITH INFORMATION, ORGANIZATIONS, AND MANUFACTURING

The FDA definition of process validation is contained in the ''General Principles of Validation'' guideline (5) as

> establishing documented evidence which provides a high degree of assurance that a specific process will consistently produce a product meeting its predetermined specifications and quality attributes.

The FDA has no formal definition of computer system validation and expects the definition of validation to apply equally to manufacturing control processes involving computers and other types of automation equipment. The Pharmaceutical Research and Manufacturers Association (PhARMA; formerly the PMA) developed a life cycle approach to computer-related system validation (6). This effort defined a process for defining, developing, and quality testing of new and existing computer systems. The Parenteral Drug Association (PDA) Committee on Validation of Computer-Related Systems report (7) defined a method emphasizing comprehensive computer-related system requirements (functional and design specifications) and computer system construction, implementation, and qualification. (See Fig. 2).

The PDA SDLC includes evaluating a vendor's development environments, support and maintenance capabilities, and change control practices for its commercial systems for meeting cGMP requirements. Computer system validation in the PDA model is defined like process validation so as to establish documented evidence that provides a high degree of assurance that a specific computer-related system will consistently operate in accordance with predefined specifications.

The life cycle methodology enables users with little or no computer skills to navigate through the phases of an integration project with the focus on system validation. Both the PhARMA and the PDA methodologies are examples of type 2 architectures. They define the life history of process and computer-related sys-

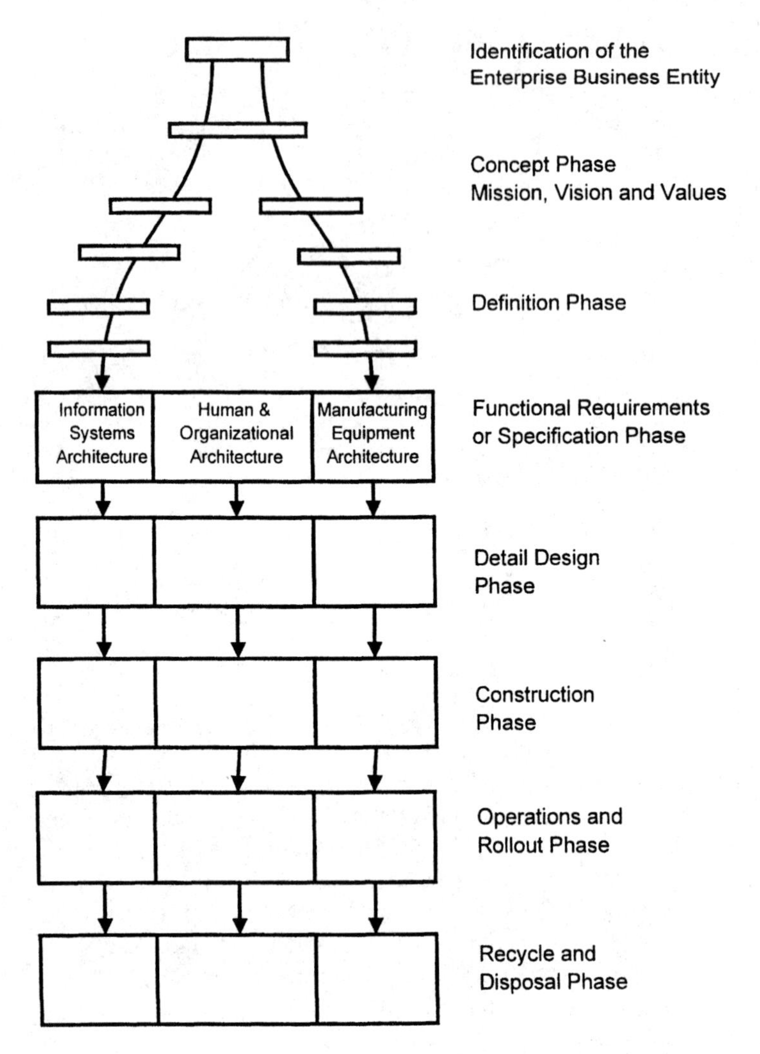

Fig. 1 Phases of the Purdue architecture in terms of the types of tasks that occur throughout the life cycle of the architecture.

tems from conception through validation and then operation and eventual disposal at the end of the system's productive life.

III. CIM ARCHITECTURE FOR VALIDATION

Using PERA, we can represent an enhanced system development life cycle for pharmaceutical manufacturing automation and integration projects. The PERA-

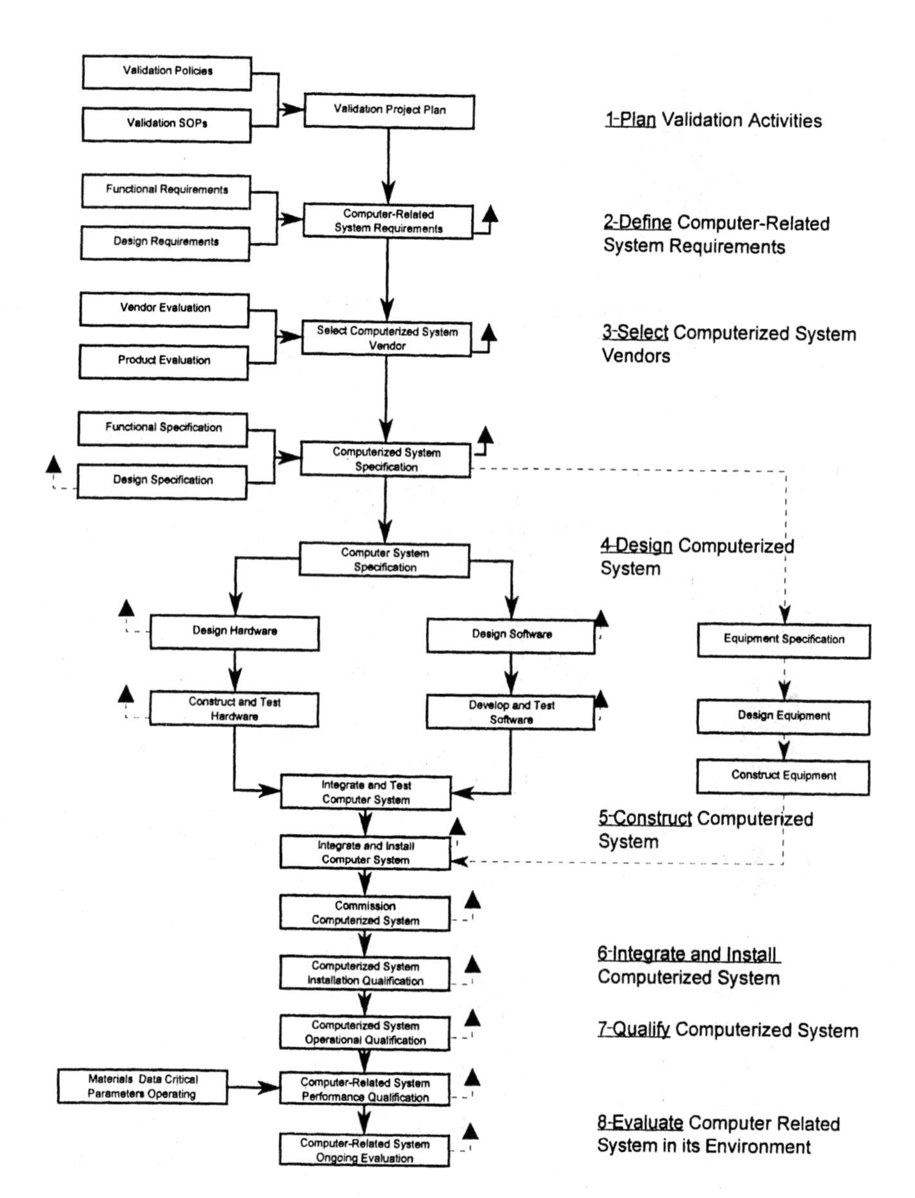

Fig. 2 Steps in validating computer-related systems.

base architecture integrates the information, human and organizational, and manufacturing equipment architectures into a unified validation master plan. The phases of the plan are the following:

PERA-based Validation Master Plan or Architecture

Concept (mission, vision, and value)
System definition
Functional specification
Detail design
Construction
Installation and validation
Operations and rollout
Decommissioning at end of life

The PERA-based validation master plan is an example of an architecture that can be used for automation projects requiring validation. Like the PhARMA and PDA methodologies, it covers all phases of system operation from conception through redesign or decommissioning. It allows the developer to integrate into a single plan the mutually independent architectures for

- Manufacturing equipment
- Human and organizational
- Information

All three components are included in each phase of the life cycle to support validation and fit for use of the resulting system.

The architecture can be used for all sizes of automation projects. Its benefits expand when used for such complex projects as integrating material and lot traceability across a complete plant, the multiplant rollout of a raw material control, and QA release or warehouse dispensing operations for multiple product lines.

Because validation represents special hurdles to FDA-regulated companies, the PERA-based validation master plan helps answer primary questions, including the following:

- How is the computer-based system used in product manufacturing?
- What functionality is the system going to perform?
- How will the computer system record product production?
- Does the system meet its predetermined specifications and requirements?
- Do organizations have the proper education and training to manage and use the new systems?
- Have we documented the system implementation in a manner that supports validation guidelines?

The PhRMA and PDA validation master plans fit very well within the PERA system architecture. The manufacturing component contains the physical process equipment lines, computer systems, networks, hardware controllers, operator workstations, control room functions, operator control panels, and software applications. The human and organizational architecture defines the involvement of people in the new system. The boundaries of how much automation will be implemented on both the physical and information sides of the system are fully defined and documented. Often the changes in the people skill sets needed to support the new systems are not addressed during the early life cycle phases. The information architecture catalogues the validation documentation needed to describe each phase of the project; the information systems needed to support the process (e.g., batch record recording, standard operating procedures [SOPs], quality control [QC] test results); and the system performance parameters, production batch record information, and operator instructions. We have all of the information for a successful and complete validation of the final implemented system. Nothing has been missed.

The PERA validation master plan is a set of project phases that documents WHAT business process needs are to be transformed into the required computer-based system and HOW they will be executed (activities and documentation).

IV. CONCEPT AND DEFINITION PHASES: BUSINESS PROCESS IMPLEMENTATION

The business process planning starts with the company's business plan. The vision for the proposed CIM project is considered in the context of the corporate mission and vision objectives. The concept and definition phases define and clarify the organization's business objectives and the related elements that are critical to achieving these objectives. Taken together, these constitute the "as is" of the business or where we are today and the "to be" environment that represents the enhanced business state. The analyses and documents collected, catalogued, or developed during this phase are given in Fig. 3.

The definitions are arrived at by ascertaining the company's business mission, measurable business objectives, critical success factors, and strategies. The specifics could be gathered by answering such questions as the following:

- What and how are we doing today?
- What is our business mission?
- What business objectives will achieve this mission?
- What are the critical success factors for these objectives to be achieved?
- What business strategies will need to be deployed to ensure that we achieve these critical success factors?
- How can we measure success and when can we stop?

Concept and Definition Phases		
Manufacturing, information and personnel policies	Mission, Vision and Values. Management philosophies	Present or proposed production entities including product, cGMP and operational policies
Validation Policies and SOPs Validation program plan guidelines Information technology standards, models, Project plan Cost verses benefit analyses	Organizations plan	Project identification Automation strategy

Fig. 3 Concept and definition phases.

V. DEFINING ORGANIZATIONAL SUCCESS

Performance measurements with numeric values or ranges of values are needed by the organization to monitor its progress toward success. Many different measurements can be used to monitor manufacturing and business performance. Some are primarily diagnostic tools, while others are the vital signs that allow an organization to monitor the health of the operations and the success of the overall project.

Specific measurements determined during the implementation should be viewed as "dynamic" rather than "static." They define how we are operating today. They define what educational, training, and certification plans need to be developed and executed to improve performance. As performance improves, organizations may elect to change the measurements and raise the bar on performance. Corporate measurements, which senior management will review on a regular basis, will establish a hierarchy of many other measurements within each plant or manufacturing area within a plant. Accountability should be passed down throughout the organization to support meeting the new measurements. This in turn may require additional education and skill level retraining.

Validation considerations identified by the business component would be incorporated into the information system that must support the deployed business strategies. By defining system purpose in the view of business processes with accompanying organizational plans, business scenarios can be constructed that show how the resulting system will document how products are being produced according to their predetermined specifications and quality attributes. As production practices are changed by the new system, the business scenarios can be modified to reflect these changes, keeping the organizations synchronized with the new operational model.

VI. FUNCTIONAL REQUIREMENTS PHASE: DOCUMENTING THE WHAT OF THE PROJECT

The use of computer-based systems will cause changes to occur in the core systems of the pharmaceutical enterprise that need to be integrated into prevailing standards and practices, including the following:

- Raw material and intermediate product testing and release control
- Material traceability and genealogy
- Equipment traceability
- Batch record data collection and historical recording
- SOPs, basic operating procedures (BOPs), and operating and test specifications
- Batch release criteria

Technology-based decisions will be documented during the functional requirements phase, including the following:

- System hardware trade-offs
- The extent of automation for process equipment and information systems
- Vendor reviews
- Analysis of vendor application software
- Project schedules, notebooks, etc.

This documentation will provide a high degree of assurance that the translation of the human processes and technical descriptions for the resulting system will consistently operate according to its intended use. The detail analyses, plan, and documentation for the phase are given in Fig. 4.

Addressing validation requirements throughout the SDLC will enable the resource effort needed for IQ, OQ, and PQ testing to be controlled. Time and resource benefits can be achieved if the validation testing effort can be planned and estimated accurately while still maintaining or enhancing the quality of the audit effort. Industry estimates of typical validation costs range from 20 to 100 percent of system costs, which include system purchases, developments, and internal project costs. Reference 8 shows the relationship between committing and consuming budgeted during life cycle phases. By identifying and documenting the validation testing and audit requirements early in the life cycle, costing can be included in the financial budgets. (See Fig. 5).

By the time the design is completed, 5 percent of the budget has been spent, but 85 percent has been committed. If validation costs can be part of the planning phase, then validation-testing resource requirements can be quantified and

Functional Requirements Specification Phase		
Information Systems Architecture (ISA)	Human & Organization Architecture (H&OA)	Manufacturing Equipment Architecture (MEA)
Planning, scheduling control and management reporting requirements	Organization, teams, skill sets	Physical production requirements
Validation program planning and documentation	Batch Record Re-engineering • Batch record rationalization • SOP re-engineering	Definition of existing systems • Process systems • Information networks • Product flow • Material flow • Equipment
Project plan updates Vendor audits Implement Change Control procedures	As-Is and To-Be Environment • Operator User Interface • QA, QC requirements • Batch record changes • Material, equipment and lot traceability • Batch release criteria	As-Is and To-Be environment • Unit operations • Automation equipment • Product and material flow • User interface
Document: Business scenarios • Identify business benefits at the operational level	Certification procedures Training program methodology	Application interfaces • Integration transactions • New and legacy applications
Functional requirements • Product equipment and information flow • Technical requirements • Input-Process-Output diagrams • Batch record data • Manual operations • Automation operations		Automation changes • Piping and instrumentation diagrams • Logical automation network topology • Logical workstation and data collection requirements • Product material flow
Logical data model • Product, Process, equipment dependencies • Product and material information flow • Production history for EBR • Manufacturing unit operations		

Fig. 4 Functional requirements specification phase.

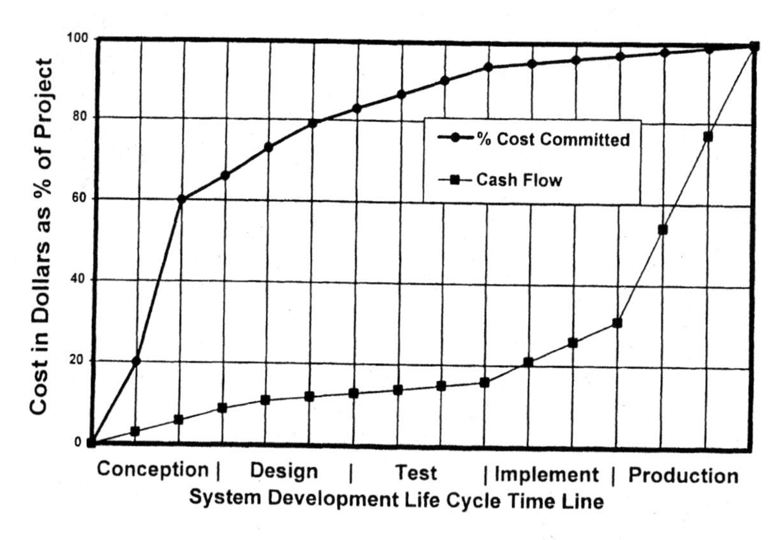

Fig. 5 Product life cycle accounting.

planned like any other resource requirement. Most system integration projects are initiated based upon a return of investment, and the quicker the system can be put into use, the sooner benefits can start accruing to the project budget.

VII. DEFINING THE LEVEL OF AUTOMATION BETWEEN OPERATIONS AND TECHNOLOGY

How much automation will be introduced by the planned project? The transition from manual operations to electronic practices are an important aspect of any pharmaceutical system implementation. Defining the business process rule changes for the to be environment will ensure that operations and product documentation still performs appropriately. The key to how much automation will be implemented (or conversely how much the operator and organization should do) depends on a number of independent factors, including the following:

- Plant size and available space
- Legacy systems that cannot be disturbed
- Budget for automation project verses potential benefits
- Skill levels of geographic job pool
- Regulatory documentation on file that cannot be changed
- Union or governmental requirements

On the manufacturing side, we are involved with physical tasks that operators must do. Examples are how much can people lift, move, stir, or mix; and operator/

Table 3 Manufacturing Investment Drivers

Prioritized list	Other drivers
FDA validation	Time to market
Document management	Cost reduction/waste reduction
Production management	JIT/capacity planning
Inventory management	Design for manufacturability
EPA regulations	Moving to make/package to order
Production optimization	Customer service
Product costing	

Source: Advanced Manufacturing Research (AMR) study, fall 1992.

product production safety dependencies. The information component represents the thinking side of the organization, such as what data will be recorded for batch record compliance, what the operators will see on the control panels, and what is required for coordinating QC results with batch release. Often the addition of a new production suite or the introduction of a new product line moves the line of automation between equipment and information. With limited project and operational resources, how much change can be successfully introduced in the organization within the project's time lines. New suite construction schedules (or a new product introduction date) often define(s) the limits of automation. Digital Equipment (9) commissioned a study that revealed some key investment drivers for pharmaceutical manufacturing. The list included the drivers in Table 3.

Validation considerations were among the top investment drivers. Document management, production and inventory management, and cost controls were in the top selection. While information technology is typically the focus of a system implementation, it was not a key business driver for pharmaceutical automation and other applications.

VIII. DETAIL DESIGN SPECIFICATION PHASE: PLANNING FOR SUCCESS

This phase transforms the functional requirements into design rules that allow any interpretation by the developer. The detail analyses, plan, and documentation for the phase are given in Fig. 6.

The functional requirements define the business processes in terms of functions that produce a product (or products) that in turn is (are) used as input or ''material'' for a subsequent process's function. The value-added business process may produce a tangible product (e.g., a compound ingredient) or an intangible one (i.e., information). Using any of a number of modeling or flow-charting techniques, we are able to identify the material flow, parameters used to control

Detail Design Specification Phase		
ISA	H&OA	MEA
Physical data model	Operator User Interface requirements	Product, Process, equipment dependencies
Detail business scenarios	User interface prototypes	Process and equipment layout
Refine business benefits	User educational requirements	Operator - Machine requirements
Batch Record information and data collection formats	Training program design	
Refine education plan	QA, QC sampling and labeling requirements	Operator station functions • Operator graphic interface
Refine training plan	Batch release requirements	Legacy system integration requirements
Unit operations design	cGMP cleaning, safety and environmental requirements	Application interface definition
Factory acceptance test (FAT) plan • Unit test plans • Integration tests	Refine skills assessment	Integration transactions data definitions
Site acceptance test (SAT) plan	Refine roll-out plans	LAN and WAN network design
Installation Qualification (IQ) plan	Training plan development	Database, access and storage applications and tools
Operational Qualifications (OQ) plan	Education plan development	Information systems network definition
Performance Qualification (PQ) plan • Test protocols • Test cases and data scripts		Computer system design • Operating system • Physical workstation and data collection locations
Traceability matrices for detail design to functional requirements		Vendor user manuals
Application interface specifications		Vendor installation manuals
Integration transactions data formats		Manufacturing Network topology and construction plan
Refined Project implementation plan		
Data migration plan		

Fig. 6 Detail design phase.

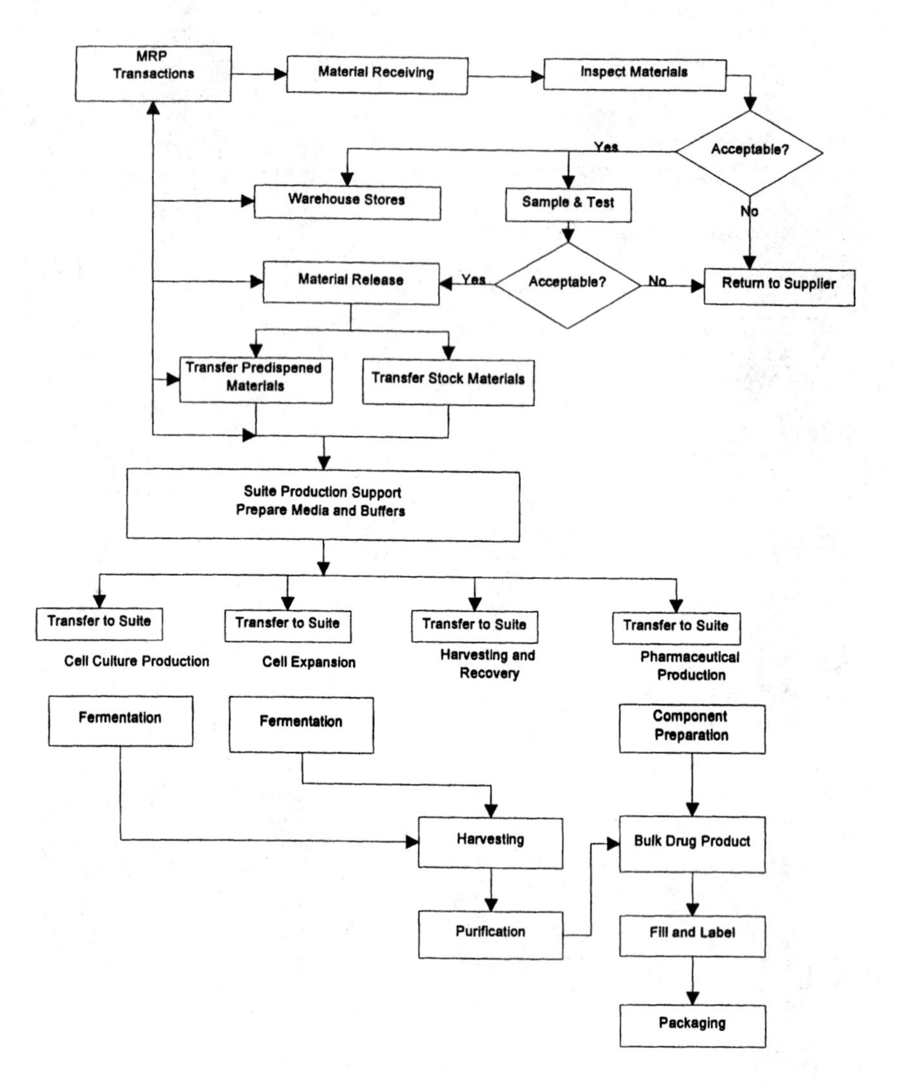

Fig. 7 Business process flow diagram for biotechnology MES operations.

the material transformation, and the planning information and the mechanisms used. (See Fig. 7).

The modeled system can be viewed as a controlled set of business functions that are executed by people and technology bounded by the business objectives and success factors. The result is an approach that not only focuses on information technology, but also the changes to the company's business processes and the way people and organizations will be affected. Functions have resources as inputs and are acted upon by controlling mechanisms. They produce one or more products. Controlling mechanisms are people, manufacturing application software, and process equipment. Resources and products are materials, energy, and information. The exchange of information that occurs when the product of one function becomes a resource for another identifies behavioral dependencies among functions. For example, a behavioral dependency exhibits itself when a raw material receiving function cannot be completed until the laboratory testing function acknowledges that it can perform the necessary tests for the incoming material. The system therefore must identify the dependency action when the laboratory acknowledges that the test can be performed. The information and control flow between and among the different functions creates the physical database model for both materials and information.

Applicable validation considerations center on how the system is used to manufacture product and manage information in a current good manufacturing practices (cGMP) environment. This phase will create the traceability matrices for each design element document to its corresponding functional requirements specification element. As a result of the design activities, the functional requirements may have to be updated as additional requirements have been uncovered and need to be documented.

The application engineering tasks identify application software, commercially available or planned for development, that is required by the functions and controlled mechanisms in the modeled system. The results describes the functions, user interface, database access and capture, and integration characteristics and standards that the applications require to execute properly. The technology tasks define the infrastructure required to support user access, data manipulation, and integration of the manufacturing application software.

The infrastructure can be broken into the following:

- User/machine interface
- Data management
- System interconnect (i.e., networked computing platforms)

Manufacturing application software allows users or machines to create transactions that manipulate data. An example of a transaction might be the dispensing of 2000 pounds of sugar to a consumption order for product manufacture and performing the necessary transactions to inventory and work-in-process files. The user interface is the most important design output for MES and process control systems, as operators can quickly relate to screen operations. In implementing electronic batch record systems, use of screen captures to support the existing paper batch record information and data collection contents is essential.

Data management is defined during the design phase. Data sharing, data ownership, and distributed data storage as well as information genealogy and traceability need to be defined before the construction phase. Failure modes and recovery procedures must be determined and planned as a part of the definitions.

The present information technology infrastructure at each location as well as within the plants along with the communication links between sites is reviewed and catalogued for its applicability in the new infrastructure.

The most common mistake made in any systems integration program is to create a detailed design specification that describes only application products and technology concerns. An advanced manufacturing research (AMR) survey on business barriers and opportunities to CIM (9) concludes that system solutions must address more than information technology. An overwhelming 70 percent of the respondents stated that people need to be included in any systemic solution. Educational and training requirements are used as the basis for designing the organizational plans to support the resulting system.

By integrating the three architectural components of the PERA validation master plan in the design phase, the project team will be able to

- Better understand the total system required to meet the plant's business objectives
- Implement the system in a phased approach based on a prioritized set of objectives and strategies
- Better understand what skills and training are required to execute the system
- Be confident that the system will meet its intended purposes at the corporate, plant, and operations levels

IX. CONSTRUCTION PHASE

During this phase, the design specifications are used to build the custom modules, modify the commercial software, and create the system management tools needed for installation and rollout. The detail analyses, plan, and documentation for the phase are given in Fig. 8.

The design phase provided the selection of commercially available applications, use of tool sets for development, or the internal coding of an application module. The scope of construction, implementation, and subsequent testing and validation will be determined by the selection of the type of application/system element or device. The decision to use a commercially available application requires the evaluation of devices and software for data collection, bar-code label generation, and electronic batch record functionality within the new automation system environment. Comparing each device/application to the functionality and operating environment defined in the functional requirements specification will be one of the tasks. Creating a matrix with weighting values for each function

Construction Phase		
ISA	H&OA	MEA
Software application development	Batch record recording verification	Programmed unit operations
Institute configuration management practices for computer environments	Skills development	Process equipment application software development
Refined validation program	Organizational planning	Equipment specifications
Refined PQ plan	Training program development	Construction drawings
Updated project plan	Certification development	Architectural drawings
Physical data model	Refine organizational design	Facilities construction
Refined traceability matrices	Refine site specific education plan	Refined IQ
Revises FAT • Unit tests • Integration tests	Refine site specific training plans	Refined OQ
Executed CC Procedures		Network specification and installation
Execute unit test plans		Refine rollout System Configuration
System and integration testing		Confirm site specific equipment
Executed FAT		Confirm site specific processes
User documentation		Equipment specifications
Executed Change control procedures		Bills of Materials
Refine rollout system Configuration		P&ID's
Refine site specific application software		
Confirm site specific unit operations		

Fig. 8 Construction phase.

can serve as an effective tool in the selection process. Operators and any other groups that will be using the system, its elements, and the external devices (scales, bar-code wands, electronic identification [eID] devices) on a daily or weekly basis should be included in the evaluation team for the final implementation options. They can provide the final variable in determining the appropriate hardware/software selection (i.e., that of "user acceptance" in the operating environment that supports cGMP compliance).

Factory acceptance testing at the system level for the newly developed software needs to follow the unit and system testing plans that have been developed in prior phases. The result of the testing will produce the documentation to support the installation qualification testing on site in the production environments. The PERA-based validation master plan will support all of the testing criteria of the PDA and PhARMA validation methodologies for structural testing of custom software.

X. INSTALLATION OPERATIONS AND ROLLOUT PHASES

The detail analyses, plan, and documentation for these phases are given in Fig. 9.

Performing the final software and system tests portion of the validation plan for the system is now in order once installation is completed. IQ and OQ testing must be performed under actual working conditions. This is a great opportunity to define and test the ongoing audit system to assure continued compliance. PQ will continue the process.

Validation of an integrated system includes the operator interface. Much of the assurance for system security rests on the integrity of the operators. Operator integrity provides the ''spirit of the cGMPs'' and is an important people asset in compliant industries. The training systems are tested to assure that operators understand what they are supposed to do and not do. The audit system is tested to verify that it can identify violations of the security systems.

Revalidation requirements are established as a part of the validation plan. A process for reviewing changes to software and manufacturing processes and to identify the revalidation needs associated with a change is established. A summary of the functions and the test plans for each function provides an easy means to determine the scope of any revalidation effort. Since it is the basis of the system and its intended use, all system documentation developed as a part of the life cycle approach is placed under revision control. Documents are modified as solution parameters change and new components, devices, and software applications are introduced into the system.

XI. SUMMARY

A PERA-based validation master plan enables an organization to integrate equipment, people, and information when implementing a new computer-based system. The plan helps achieve the organizational missions because

- The approach has identified only the value-added business processes or functions.
- The information necessary to produce the products that are in turn necessary to measure the business objectives has been identified.
- Organizations are defined by the functions they perform and the dependencies they must support.

Installation Phase		
ISA	**H&OA**	**MEA**
Installation and commissioning	Execute education plans	Installation and commissioning
	Execute training plans	Connection diagrams
Executed IQ	Install new organizational design	I/O Listings
Executed OQ	Parallel operations	Wiring and cable
Executed SAT		Location & layout diagrams
Executed PQ		Power and fusing
Parallel operations		Executed IQ
Finalized Rollout Plan		Executed OQ
Refine Site specific IQ, OQ, PQs		Executed SAT
		Parallel operations
Operations and Rollout Phase		
ISA	**H&OA**	**MEA**
Continuing documentation	Continuing organizational development	Distribution of functions
Maintenance	Continuing skill training	Unit operations
Executed Revalidation plan	Human-Machine operations	Equipment requirements
	Revise performance measurements	System maintenance
Instituted CC procedures	Continual quality enhancement	Continuing system development
Executed Rollout Plan by site	Continuous improvement of organizational development and skill set training to enhance compliance and quality	Rollout System Configuration
Site executed IQ, OQ, PQs	Performance monitoring	Site specific equipment
Site parallel operations		Site specific Installation and commissioning
Performance monitoring		Site executed IQ, OQ and PQs
Continuous improvement of quality and compliance		Performance monitoring
		Continuous improvement of quality and compliance

Fig. 9 Installation and operations and rollout phases.

- The mechanisms and controls are defined to execute the business process function.
- The integration requirements among the functions are collected.
- The information flow between the functions and to and from external sources supporting the business objectives is known.

The PERA validation master plan can be viewed as a controlled set of business processes bounded by the business objectives and success factors that are executed by people, equipment, and information technology. The result is a methodology that not only focuses on information technology, but also on the changes to the company's business processes and the way in which people and organizations will be affected. Validation testing can then assure that the new system meets its intended purposes, as many issues have been resolved during the life cycle development and documented for later verification.

REFERENCES

1. T. J. Williams and H. Li, eds. *A Specification and Statement of Requirements for GERAM (the Generalized Enterprise Reference Architecture and Methodology) reference*, report 159, version 1.0, Purdue Laboratory for Applied Industrial Control, School of Engineering, Purdue University, West Lafayette, Indiana, Sept. 1995.
2. *A Reference Model for Computer Integrated Manufacturing*, T. J. Williams, ed., Instrument Society of America, Research Triangle Park, North Carolina, 1989.
3. T. J. Williams, *The Purdue Enterprise Reference Architecture*, Instrument Society of America, Research Triangle Park, North Carolina, 1992.
4. G. A. Rathwell and T. J. Williams, *Use of the Purdue Enterprise Reference Architecture and Methodology in Industry*, EI95, Working Conference on Models and Methodologies for Enterprise Integration, Heron Island, Queensland, Australia, Nov. 1995.
5. *General Principles of Validation*, Food and Drug Administration, Center for Drug Evaluation and Research, Rockville, Maryland, May 1987.
6. Validation concepts for computer systems used in the manufacture of drug products, PMA's Computer Systems Validation Committee, PMA Proceedings: Concepts and Principles for Validation of Computer Systems Used in the Manufacturing and Control of Drug Products, Chicago, 1986. Reprinted in *Pharm. Tech.* (May 1986).
7. Validation of computer-related systems, technical report no. 18, *PDA J. Pharm. Sci. Tech.*, supplement, *49* (SI), (1995).
8. J. P. Campi, Corporate mindset: Strategic advantage or fatal vision, *J. Cost Mgt.* 5 (1), (1991).
9. Digital Equipment Corporation study by Advanced Manufacturing Research, Boston, Massachusetts, Fall 1992.

10

System Implementation Plan for Validated Manufacturing Systems

Joseph F. deSpautz

INCODE Corp., Herndon, Virginia

I. SYSTEM INTEGRATION PROJECT PLAN

Using the Purdue Enterprise Reference Architecture (PERA) master validation plan, a detailed project plan can be defined for system integration projects for pharmaceutical manufacturing automation. The plan defines the activities, activity objectives, and tasks for each project phase using the PERA phase definitions, as follows:

Concept and definition
Functional requirements specification
Detailed design specification
Construction
Installation
Operations and rollout

For each of the phases, a set of activities is defined. These activities have specific tasks that need to be executed for a successful project. Specific system and documentation deliverables have been defined for each phase. The documentation forms the basis of installed system validation as well as planning tools for the next phase. The documentation can also focus on the potential system benefits that demonstrate project progress. Demonstrating progress is an important element of a successful manufacturing project implementation. The project plan will support the Parental Drug Association (PDA) and Pharmaceutical Manufacturers Association (PhARMA) methodologies and is an example of a plan that will support regulatory compliance and system validation.

II. PHASE I: CONCEPT AND DEFINITION

The concept and definition activities of the system integration project plan are:

Project start-up and preparation
Business systems requirements analysis

The activities, deliverable results, and roles and responsibilities of this phase are given below.

A. Activity 1: Program Preparation and Start-up

This activity formally starts the project by communicating the objectives, scope, approach, life cycle methodology, organization, deliverables, and proposed work breakdown structure (WBS) to the organization, executive management team, and the composite project team. It generates enthusiasm for the project. The project environment is established (i.e., facilities, systems engineering hardware and software). Typical activities include the following:

Form the project team. Form the project teams and identify the program manager and team leaders. If you are going to use outside resources, confirm the system team's program manager and his or her additions to your teams. All team roles and responsibilities should be clearly defined and the results of this task documented in the project program plan.

For multiplant rollouts, the management steering committee will need to support the plant implementation plans.

Kick Off the project. The project's executive sponsor formally initiates the project for key users, information systems management and personnel, and appropriate staff personnel and selected vendors. Prepare orientation materials and conduct an orientation for all stakeholders and team members to develop an in-depth understanding of project objectives, tasks, and deliverables. The proposed orientation should include a fundamental understanding of the different systems to be deployed, including enterprise resource planning, manufacturing execution, process control, document management, and a technology overview (client/server, network architecture, etc.).

Establish project environment. Establish the project environment by preparing the facilities, systems engineering hardware and software tools, and project control standards and procedures.

Finalize work breakdown structure. Finalize and communicate the detailed WBS to project personnel and appropriate personnel from the user organization(s).

Team orientation and training. Members of the project team are trained as needed on architectural principles and techniques and Computer Aided Software Engineering (CASE) tools to be employed during this phase of the project.

Assemble related documentation. The project team collects materials on business processes, functions, goals and objectives, and other related documentation that has been produced in conjunction with the project, current systems, and other project initiatives.

B. Activity 2: Business System Requirements Analysis

Most organizations have already defined their business system requirements. It should not be the intent of the project to reinvent these requirements, but rather to leverage the existing work. The business system requirements are gathered from the various studies, analyses, and reengineering projects. Using these initial business system requirements as the baseline, joint meetings are held with user personnel to provide a clear understanding of everyone's business system requirements.

A clear definition of the requirements provides the essential foundation for the functional requirements specification. The definition of requirements will be iterative with the specification activity. Often, requirements change or are added and/or deleted based on the specification.

1. Tasks

Define business architecture. Review existing requirements documentation, cost/benefit analyses, and other related documentation. Conduct working sessions with users to verify, clarify, and/or modify business system requirements. Develop a document that lists corporate objectives and business process improvements and their impact on manufacturing product requirements, manufacturing environment, and requisite strategies. Typical key business processes are lot release, lot tracking, change in control, and document management.

The results are summarized and reviewed with working session participants to verify that comments and concerns are properly documented.

Review existing systems. Review existing information technology systems to develop the information technology environment, validated systems, and new system needs. Often, existing systems, both manual and automated, are not adequately documented or completely understood within the organization. Examples of these types of systems are the methods and lists of individuals for routing and approval of engineering and document changes, criteria for what needs to be reviewed, and what the existing sources and types of information used for product approval decisions are.

The results are summarized and reviewed with working session participants to verify that comments and concerns are properly documented.

Identify process improvement opportunities. Identify, collect, and review business process change opportunities for existing business processes.

Document and approve the business achitecture. Define the business architecture by building a consensus on the organization's mission, objectives, and critical success factors. Based on the success factors, identify the appropriate business strategies and define the business system requirements. Through a set of presentations for accuracy, clarity, ranking, and completeness, resolve outstanding issues. Obtain the business system requirements approval from the appropriate management and validation/quality control group and then distribute to all program personnel.

C. Phase I: Deliverables and Milestones

Each deliverable is based on the task outputs from the phase and becomes part of the project documentation. The deliverables are as follows:

Program team matrix. Identifies program team members, mission, responsibilities and roles, and communication vehicles.

Business system requirements. Contains a prioritized list of business, data, and automation needs to meet the business objectives. This report will identify any short-term business improvement opportunities that may have been discovered during the course of the study.

D. Phase I: Roles and Responsibilities

The roles and responsibilities for phase I are given in the following table.

Team	Roles	Responsibilities
Organization	Senior management Functional managers as process experts Management steering Committee	Senior management for project Kickoff Project organization Project management Documentation approval and sign-off
System team	Project manager Validation consultant Solutions architect Process manufacturing Business process Reengineering consultant	Project organization coordination Project management Business process decomposition Material, information, and control flows

III. PHASE II: FUNCTIONAL REQUIREMENTS SPECIFICATION

The functional requirements specification is as follows:

Develop PERA architectural components for functional requirements
Create multiplant rollout plan
Define conference room pilot for multiplant operations
Develop validation program plan guide

The activities and deliverable results of this phase are given below.

A. Activity 1: Develop Information System, Human and Organizational, and Manufacturing Equipment Architecture

By incorporating the business system requirements into the architectural components of the PERA plan, all of the functional requirements of the new system will be defined.

Model manufacturing business processes. Model (process and information flow diagrams, input-process-output charting, etc.) mission-critical business processes and functions using any chosen modeling techniques. The models will depict the business requirements, business process change opportunities, products, resources, logical database requirements, product/process/equipment dependencies, behavioral dependencies, and the mechanisms used to execute the business functions.

Identify process improvement opportunities. Identify business process improvements from the business, process, and information architectural components. These improvements will include cost/benefits, risk analyses, work flow changes, change management requirements, and implementation ramifications.

Define process requirements. Define the functional requirements that satisfy the business requirements and their perceived functionality. Identify risks associated with selected products and develop recommendations.

Define technical requirements. Define the technical architecture required to support the system requirements and applications software. The technology environment includes hardware, network, database, user interface, network application services, and system management services.

Review functional requirements. Review the requirements through a set of presentations for accuracy, clarity, and ranking of critical success factors, resolving all outstanding issues.

Revise business system requirements. Reconcile the business systems requirements.

Approve and publish functional requirements specification. Obtain approval from the appropriate senior management and from quality assurance as required for validation and quality considerations. Distribute the document to all appropriate personnel.

B. Activity 2: Create a Rollout Plan for Multiplant or Multiproduct Operations

A rollout plan will be required equally for extending the system across multiple business units or product lines as well as across plants. Measurements are a critical part of the rollout and management processes. Setting goals and objectives, measuring performance for feedback and corrective action plans, and assigning responsibilities are all part of the closed-loop manufacturing management process that is used in successful manufacturing operations. The rollout plan should include a performance measurement process for determining the success of the manufacturing systems in operation.

For large plant systems or multiplant rollout strategies, one approach is to develop a conference room pilot system. A conference room pilot is a ''four-wall'' controlled analysis of how the system will behave in production using real products, actual batch record recording practices, and other manufacturing functions. The project team will define which product lines from the different plant sites will be used in the testing, which users will be involved, the characteristics and media for documentation, and an approach for addressing organizational and multiplant issues.

Identify common system elements. There will be a large number of common system elements across the different plants. These common elements must be identified and a consensus must be developed that functional requirements should support each operational environment. The unique requirements are identified and tabulated for future development.

Establish performance measurements and success factors. Establish the performance measurement process for achieving success. The first step will be to establish performance objectives of operations that are clear, easily understood, and measurable. Present performance against these measurements will be determined during the rollout phase. All problem areas and issues will be identified. As the next step, develop action plans with resources and responsibilities for solving the problem performance areas.

Establish a rollout strategy. The combined team should establish overall implementation goals and performance measures. This will result in a detailed phase-in strategy to manage the entire rollout process across plants that will yield the most benefits to each plant. The implementation plan will be organized to clearly describe the sequence, timing, resources, cost, improvement opportunities, and risk factors for the rollout strategy.

Define conference room pilot scope. The team can define the scope of the conference room pilot, including what common modules, application packages, or custom modules will be tested. The scope will account for time, ROI, and the critical success factors identified in the business architecture.

Define rollout team responsibilities. The plant implementation team members will be selected and individual roles and responsibilities defined. Working with the internal plant-level managers and sponsors, a plant-level implementation steering committee will be formed. This committee should include three or four members of plant operations management as well as individuals specializing in documentation and validation activities at the plant.

C. Activity 3: Conference Room/Prototype Pilot (Optional)

The principal objective of this activity is to verify any assumptions made during the modeling activities using the selected application software product(s). This is achieved by reviewing key business transactions of specific product lines and using the application in a four-wall operational environment. The team will learn how to navigate through the application and how the application transactions and functions support the key data and system behaviors. User interface requirements will be an output of this activity. Summarize risks and issues associated with the conference room plan and develop strategies to help control or reduce the risks.

1. Maintain Conference Room Test Environment

Develop and maintain a conference room pilot of the selected software application(s) using the targeted hardware. The pilot will be synchronized with actual plant operations. Load, configure, and set paremeters (through direct support from each application software vendor's consultants) of the application software and layered products for plant operations using specific product lines. The Management Information Systems (MIS) staff should provide the program team members with access to the environment, security clearance, access to printer services, and application software. Review the vendor-supplied user documentation and identify key transactions required by business process functions.

2. Conference Room Analysis of Common System Elements

Conduct a structured conference room analysis of the application(s) using the actual operational documents, paperwork, forms, batch records, lab analyses, logs, and so forth for the selected products from the different plants. FDA compliant documentation will be used wherever possible and necessary during the testing. Specific business process scenarios will be run or recreated using the software. Prototyping may be used for critical functions where required. All test results will be recorded during the pilots.

Conduct a structured walk-through of plant operations to ensure that all plant business processes and requirements have been captured in the pilots and business system requirements. Integrate results of the conference room pilot into the functional requirements specification to make one composite document.

3. *Review the Composite Specification*

Through a set of presentations, review the resulting specification for accuracy, clarity, ranking of critical success factors, and outstanding issues to be resolved. Reconcile the business systems requirements, application requirements, business redesign considerations, validation issues, and other requirements. Obtain sign-off from the quality assurance group for validation/quality considerations. Distribute the requirements specification to all program personnel.

D. Activity 4: Validation Program Plan and Acceptance Test Planning

Throughout the project, there must be cooperation with the quality assurance group to define its validation efforts and plan. The manufacturing program validation protocol has to be structured to conform the validation/quality assurance group's requirements. The system acceptance test plan will be developed as part of this effort. It is important for all program personnel to understand that it is their responsibility to be concerned with validation to achieve testing and validation objectives. The factory and site acceptance test plans will be developed to demonstrate that the system will consistently operate in accordance with pre-determined specifications and that it passes performance tests.

1. *Validation Planning*

By using the documentation developed in the different phases together with the quality assurance group's validation requirements, a congruent manufacturing validation plan may be defined. The validation program plan will support which current Good Manufacturing Practices (cGMP) guidelines apply to their production and laboratory environments.

Identify and develop the configuration management environments to address the different phases of the project and the system in operation. All of these environments are required to support different configurations, tests, and controls. They do not, however, need to be implemented all at once and can be phased in over time to support the program as required.

2. Change Control Procedures

Identify change control procedures, including: change control tracking, the change request process, the review process, the approval process, and the distribution of approved changes. Identify document management procedures for all documentation deliverables. Identify and collect the current information from the software application and layered products to form the baseline set of documentation. Put all documentation under document management control.

E. Activity 5: Refine System Rollout Plan

The team will need to develop an accurate scope and plan for the plant system that represents the actual system to be used in operation. Activities will include design, construction, and execution phases. Strategies will be determined to address such issues as which users will be involved, the documentation's characteristics and media, and what approach(es) will be used to address organizational issues.

1. Define and Refine the System Rollout Plan

It is time to quantify system benefits, ROI, and critical success factors for the project. Identify the technical, hardware, and software requirements needed to support the system during the rollout to different sites. Update the schedule, resource effort, and projected system costs required to complete the different rollout configurations. By summarizing the risks and issues associated with the project plans, you will be able to develop strategies to help control or reduce the risks.

Finalize, package, and distribute the plan to appropriate management and key personnel. Present the plan to the executive steering committee and obtain approval.

F. Phase II: Deliverables and Milestones

1. Functional Requirements Specification

The functional requirements are typical in four categories. The business component defines the business objectives, critical success factors, and business process rules to be used in the system. The process and information component defines the mission-critical business processes, functions, resources, products, mechanisms, and behavioral dependencies used to achieve the business strategies. The application component defines the commercial products to be used or the products to be modified during construction. The technical component defines the information systems infrastructure required to support the applications.

Conference pilot room plan. Defines the scope and resources for the conference room pilot.

Validation project plan guidelines. Documents the quality assurance guidelines for the project.

Factory and site acceptance test plan. Describes the testing guidelines that will demonstrate the system fitness for production use and meet its performance criteria.

Business process improvements plan. Consists of project profiles for each potential improvement area, including cost/benefits, risk analysis, change management requirements, and implementation ramifications.

Project plan. The revised time-phased project plan for the remaining life cycle phases. It includes project and resource schedules, implementation priorities, and cost. The plan will be updated during the remaining phases.

G. Phase II: Roles and Responsibilities

The roles and responsibilities for phase II are given in the following table.

Team	Roles	Responsibilities
Organization	Project manager Functional managers as required QA audit team member IS system consultant	Operational fit of application software in conference room pilot determined by computer systems management Performance measurements development Validation planning requirements Documentation approval and sign-off
System team	Project manager Validation consultant Solutions architect Process manufacturing consultant Case consultant	Project organization coordination Material, information, and control flows Legacy system definition Integration requirements Performance measurements development Technical infrastructure requirements Validation planning requirements
Application vendor(s) if required	Project manager Technical consultant Financial consultant Manufacturing consultant System engineer	Project organization Vendor project management Install, test, and make operational application software Support conference room pilot Functional specification for deficiencies and changes Support document development

IV. PHASE III: DETAIL DESIGN SPECIFICATION

The plant system design activities are as follows:

- System design
- Application proof and concept
- Data conversion and configuration
- Design testing
- Training procedures
- Refine project plan

A. Activity 1: System Design

The system design defines the specific internal behaviors of the manufacturing applications, layered products, and system management software that are required to achieve the functional requirements. A traceability matrix is developed so that each functional requirement is identified with its corresponding design requirements.

During this phase, the physical computing system, data storage, user display devices, network configuration, and manufacturing processing equipment (e.g., DCS, PLCs, scales) will be defined. The physical data model will be defined from the functional requirements and the logical data model developed during the prior phase.

Transform functional requirements into design requirements. All of the functional requirements are transformed into internal detail design specifications. The specifications will include transaction design, user interface design, and database management access for custom modules, vendor-supplied application modules, and internally developed or existing software. Identify integration protocol design for modules involved in business transactions that span multiple applications.

System startup, backup, and recovery procedures. Design system management procedures and routines required to start up or shut down the system, backup/restore the database, and recover the system from shutdowns. Identify performance monitoring tools.

Physical database design. Design the physical database, database access routines, network application service modules, network communication modules, interprocess communication, and user interface modules.

Information technology infrastructure. Detail the specifications for hardware, system software, network, database technology, and topology of application and infrastructure software on the physical computing platform.

Review and document design specification. Review the system design through a set of business scenarios for accuracy, clarity, and completeness. Identify and reconcile outstanding issues. Obtain the system design sign-off from program management and the validation/quality control group. Distribute the approved design to all program personnel.

B. Activity 2: Application Proof of Concept

This activity will verify any assumptions about internal behaviors for the selected applications made during system design. Learn the database commit and recovery behaviors of the manufacturing application software modules when integrated with one another. This activity complements the system design activity.

1. *Test Business Scenarios*

The IS staff must provide the program team members with access to this environment, security clearance, access to printer services, and application software. Review the vendor-supplied user documentation and identify key transactions required by business process functions defined in the specification and verified by the conference room pilots. Through cooperation with software vendor personnel, test application software with layered products integration routines. Conduct business scenarios of specific business process integration requirements using the application software.

C. Activity 3: Data Conversion and Configuration

Existing system data tables need to migrate to the new systems. The team will have to design the conversion routines required to translate and migrate current system data to new applications. The new logical and physical data models are needed for this development. Additionally, the data required to configure the package software will be defined to support the functional requirements. All documentation will be updated.

D. Activity 4: Design Testing

1. *Objectives*

Test scripts, testing routines, emulators, and test data required to adequately test the system must be designed. Additionally, test environments, directories, and tools required for proper configuration and control will be designed. Using the factory and site acceptance test plan defined in phase I, all routines, emulators, and test data backup/restore procedures are designed. The proper methods, tools, and procedures needed to test the system will be documented.

E. Activity 5: Training Procedures

1. *Objectives*

Training methods and procedures will apply to both plant system pilot execution and production. Identify current training material available for legacy systems supplied by application vendors. Define the training procedures and methods to be used by operators and end-user personnel. The methods should include manuals and online accessible documentation.

F. Activity 6: Refine Project Plan

At the completion of this phase, the team will have a detailed count of programs to be coded, interfaces to be developed, and the hardware, layered software, configuration management tools, and other equipment to be purchased. The current plan should be refined and submitted for approval to the executive committee, if required.

G. Phase III: Deliverables

Each deliverable is based on the expectations of the task activities and an understanding of the program scope. The deliverables are as follows:

Design requirement specification. Defines the internal design required to achieve the product functionality identified in the specification. It will describe standard package transactions, customized package transactions, database design, system management, physical computing platform, and network.

Data conversion and configuration. Defines the data, data conversion routines, and design required to translate and migrate current system data to the new applications. It will also include the data required to configure the application software.

Test design. Identifies the test scripts, testing routines and design, emulators and design, test data, test environments and tools, and configuration and control required to adequately test the system and support the system acceptance test plan.

Training materials. Describe operator and end-user training procedures, manuals, and access methods to be used in both the pilot execution and production phases.

Refined project plan. Updated to reflect our increased understanding of the factors involved.

H. Phase III: Roles and Responsibilities

The roles and responsibilities for phase III are given in the following table.

Team	Roles	Responsibilities
System team	Project manager Validation consultant Solutions architect consultant Process manufacturing consultant System engineer(s)	Project management Integration design Technical infrastructure design Test design System training design Validation planning
Application vendor(s)	Project manager Technical consultant Financial consultant Manufacturing consultant System engineer	Vendor project management Application software support Functional design Application training design Support/documentation development
Organization	Project manager Functional managers as required QA audit team member IS system manager	Project management Computer systems management Application software maintenance Consultation on operational areas practices and procedures Organization and measurements implementation design Validation design support Documentation approval and sign-off

V. PHASE IV: SYSTEM CONSTRUCTION

System construction activities consist of the following:

Software components
Acceptance test package
Training materials

During this phase, the design specifications are used to build the custom modules and interfaces and packaged software is modified if needed, the configuration data are loaded, and the system management utilities are developed. These modules, interfaces, and configurations are tested at each stage of the development to verify functionality and performance accuracy. Procedure manuals are developed and acceptance tests are conducted by users and IS personnel. Further, a program is developed to train the users and IS personnel to work with the package and custom modules. Schedules are made for development, testing, and training.

Upon acceptance of the modules and completion of the required training, system data are converted and the new system is ready for plant installation or rollout to multiple sites, if applicable. This phase culminates in a pilot-ready group of manufacturing system elements that closely match the daily operations of the enterprise. Revisions to the design of procedures or system will be reflected in the validation documentation as well as in the test plans.

A: Activity 1: Software Components

1. Construct Software Modules

Develop, modify, or configure each component of the system design specification. Upon completion, these components are unit tested in accordance with the test specification. Develop test routines, emulators, and data backup and restore procedures. Upon completion, the components are unit tested in accordance with test specification. Construct pilot data conversion software. Once conversion has been initiated, the data conversion process is validated for data integrity.

B. Activity 2: Acceptance Test Package

1. Set Up Integration Environment

Using proper configuration control, migrate the unit test components to a system and integration environment. Test components in accordance with the test specification. Test platform and network in accordance with the test specification. Revisions to the design are noted and reflected in the validation documentation along with the test results.

2. Perform Acceptance Tests

After systems integration and platform and network testing, migrate the system to the system test environment, where IS personnel, key users, and quality assurance (not to include developers) test the system in accordance with the user-acceptance test specification.

C. Activity 3: Training Materials

1. Further Develop Training Documents

Develop procedures manuals required to implement and operate the system according to the outlines generated and approved during the design phase. These procedures cover such areas as user procedures, security and control, backup and recovery, disaster recovery, startup and shutdown, and operations.

2. Train the Trainer Program

Secure training facilities and hardware. Train course instructors and core team users. The training program includes participant manuals, instructor guides, and presentation materials for each course defined during the design phase.

D. Phase IV: Deliverables

Tested system. Ready for installation into the pilot execution environment. All test results, progammer documentation, and any updated design documents are modified and made available. The system will be tested by developers, vendor consultants, IS staff, or users who were designated to assist in testing.

Data conversion. Data conversion software has been tested and is ready for use.

Procedure manuals. Required to implement and operate the system. They cover such areas as user procedures, security and control, backup and recovery, disaster recovery, startup and shutdown, and operations.

E. Phase IV: Roles and Responsibilities

The roles and responsibilities for phase IV are given in the following table.

Team	Roles	Responsibilities
Organization	Project manager QA audit team member IS system manager	Project management Computer systems management Application software maintenance Organizational change management Validation design support Documentation approval and sign-off
System team	Project manager Solutions architect consultant as required Software engineer(s) as required	Project management Integration development Technical infrastructure development/installation Test development System training material development Validation documentation
Application vendor(s)	Project manager Application consultant(s) Technical (4GL) system engineers Software engineer(s)	Vendor project management Application software support Functional development and test Application training material development Support documentation

VI. PHASE V: INSTALLATION

Installation consists of the following steps:

Test accepted system
Training materials
Validation approach
Rollout plan

A core team of users from each of the plants will be trained on the system with appropriate subsystems for their operations. They will use the system to simulate the production of specific product lines. They will be supported by the program team to verify the operation of the system and to identify necessary changes or corrections to the software, procedures, and/or training materials. The plant roll-out will be planned.

A. Activity 1: Test Accepted System

Test the mission-critical business processes identified in the specification. This will establish enhanced processes as well as develop performance improvement measurements to track system effectiveness. Conduct system pilot testing and initial validation testing. The primary objectives of the systems validation testing are to verify the following:

- That the system does what it purports to do
- That the system is operationally reliable
- That the system's overall quality is acceptable
- That development, documentation procedures, and validation strategies have been followed

Establish data center operations right from the start. The data center will be responsible for starting up the system, initiating backups shutting down the system, and restoring the system when required. Documentation of policies and procedures are updated when required.

B. Activity 2: Training Materials

Establish a ''train the trainer'' program for key users. The participant trainees will be used during the rollout phase to train new users.

C. Activity 3: Validation Project Plan

Perform validation activities as defined in the installation qualification (IQ) and operational qualification (OQ) test plans. These tests are performed by the users and test validation members under the direction of the quality assurance group.

D. Activity 4: Rollout Plan

The plant implementation team members have been selected during phase I and are an integral part of the program team. Working with individual internal plant-level managers and sponsors, a local plant-level implementation steering committee will be formed. This committee should include three or four members of plant operations management as well as individuals specializing in documentation and validation activities at the plant.

Measurements are a critical part of the rollout and management processes. Setting goals and objectives at a plant level has to occur. Measuring performance for feedback and corrective action plans and assigning responsibilities are all part of the closed-loop manufacturing management process that is used in successful manufacturing operations. The rollout plan should include a performance measurement process for determining the success of the manufacturing systems in operation. The management steering committee will be briefed to gain input to, approval of, and commitment to the implementation plan and performance measurement process.

1. Define Individual Plant Systems

Identify the system elements that will be contained in each plant's operational system. Establish overall implementation goals and performance measures. The implementation plan will be organized to clearly describe the sequence, timing, resources, cost, improvement opportunities, and risk factors. Establish the performance measurement process for achieving success. The first step will be to establish performance objectives of operations that are clear, easily understood, and measurable. After commissioning and validation is performed successfully, the plant should measure performance to monitor performance and continue to take action to achieve and maintain satisfactory performance levels on a continuing basis.

E. Phase V: Deliverables

Each deliverable is based on the expectations of the task activities and an understanding of the program scope. The deliverables are as follows:

User accepted system. Ready to be installed into each plant production environment. All test results, programmer documentation, and any updated design documents that required modification will be completed.

Updated procedure manuals. Required to implement and operate the system updated from the activities of phase IV.

Rollout plan. Contains implementation goals, performance measures, and a detailed project plan with a phased implementation strategy to manage the entire implementation process. A detailed performance measurement process is included.

F. Phase V: Roles and Responsibilities

The responsibilities and skills for phase V are given in the following table.

Team	Roles	Responsibilities
Organization	Project manager QA audit team member IS system manager Functional areas as required	Project management Computer systems management Application software maintenance Validation activities System and documentation approval and sign-off
System team	Project manager Validation consultant Process manufacturing consultant Software engineer(s) as required	Project management System test support System training Validation activities Complete documentation Validation documentation
Application vendor(s)	Project manager Manufacturing consultant Software engineer(s) as required	Vendor project management Application software support Functional test support Training updates Complete documentation

VII. PHASE VI: OPERATIONS AND PLANT ROLLOUT

The operations and plant rollout activities in phase VI are as follows:

Establish production environment
Train users
Monitor system rollout
Validate

We are now ready to roll the system into plant production environment and perform validation testing on the installed systems. Production data will be converted, plant users trained, and production operation initiated. Process validation and performance verification is a second objective that will be completed in conjunction with the rollout. The performance measurement process will be initiated and become part of operations management.

A. Activity 1: Establish Production Environment

Establish the production database with attention to the details of sizing, data integrity, and version control. From the onset, proper maintenance and backup procedures must be established. Adequate security is also mandatory, as are reliable tested recovery procedures. Convert any necessary production or configuration data through the use of conversion routines or manually keyed entry. Prior to execution, the data will be verified for accuracy. Complete all preparations required prior to actual implementation and start-up. These activities include the final setup of the production environment, introduction of new or reengineered business processes, establishment of the new organizational structure and communications, and the institution of new performance measurement processes.

B. Activity 2: User Training

Train users on the new system prior to start-up. Training materials developed previously will be utilized. The sessions should be conducted by users who have received the train the trainer programs.

C. Activity 3: Accepted System Rollout

Monitor the systems as they are put into full production to verify that nothing has been overlooked. This often includes such tasks as additional one-on-one training, enhancement of documentation, and correction of minor software problems. Establish proper configuration and control procedures, help desk, and sustaining production environment. It is important to establish this production-sustaining environment separately from the next system version.

D. Activity 4: Validation

1. IQ/OQ/PQ Testing

Perform IQ/OQ efforts according to the validation plan. Establish successful operations of systems in actual environments using parallel operations or other acceptable techniques. This will provide the performance qualification (PQ) steps of the validation plan. Establish and put in place the application support and maintenance system, practices, environments, and policies to support any program changes, bug fixes, or other changes that will occur during actual operations. Institute and use change management and document management practices to support the revalidation plan.

E. Phase VI: Deliverables

Each deliverable is based on the expectations of the task activities and an understanding of the program scope. The deliverables are as follows:

Installed system(s). User-accepted system(s), completely tested, will be ready for operation in the production operating environment. Procedures covering user operations, security and control, backup and recovery, disaster recovery, start-up and shutdown, and operations will be in place.

Documentation management schema. A documentation management control schema will be installed that supports the validation plan.

System documentation. Updated procedure manuals, user documentation, design specifications, and so forth will be released under documentation management control.

Implementation plan goals. Implementation goals and performance measurements to measure operational effectiveness will be put in place and communicated to all operational personnel.

F. Phase VI: Responsibilities and Skills

The responsibilities and skills for phase VI are given in the following table.

Team	Roles	Responsibilities
Organization	Project manager QA audit team member IS system manager Plant management teams	Project management Systems management Validation activities Ownership of project documentation
System team	Project manager Validation consultant as required Process manufacturing consultant as required Software engineer(s) as required	Project management System functional support Validation activities Complete documentation Validation documentation
Application vendor(s)	Project manager Manufacturing consultant as required Software engineer(s) as required	Vendor project management Application functional support Application training as required Complete documentation

11

Enhanced Regulatory Compliance Using Manufacturing Execution Systems

Frederick R. Bickel

Kineticon Group, Inc., Loveland, Colorado

Richard E. Blanchette

Green Mountain Technology Inc., Boulder, Colorado

I. INTRODUCTION

In order to address various needs, many pharmaceutical and process-oriented companies are installing a manufacturing execution system (MES) to improve efficiencies, reduce cycle times, and facilitate the control of manufacturing processes. Since these functions potentially impact the identity, strength, quality, and purity of the products, these functions are regulated by current good manufacturing practices (cGMPs) requirements defined in the Code of Federal Regulations (CFR), title 21, chapter I, parts 210 and 211. The purpose of this chapter is to discuss the regulatory compliance benefit of an MES rather than the business or technical drivers.

II. PURPOSE

The reasons for implementing a computer-based control system are varied. Certainly, improved manufacturing performance, production efficiency, and enhanced regulatory compliance are at the top of the list. To determine the state of regulatory compliance, the cGMPs must be examined.

The cGMPs provide a guide for the minimum standards for such a system. Section 211.68, Automatic, Mechanical and Electronic Equipment, states:

> (a) Automatic, mechanical, or electronic equipment or other types of equipment, including computers, or related systems that will perform a function satisfactorily, may be used in the manufacture, processing, packing, and holding of a drug product. If such equipment is so used, it shall be routinely calibrated, inspected, or checked according to a written program designed to assure proper performance. Written records of those calibration checks and inspection shall be maintained.
>
> (b) Appropriate controls shall be exercised over computer or related systems to assure changes in master production and control records or other records are instituted by authorized personnel. Input to and output from the computer or related system of formulas or other records or data shall be checked for accuracy . . . A backup file of data entered into the computer or related system shall be maintained.

Therefore, the regulations specifically accept the use of computers and related systems, providing certain conditions are met. These conditions are routine inspections, secure access, accuracy of data, and backup files.

Routine inspections can be accomplished initially and periodically thereafter, by printing all of the directories and files associated with the computer system and verifying the file name, size, and time/date. Any changes to the file structure should be supported by a change request or system upgrade documentation. The results of this review must be documented, approved, and stored as the benchmark for the next review period.

Access to the computer system can be controlled through both electronic and physical means. The use of password-restricted access will prevent unauthorized software access, while physical restrictions will prevent access to the computer system (server) or drives on the system. Both approaches are usually employed. Additionally, access to the database for the purpose of additions, changes, or deletions must be restricted to knowledgeable individuals.

Accuracy of data is the most critical task in setting up and maintaining such a system. If the data input to the system are not true and accurate, there should be no expectation that the data being returned will be valid. The sources of data should be examined to determine the accuracy of the information prior to populating the system database. If data are imported directly, the structure of the import statements must be reviewed to ensure that the desired data are imported. If data are manually entered, a second person review is recommended.

The process of backing up the system files, logs, and data should be established early in the process. A prototype built prior to the actual implementation can provide much of the information concerning what needs to be subject to recovery. These processes should define the needs for recovery from an isolated failure—for example, one workstation—or from a catastrophic site failure. It is important to remember that the files are the historical record needed for regulatory review.

III. OBJECTIVES

Although business and technical benefits will be discovered, the primary objective of a computer-based system is improved compliance. Any system must meet the current regulatory position without regard to any technical or business benefit. Additionally, pursuing a state of improved compliance is not an admission of compliance deficiencies, but the desired progression of a regulated business. It quickly becomes obvious that compliance with cGMPs not only satisfies regulatory aspects, but has economical and technical benefits as well.

Regulatory compliance is usually approached at several levels. Systems must be designed to comply with each part of the cGMPs and cumulatively comply with the intent of the regulations. This analysis of enhanced compliance will show the regulation and how a computer-based system may further satisfy the requirements.

IV. BENEFITS FROM IMPLEMENTATION

The benefits of an MES implementation are varied. Each company, based on its current environment, will weigh each improvement as it applies to it. Generally, the benefits are

- Eliminate deviations from current operating standards
  - Improve regulatory compliance by automatically generating accurate reports
  - Reduce levels of nonconforming product as the result of better enforcement of cGMPs
  - Improve safety awareness through better information
  - Improve efficiency and overall accessibility to standard operating procedures (SOP) and material safety data sheets (MSDS)
- Generate savings through optimized processes
  - Reduce quantity of off-target product
  - Precisely control production and deliver real-time data from those processes
  - Improve control and quality of operator training
  - Improve yields
  - Simplify functions or processes by reducing or eliminating
    - Paperwork and redundant data entry
    - Manual review and approval
    - Manual procedures and administrative tasks

Eliminate costs associated with paper systems
Reduce storage space needs
Improve ability to retrieve or recover documents
Improve interdepartmental communications
Achieve strategic benefits by increasing levels of quality and consistency
Decreasing regulatory exposure
Improving competitive position

V. ENHANCEMENTS FROM MES

Computer-based systems provide enhancements from paper-based systems. Three of the benefit categories, data capture, process administration, and record compliance, are discussed in detail. Several examples are given, but these examples are not meant to be all-inclusive. Each company needs to determine the current state of compliance and the improvements that can be obtained with a computer-based system.

VI. DATA CAPTURE

Section 211.188 of the cGMPs, Batch Production and Control Records, states as follows:

> Batch production and control records shall be prepared for each batch of drug produced and shall include complete information relating to the production and control of each batch. These records shall include:
>
> (b) Documentation that each significant step in the manufacture, processing, packing, or holding of the batch was accomplished, including:
>
> (1) Dates;
>
> (2) Identity of individual major equipment and lines used;
>
> (3) Specific identification of each batch of component or in-process material used;
>
> (4) Weights and measures of components used in the course of processing;
>
> (5) In-process and laboratory results;
>
> (6) Inspection of the packaging and labeling area before and after use;
>
> (7) A statement of the actual yield and a statement of the percentage theoretical yield at appropriate phases of processing;
>
> (8) Complete labeling control records, including specimens or copies of all labeling used;
>
> (9) Description of drug product containers and closures;
>
> (10) Any sampling performed;

(11) Identification of the persons performing and directly supervising or checking each significant step in the operation;

(12) Any investigation made according to Section 211.192;

(13) Results of examinations made in accordance with Section 211.134.

The intent of this section is to require the collection of information and data so that the process is understood and the impact of the changes can be predicted. It is important to collect the right data at the right times using the right methods of collection and analysis. A computer-based system can assist in the information and data collection and analysis.

Once the plan for the data collection has been established, a computer-based system can assure that the data are collected. The data could be obtained directly from the equipment or process (if a physical attachment is in place) or through an operator interface screen. The system can be configured so the operator cannot proceed until any required entry has been completed.

After the data have been gathered, the system can perform a statistical analysis of the data, if necessary. This analysis leads to data accuracy, trending, range checking, or error trapping. The following sections describe each of these areas.

A. Data Accuracy

A computer-based system, particularly coupled with data input devices such as bar code readers, can significantly improve accuracy. Studies show that manual data entry has an average error rate of 1 in every 300 characters. Automated (bar-coded) entry error rate is less than one in 1,000,000 entries. The further the data entry activity is from the source of the data the more entry errors result. Additionally, if data are gathered, compiled, and then keyed into a system, the chances for transcription errors increase dramatically. Only with a computer-based system can data be collected, reviewed, and evaluated at the time of processing. This data review does not replace the quality assurance review required in section 211.192 or section 211.180. (These sections are addressed later.)

B. Trending

Although not a specific requirement within the cGMPs, trend analysis can lead to a better understanding of the process. For example, examine the collection of tablet weights where the values are observed sequentially. Generally the observations are considered to be random; that is, varying about the central value (the median). However, if the process is not random, we would expect to see trends in the data. A series of high or low values is unlikely to occur by chance and could therefore be attributable to some variable in the process. Observing such trends can allow operators to correct problems as they occur. Also, understanding this part of the process can lead to further studies that may determine the source of the variability. Computer-based systems also allow the rapid analysis of real-time data. It is no longer necessary to retrieve filed or archived copies of paper records and compile data from them manually. The data from electronic log files can be accessed, sorted, compared, and studied.

C. Range Checking

Using minimum and maximum specifications that have been established for a parameter in the process, range checking can be an important tool. If data from an operation exceed the established range, notification can be immediately sent to the operator or other interested individuals. This allows intervention before the operation is completed.

For noncritical parameters in cases in which specifications are not necessary or have not been established, the product history can be quite helpful. A computer-based system can compare product history with the current batch. This comparison can provide insight into the process. This comparison also allows the operator the opportunity to view actual historical data to assess the degree of variation.

D. Error Trapping

Unlike paper-based systems, computer-based systems can be designed to prevent errors. These systems are also capable of expanding the field of information that can be tracked. In the event that an error is made in the entry of data, a computer-based system can easily compare the entered value with the expected value. Based on the type of entry, the operator may correct the entry, verify that the error was made and correct the entry, or verify that the entry is correct but did not match the expected value. Exceptions can be completed in real time and supervision notified immediately. Data security can be established so that all original data are maintained and no entries are ever removed from log files. If required, the system can enforce supervisory approval before proceeding.

VII. PROCESS ADMINISTRATION

Section 211.100 of the cGMPs, Written Procedures; Deviations, states as follows:

> (b) Written production and process control procedures shall be followed in the execution of the various production and process control functions and shall be documented at the time of performance. Any deviation from the written procedures shall be recorded and justified.

The intent of this section is to require the adherence of the processing to the master production record. Many factors can be presented to demonstrate compliance. As examples, signatures, calculations, and timing are discussed.

A. Signatures

The issue of electronic signatures has been discussed in many papers. Another aspect of signatures is the role of signatures for compliance. In any processing plant, there are many standard procedures that must be followed. These procedures are required by the cGMPs. The standard method to acknowledge that the procedure was indeed followed is through a signature. The cGMP section referred to earlier (section 211.100) requires documentation ''at the time of performance.'' Looking at the intent of this requirement, if a signature is not affixed immediately, an argument could be made for noncompliance. A computer-based system can block the operator or other individual from proceeding until the required signature is completed. By recording the operator identity and password with a date and time stamp, you can actually demonstrate that the procedure was followed and documented.

Furthermore, if the computer-based system monitors or controls the process directly, the requirement for an operator signature as a means of documenting compliance with procedures disappears. The computer-based system documents the execution of the procedure.

B. Calculations

Processing frequently requires many operator calculations. These calculations usually are of such a nature that they can affect the quality of the product being produced. A common and recurring calculation is the yield determination. Section 211.103 of the cGMPs states this requirement. With a computer-based system, the yield calculation can be automated with a scale interface (weight in/weight out) so that the yield is determined online, eliminating one source of potential error. The actual mathematical calculation, which is even more difficult for the operator, can also be automated. Again, transcription errors or calculation errors can be prevented.

Time calculations are difficult and error-prone even in the simplest cases. With a computer-based system, the internal system clock can be utilized to enhance accuracy and eliminate the need for an operator calculation.

C. Timing

Along with the requirement to document the performance of procedures at the actual time, the cGMPs also require companies to establish ''time limits for the completion of each phase of production'' (section 211.111). If the process is continuous or performed in a short time frame, compliance with this requirement is not difficult. However, if the process is lengthy or interrupted, elapsed timing may not be as evident. With a computer-based system, the system clock can be employed to maintain the actual time and alert appropriate individuals.

VIII. RECORD COMPLIANCE

The cGMPs state in section 211.192, Production Record Review

> All drug product production and control records, including those for packaging and labeling, shall be reviewed and approved by the quality control unit to determine compliance with all established, approved written procedures before a batch is released or distributed.

The intent is to require that the records and therefore the processing of the drug product comply with the regulations. As each company has designed its systems to address the regulations, the cGMPs require a final check to assure that all records follow requirements and are cGMP-compliant. This review requires significant effort, and in the event of an omission or error, requires an investigation. In the worst case, the product may be considered adulterated and may need to be destroyed. A computer-based system monitors each step as the product is processed so that omissions cannot occur and errors are corrected as they occur. Obviously, if a serious problem occurs, supervision is notified immediately and processing may be halted without incurring further costs.

Further, section 211.180, Records and Reports, General Requirements states

> (a) Any production, control, or distribution record that is required to be maintained in compliance with this part and is specifically associated with a batch of drug product shall be retained for at least 1 year after the expiration date of the batch. . . .
>
> (c) All records required under this part, or copies of such records, shall be readily available for authorized inspection during the retention period at the establishment where the activities described in such records occurred. These records or copies there of shall be subject to photocopying or other means of reproduction as part of such inspection.

Record retention has become a more critical and difficult function. The requirements are clear that the records produced must be available for inspection. With the growing number of documents needed to comply with the regulations, the management of the record files or archives becomes more challenging. The organization and filing/archiving of computer-based records is viewed in the same light. It is recognized that record retrieval is quicker and more accurate from a computer than from a document warehouse. Additionally, few companies provide for a set of duplicate paper records to protect against a disaster. A computer-based system that holds records to demonstrate compliance can be easily maintained. Additionally, off-site storage is no longer a major warehousing effort.

IX. VALIDATION

As with any system that is upgraded or installed within the regulated industries, validation is a major concern. Although validation is the specific topic in another chapter, there are certain aspects of enhanced compliance that are worthy of mention.

Any reduction in the review cycle or prevention of a noncompliant situation has significant payback. Once validated, a computer-based system can provide such a reduction in effort by tracking the process and providing documentation at a level not previously attainable. Not only can the number of reviews be decreased, but the required reviews are faster and more assured.

The effort to validate the process may also be reduced. The major contributor to validation effort (costs) is variation. If the variation is reduced, then the test cases needed to support the variation can be reduced. For example, to validate a mixing time, several studies must be performed. These studies are usually designed to predict the impact of shorter or longer mixing times to accommodate operator variation. If, however, the system controls the mixing process, only the optimized mixing time needs to be validated.

X. SUMMARY

The regulations (cGMPs) explicitly permit the use of computer-based systems for the control and manufacturing of drug products. There are significant enhancements to compliance that may be obtained through the use of properly designed and implemented computer-based systems. These enhancements provide justification of the costs for such an implementation. There can be major improvements in the way a company approaches regulatory compliance.

12

Investing in Education and Training

James L. Vesper

LearningPlus, Rochester, New York

I. INTRODUCTION: THE CASE FOR TRAINING

Along with developing and executing a validation protocol, training is one of the largest expenditures associated with a new information system. When one considers the direct (e.g., course development and production, instructors, travel, coffee and donuts) and indirect costs (time away from the job, internal facility use, administration, etc.) the numbers add up very quickly.

The overarching goal for training expenditures is to transform them from costs into an investment that pays a high return. The training should have a significant, measurable impact on those using and supporting the information system, yet it is wasteful to overload the users with facts and skills they don't need.

This chapter presents an overview of what education and training can do to support the introduction of a new technology or computer system into a work environment. Specifically, it provides information on a process that should be used to design and implement an effective training program.

A. Changing Work and a Changing Workforce

In all industries, there is a change from the nineteenth century labor model that had discreet categories of ''doers'' and ''thinkers.'' There are now fewer jobs that require unskilled or low-skilled personnel. Recently, the number of professional and managerial jobs increased 32 percent in the United States; the number of operations and laborer jobs increased by 6 percent (1). There is also now less of a distinction between ''doing'' and ''thinking.'' For example, a maintenance person servicing a labeling machine needs to have a highly developed set of problem-solving skills (a type of ''intellectual'' or cognitive skill) as well as skills in taking apart the machine to diagnose and correct the problem (i.e., motor skills). Because of E-mail systems, more managers do work that was recently considered strictly clerical; now they compose their correspondence as they type it on the screen. When automation is introduced, or when there is a significant change in the type of automation used, an additional challenge is ''reskilling'' the workers to help implement the innovation.

Education and training are tools that not only help prepare people to use the new technology, but help achieve optimal performance.

Training is also important in protecting the investment made in technology and automated equipment. Computer-integrated manufacturing systems and automation can cost ten to 100 times more than nonautomated systems used twenty-five years ago. An engineer who improperly overrides the programmable controller of an autoclave can not only damage it, but cause a significant disruption in a facility and its operations.

A paradox of increasing workplace technology is that when things are working correctly, when the equipment is ''humming along,'' there is little need for human intervention; people simply monitor the process, making sure it runs properly. In these situations, a minimal amount of training suffices. The challenge comes when something goes wrong or an unusual pathway is followed; then people must make fast and correct decisions. This is where training and coached practice have an extremely important payback. Examples of this are found in the new commercial jets that are highly automated and in chemical manufacturing facilities in which the operators monitor the process on a computer monitor while seated in an air conditioned control room. There is far less user involvement in normal operations, but when something goes wrong, having trained, skilled performers who can react quickly is essential to protect lives, the environment, and property.

B. Definitions

To provide more precision to our discussion, some definitions may help.

Instruction: The formal or informal process of providing a learner with knowledge and skills. This can be done by people (e.g., instructors, mentors) or by such technology as multimedia instructional programs. Instruction must include a method to assess if learning has taken place.

Education: Information, knowledge, and skills provided to a learner as a resource and long-term foundation for other learning and development. An example may be a course in the basics of how computers work.

Training: Knowledge and skills provided to a learner to help the learner accomplish a defined set of activities, closely related in time to when the training is provided. An example may be a course on the programming of a specific programmable controller.

Learning: The assimilation of knowledge and skills that result in a verbal/nonverbal change in the learner's behavior. When training involves information and facts that are "internal," the only way to determine if learning has occurred is by a change in behavior. Using a properly designed assessment tool, one can determine if a person has learned specific information.

Information sharing: The process of communicating for purposes other than providing a foundation of knowledge and skills or helping accomplish a set of activities. It can be used to prepare, inform, persuade, and so forth, but the process does not assess if a behavior change has occurred.

Practice: The opportunity of using knowledge and skills in a risk-free environment that provides feedback on the learner's performance so the learner can improve.

C. Who Needs to Be Trained?

Identifying who needs to be trained is a critical step in implementing a rational training strategy. Training needs to be provided to the people who must have the knowledge and skills to safely and efficiently operate, support, and maintain the system. Training may also be appropriate to those who more peripherally interact with the information system whose performance would benefit from additional knowledge and skills, such as management.

Not all system users need to be taught the same thing; the needs analysis process (described below) is used to identify what various audience members need to be trained in.

A distinction should be made between information sharing and instruction. Information about the system, its effects, how it will help accomplish organizational goals, and so on should be communicated to a broad audience. This would include people who would later receive training and education on the system. The early communication can help prepare the way for the system and reduce anxieties and fears. Since there is no assessment or feedback loop in this type of communication, it is not strictly defined as training or education. However, it is important to the overall success of the project.

There may be situations in which very little training is needed such as when, paraphrasing Mager (2), "people could do it if their lives depended on it." In these situations, users might only need the opportunity to practice. This type of situation is found in very simple, well-designed, intuitive systems.

An example of an information system for which most users have not needed formal training is in operating an automated teller machine (ATM, or "money machine''). Most of us were able to use one the first time without difficulty. The device provided its own instructions and feedback (called ''electronic performance support'') that we were able to understand. Errors, such as putting the ATM card in upside down, were detected by the device and appropriate messages were given. As we used the devices more often we became more proficient. Practice improved our skills at accomplishing the task. If a system is as simple and easy to use as this, users may not need formal training.

A needs analysis will identify situations in which training is not required because the task is simple and the system itself provides the necessary performance-supporting tools.

II. ACCOMPLISHING THE PROJECT

At the very beginning of the project, the planners and users need to develop a common vision of how training is to fit into the broader project. Certainly the problem and the solution will shape the vision in determining the type and amount of training required. For example, how will users interact with the system, using special language or commands or following a series of menus? Simply using command lines will be easier to build from a programming standpoint, but much more complicated to train people on compared to a menu-driven system. Also, how much ''help'' will be provided by the system itself? Will there be context-sensitive help capabilities, or will there only be a thin user's manual?

Another part of the vision would be an understanding of what failure of the system would mean to the organization, the workers, and the community. If failure could cause a serious business, regulatory, safety, or environmental problem, the costs of a comprehensive training program with sophisticated simulators would be easier to justify.

The strategic role of training should also be factored into the vision. Some technology-intensive organizations are realizing the only way they will remain leaders in their industry is to provide training to their personnel that is superior to that given by their competitors. Training is becoming a distinguishing feature of successful firms. For example, at General Motors' Saturn motorcar facility (one of the most automated in the world), each employee participates in 300 to 600 hours of preproduction training plus thirteen days of training each year. Motorola Electronics has committed that each employee receive a minimum of forty hours training per year at a cost of $60 million (1990 dollars) (3).

To help address the training aspects, most successful projects use a cross-functional team that includes users, technical personnel, developers, and training professionals. All members should have an understanding of the goal and scope of the project and an overview of the process that will be used to define and produce the training solutions.

Some people are much better suited than others in being part of a training

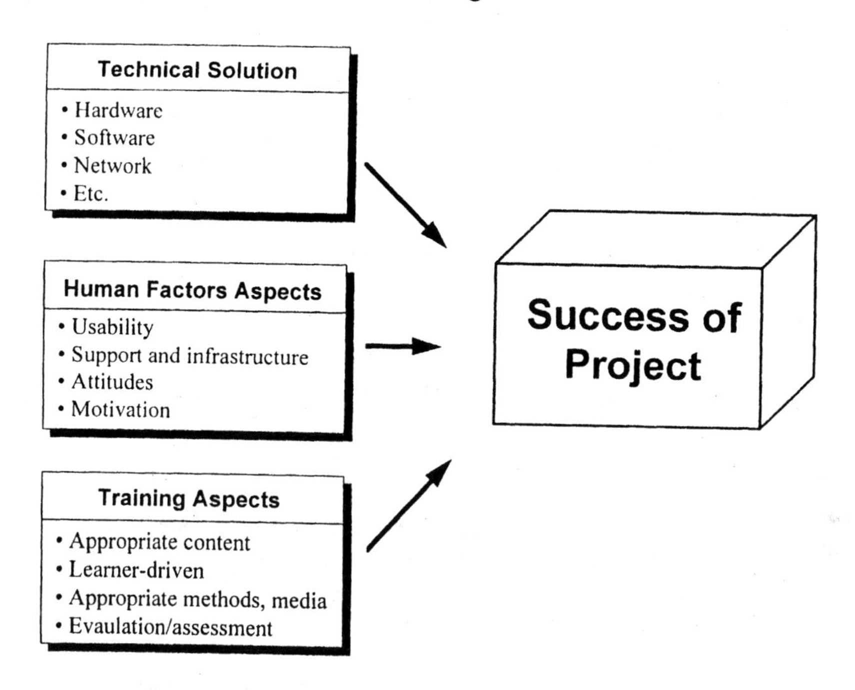

Fig. 1 Factors that contribute to a successful project.

project. There are some people who can perform a probing and insightful analysis; however, as classroom instructors, they cannot effectively share information. More so than in other endeavors, forcing a person to be involved in training activities against his or her will or capabilities will have negative effects in the final product.

As shown in Fig. 1, there is a relationship between the people issues and training required for the success of the project. There is not necessarily one best way of accomplishing training; the team and management need to find the best combination of ways to accomplish the goals given the particular situation and their vision. There are, though, certain approaches that are much more successful than others and will have more satisfactory long-term results.

Producing effective training takes time, qualified people, and money. If it is shortchanged, it will impact the success of the entire project.

A. The Role of the Vendor

If a system is purchased from a vendor or custom designed by technology experts, they should be an educational and training resource. Whether they provide quality instruction that will meet the users' needs largely depends on how the purchase agreement or contract was written as well as on the supplier's own capabilities.

More and more equipment purchasers (e.g., drug and device manufacturers) are wanting vendors to provide quality training instruction as part of the "package." As we will discuss below, the instruction must go much farther than a typical "how-to" manual. When evaluating a supplier's instructional materials, actual programs or the design/development strategy that will be used should be carefully reviewed by someone knowledgeable in instructional systems design before they are implemented.

Several vendors of information systems have seen the benefit of developing and supplying high-quality, effective training programs and have even created subsidiaries to do just that.

III. THE INSTRUCTIONAL SYSTEMS DESIGN APPROACH

The approach that is recognized as the most effective method in producing successful instructional interventions is called "instructional systems design" (ISD). (An instructional intervention is the education and training programs that will be produced in any of a variety of forms, from written self-study materials to workshops to multimedia simulations, in order to accomplish the goal.) The ISD model has several slight variations, but basically it includes the five basic steps shown in Table 1. (Note: There are a number of books that describe the ISD process in more detail. Two suggestions are: M. Craig, *Analyzing Learning Needs*, Ashgate Publishing, Brookfield, VT, 1994, and J. L. Vesper, *Training for the Healthcare Manufacturing Industries*, Interpharm, Buffalo Grove, Illinois, 1993.)

Some comments about the ISD model of training include the following:

- ISD is a systematic, iterative approach. The output of one phase provides the input to following phases.
- Analysis is critical. The results from the analysis phase form the foundation to the instructional activities. If a poor job is done here, the results will be obvious later on with courses that do not meet the learners' needs.
- A variety of skills is needed to produce an effective training program. Very few people have strengths in accomplishing all of the ISD tasks. Teams of people are usually used, with some team members focusing on data gathering and analysis, course design, and so forth.
- Creating effective training takes time. Conducting an analysis on one job position can take more than several hundred person hours and identify dozens of lessons. Producing lessons can take thirty to 100 person hours for each hour of instruction.
- Management support is critical. Management must share the vision of the value that training can add to the project and the organization.

Table 1 An Overview of the Instructional Systems Design Process

Phase	Description	Final output
1. Analysis	Define the goal and scope of the project; collect and analyze data about the job, task, problem, and audiences.	Prioritized list of training needs and other performance-related needs.
2. Design	Plan what the instructional intervention will look like. The plan, or "blueprint" includes learning objectives, requirements, constraints, strategies for course delivery, and evaluation. The plan is reviewed and approved by appropriate personnel and management.	An approved instructional plan.
3. Develop	Produce the instructional courses and lessons with leader-led materials, videotapes, activities, simulations, etc. as per the plan; conduct pilot programs and make modifications as needed. Courses are reviewed and approved by appropriate personnel and management.	Approved courses ready for delivery.
4. Implement	Prepare the instructors as needed and deliver the courses to the learners; collect evaluation data.	Learners who have been trained and meet the objectives of the courses.
5. Evaluate and maintain	Fine-tune and update the course as needed to more efficiently meet the learning objectives and the goal of the program.	Summaries of evaluation data and improvements to the courses, as needed.

IV. THE ANALYSIS PHASE

The purpose of the analysis phase is to define the problem and identify, describe, and quantify the parameters to be considered when preparing the solution. Specifically, the analysis will examine the following:

- Why training is needed
- How the success of the training efforts will be measured
- What the goals are
- Who needs to be trained
- What the users actually do in using the (new) system or technology
- The outputs of the tasks
- How they do it
- What the users need to know to accomplish their role in using the system
- What the users know, what are they able to do now
- What the considerations and issues are in instructing the users
- What else needs to be done for the users to be successful in using the system

In business today, the most frequent initiators for an analysis are performance problems (e.g., people not documenting their work according to the expectations of the quality control auditors) or formalizing existing practice (e.g., develop a curriculum for new employees). Recently there has been a trend in many pharmaceutical and medical device firms to establish mastery programs that generate evidence showing that people in the jobs (i.e., ''incumbents'') perform the jobs according to objective, documented standards. (Assessing an employee's performance is discussed in Chapter 14.)

Implementing a new information system or technology can also initiate an analysis; this will be our focus.

A. Analysis for a New Information System or Technology

In this phase, the analysts want to understand the goals of the project. This is important so all the efforts are focused and there isn't wasted effort. Also, they will identify the tasks that people perform and the knowledge and skills that they need so they can efficiently and safely perform the tasks. For a new system that is being implemented, this is made more complex because the facility doesn't have any (or many) people who are expert performers; the technology or system does not yet exist. Oftentimes the new tasks have not been formalized into standard operating procedures (SOPs) that define who does what, when, and in what sequence. Additionally, in areas that have not used computer systems before, there are additional basic training needs (e.g., signing on, using passwords, deciding what to do when the system doesn't immediately respond).

Often automation and high technology projects have their own jargon and sets of acronyms. These should be collected and assembled into a glossary that is available to learners during the training and to users of the system as a reference.

B. Audience Analysis

Besides the knowledge, skills, and tasks that are analyzed, the audience needs to be considered. This includes examining their characteristics, such as the following:

- Educational background
- Literacy levels
- Previous experiences with the technology
- Examples of training that have and have not been successful in the past
- Age and sex of the learners
- Situations in which the learners have special needs
- How many people need to be trained
- When training needs to be given/scheduling constraints
- Geographical considerations
- People or environmental conditions that could influence how the learners will perform the skills and tasks

These data will not only help shape the content, but also how the instruction will be provided to the learners.

C. Techniques for Collecting the Data

There are several techniques that are helpful in collecting and analyzing data in situations in which a new technology or process is being implemented. To improve the completeness and quality of the resulting information, at least three different sources of data and/or methods should be used. This way, there is less chance of singular points of view biasing the results.

There is not one uniform sequence of when to do what. It will depend on the situation as well as when information and people are available. The process is also iterative; that is, it is helpful to talk with the same people several different times so they can clarify and correct the information that is collected.

If at all possible, feed the collected information (whether it be from interviews, focus groups, observations, etc.) back to the people who provided it for their review. Doing this will greatly improve the quality of the resulting information and also build trust and credibility with the people the team is working with.

More details on using these techniques can be found in the references mentioned above.

1. *Tools That Can Be Used*

Table 2 can be used (or modified as needed) to help collect and organize data while using the methods below.

2. *Document Review*

A side benefit of an information project meeting GMP or ISO-9000-3 expectations is the documentation that is available. Requirements documents, flowcharts, SOPs, protocols, test results, and so on can be sources of information to find out what system users will be required to use. Also, flowcharts are very useful in developing SOPs and training materials.

3. *Finding and Talking with the "Experts"*

You may be able to find people with experience in the system. They could be the developers, pilot-program teams, vendor personnel, or even other firms that have previously installed the system. (You may be able to gain access to experts at another firm if you supply the firm with the results of your analysis.) One-on-one interviews and focus groups (with four to six people) are ways of extracting information. Questionnaires are often used, but they have limited utility because good ones are difficult to construct. Also, questionnaires do not allow for immediate clarification on the part of the analyst or respondent.

For new technologies, some particular questions that may be helpful include the following:

- What was most difficult in learning the new system? Why?
- Of all the tasks performed, what is most critical? Why?
- If we only had time to teach three things, what would they be?
- How is your job different now using the new system from the way it was before?
- What were you most uncomfortable with when you began using the system? What is your comfort level now? What caused it to change?
- What would you tell a new person coming into this job?
- What knowledge and skills would make it easier to learn this job?
- How can new users be prepared for the change?

Additionally, the analysts will define the duties, tasks, and subtasks of the performers. Lists, with phrases starting with action verbs and flow diagrams, are useful ways of documenting this.

4. *Observing the "Experts" Perform a Task*

If you can find people who are currently performing the task, they can be a source of information. Gayeski, Wood, and Ford (4) describe several different methods of having an expert explain what he or she is doing to an analyst.

Table 2 Sample Data Collection Form

Task Analysis Worksheet

Job/position ______________________ Date ______________________

Duty ______________________ Analyst ______________________

Outcome ______________________

Task Step Substep	Description	Knowledge required	Skills required	Tools, information used	Safety, environmental concerns	Difficulty of performance	Frequency of performance	Criticality of performance

5. Observing Naive Individuals Using the System

This technique can be one of the most powerful methods to determine what basic skills need to be taught. There are many variations on the technique, but they all involve asking several different people to try and use the system or technology to solve an actual problem. Typically they are given no or little help (e.g., the instruction book) and are observed as they work toward the goal. A wealth of human factors information will also be discovered. Carroll and Mack (5) give both a methodology and examples of resulting transcripts as they applied this method with users of a word-processing application.

Defining and selecting ''naive'' users is critical to the success of this method. The group needs to be large enough to cover individual differences in learning approaches, but also similar to those who will receive the ultimate training.

D. Analyzing the Data

While the data are collected, the immediate findings shape the follow-up questions that are asked and other data that are gathered. For instance, if the analyst discovers contradictory statements between groups or between what is written and how something is actually done, the issue must be resolved. As the data are examined in more depth, the analyst will be looking for themes, patterns, similar responses, and inconsistencies. Also, the analyst wants to find ways of supporting the learners' performance in ways that do not involve instruction.

The performance frequency, difficulty, and criticality of tasks and skills should be noted; this influences the priority and emphasis given to these topics.

Standards or performance requirements should also be determined, as they will be used in developing the learning objectives and evaluation criteria.

The output of this phase is a prioritized list of training needs that includes knowledge, skills, and tasks for each audience considered.

E. Using the Information to Generate Procedures

From the interviews and observations with the experts and a review of the documents, the analysts should have enough information to create an SOP. SOPs are required to meet GMP and quality system requirements, but they also help provide people with the information they need to do their jobs. SOPs and training should not be viewed as two separate endeavors; they are and should be closely related.

The instructions contained within an SOP can range from a low to high level of detail. For instance, the word *wash* is a function word that includes a variety of individual tasks and subtasks, such as load, close door, turn on, and set controls.

It is much simpler and faster to write an SOP with a low level of detail (i.e., that includes many function words), but there is a down side. Function words

Table 3 Example of a Multicolumn SOP
(Task: Signing on to the World Wide Web using NETSCAPE)

Step	Task	Additional detail
1	Turn on computer.	Switch located on front of CPU box. System will automatically boot up. WINDOWS will be invoked. Main window with application icons will appear.
2	Double click on INTERNET TOOLS icon.	New window will appear.
3	Double click on NET DIAL icon.	New window will appear. Commands from script will automatically execute. Phone link will be established. WINSOCK program will be started.
4	Close WINSOCK screen.	Use ''Close'' command found under FILE pull-down menu. Internet tools window will reappear.
5	Double click on NETSCAPE icon.	NETSCAPE application will be invoked. Default home page will appear.
6	Enter the URL address: http://www.cgmp.com	Type text in box labeled ''Location:__.''

can permit more variability in how the task is performed since the steps aren't detailed in the SOP. Also, function statements assume the SOP users have the experience or are given the training to properly execute the function. Therefore, using function words can increase the variability of performance or require more training in how to perform the task. This is where SOPs, training, and performance need to be viewed as a system and not in isolation. Saving time by writing SOPs without much detail may greatly increase the time required to train people.

Another element related to training and SOPs is how the SOPs are written. There is a variety of ways, but the goal should be writing SOPs that help the user perform the task. Table 3 shows an example of an alternative style for an SOP. In this version, if a person needs extra detail (such as during training or if he or she hasn't performed the task in a while), he or she can use both right-hand columns. Experienced users only need to use the center column. Other formats using ''structured writing'' methods, such as Information Mapping, are also beneficial.

A key point regarding SOPs is that different people use them at different times for different purposes. A well-designed SOP should support the needs of all of them.

V. DESIGNING THE TRAINING PROGRAM AND COURSES

Designing the training intervention is similar to producing blueprints for a building. The users' needs and requirements that were identified in the analysis phase are now used to specify the instructional content, sequencing, methods, and media. The resulting document from the design phase, called the instructional plan, will guide the development and implementation of the instructional efforts.

The length of the instructional plan can range from three to 100 pages, depending upon the scope and complexity of the project.

Another use of the instructional plan is to produce a cost estimate for producing the program.

A key activity of the design phase is taking information that was collected during the analysis phase and shaping it into manageable ''chunks'' of instruction or instructional units. Each instructional unit has a goal, along with objectives and topics. An instructional unit could be a course or a lesson.

A training course is made up of one or more lessons; each lesson is an instructional unit focused on a particular topic (that includes one or more chunks) that can be completed by the learner in one sitting. A lesson may range in time from fifteen minutes to several hours.

A. Adults as Learners

Before going into detail about the instructional plan, it will be helpful to quickly look at the special needs of adult learners.

Our previous education, job, life experiences, knowledge, and skills make each of us unique as we approach an instructional program. We learn at different rates, have different interests, and have different preferred learning styles. While some audiences may be more heterogeneous than others, there will always be diversity in the learners that should be considered. Table 4 lists some of the differences of adult learners as compared to children.

For training to be successful, it needs to build on the opportunities presented by adult learners.

Work by Knowles (6) and Rogers (7) provides guidance as to how courses for adults should be designed, produced, and delivered.

- Involve the learner during all phases of course development and delivery. Having learners participate in the development phase can help build not only quality into the final program but also the buy-in of the learners. During the training sessions themselves, pouring information onto them is not effective; having the learners participate in discovering answers for themselves is effective.
- Have the learner become a partner in the process. Since the adult learners come in with knowledge, let them use it whenever possible. Giving them some control of the program, whether it is when to take a break or the

Table 4 Comparison of Children and Adults as Learners, Based on Work of Knowles (6)

How children are traditionally taught (pedagogy)	How adults learn best (andragogy)
Teacher makes the decisions; students accept this.	Adults want to know why they need to learn material.
Teacher considers all students dependent on him or her; students believe and accept this.	Adults have the self-concept that they are adults, want to have control over their lives, and wish to be viewed as being capable of self-direction.
Students have little experience to contribute as a resource to learning; experience they have is not valued.	Adults have considerable experience of many different types: positive and negative (that can impede learning).
Students are ready for the next level when the teacher says so.	Adults learn when they can apply the knowledge or skills to a real-life situation.
Learning experiences are organized according to subject matter units and the logic of the subject matter.	Adults are "life" centered; learning is arranged around tasks or problems that the learner encounters.
Students are primarily externally motivated (by teachers' and parents' approval/disapproval).	Adults are motivated both externally (supervision, promotions, more money) and internally (satisfaction, responsibility, etc.); internal motivators are considered to be a stronger force.

sequence to cover things in a multimedia program, will create a better learning situation.

- Respect the individual. Separate the behavior from the person. Encourage. Coach.
- Focus on real life. Use problems, terms, and examples that the learners can relate to.
- Include the whys. Don't simply state how to do something. If people understand the reasons behind a task and what the goal is, they are more likely to consistently accomplish it.
- Allow for failure. If you create simulations, activities, or other interactions, there is tremendous value if people are allowed to safely fail and have an opportunity to learn why and how to recover from a failure.

B. Elements of an Instructional Plan

The contents of a complex instructional plan are shown below. The plan for a simpler project may only include the goal, objectives, detailed instructional outline, and evaluation strategy. Several of the elements are discussed in more detail.

Goal: A specific and measurable statement about the desired outcome of the training program, course, or lesson.

Scope: A statement of who will be trained, including the names of positions, departments, locations, numbers of people, and so forth.

Requirements and constraints: Special needs related to the audience, organization, project, and so on that must be considered as the instructional intervention is developed and implemented. This could include the implementation schedule, budget, equipment requirements, availability of personnel, and language.

Curriculum: A sequenced listing of courses and lessons that participants are expected to complete. Prerequisite courses or experiences are noted. The curriculum is useful in planning the development of courses as well as scheduling the participants.

Objectives (also known as learning objectives or performance objectives): Behaviorally based statements describing in specific and measurable terms what the learner should be able to do after completing the training program, course, or lesson. If the learner completes the objectives, he or she should be able to attain the goal.

Detailed instructional outline: A document that includes course titles, objectives, and topics that would be covered in a particular course or lesson. The arrangement of the content is determined by what learning domain is being affected; for example, influence attitudes or teach information (i.e., facts), or motor, cognitive (''thinking''), or perceptive skills.

In addition, based on the content, audience needs, and work-environment considerations, instructional methods and media are chosen.

Evaluation strategy: A description of how the success of the program and learner will be assessed. (For more detail, see Chapter 14.)

1. Objectives

Objectives are important to the success of an instructional program because they give the developers as well as the learners detail on what is important in the training. Objectives, if successfully attained, will help accomplish the goal or subgoal. Objectives describe outcomes, not the process used to achieve the outcome.

Objectives help developers select the best instructional content, decide how the content will be presented, determine if the instruction has been successful, and communicate to management and others about the course.

Learners use objectives to organize and focus their efforts on what is considered to be important in achieving the goal and as a standard to which the learners' performance can be compared (8).

Objectives are also useful in helping to determine what ''learning domains'' are to be taught; that is, whether the training involves information, attitudes or motor, intellectual (''cognitive''), or perceptive skills. This information will help determine the way the content of the training course is arranged.

A useful question to ask when creating or reviewing objectives comes from Mager (9): ''What should the student be able to do at the end of the course so that all that stands between the student and skilled performance is practice?''

A properly written objective usually has three parts: performance, conditions, and standards.

The performance is a behavioral description of what the learner should be able to do. It should be action-based as well as observable and measurable.

The important conditions under which the activity is to be performed should be included; for example, the type of software or hardware that the learner would use in performing the task.

The criterion (or ''standard'' or ''degree''), which may not always be included, gives the level or performance or quality that is expected of a successful performer. This could be in units per hour, allowable errors, and so on. The standard will be useful when assessing the performance of the learner (as discussed in the following chapter).

Some objective writers also define the audience in the objective; that is, who is to perform according to the description.

An example of an objective, with the three elements identified, is as follows:

> Using a Macintosh computer and a job aide (if desired) [CONDITIONS], the learner will be able to log on and log off to the corporate E-mail system [PERFORMANCE] without receiving an error message [CRITERION].

The source of information used in preparing objectives comes from the analysis phase and from the goal and subgoals.

Table 5 shows an example of the goal of a particular lesson and the objectives that relate to it.

A useful reference in preparing objectives is by Mager (9).

2. *Arranging the Instructional Content*

The organization of the information or instructional content affects how easily the information is learned. Studies have shown (10) that, based on the type of content (i.e., learning domain), there are preferred ways of arranging it.

Besides the sequence of the content, there are several other things that facilitate learning.

- Seeing the big picture. Learners should understand early on how they fit into the overall information system or automated process, including the concept of vendors and customers. This is especially important in infor-

Table 5 Example of the Relationship Between the Goal and Learning Objectives for a Lesson (Goal: Use an Internet Web Browser to Efficiently Gain Access to the Internet's World Wide Web)

Objective 1: List three situations when you would want to use a browser.
Objective 2: Describe what a browser does.
Objective 3: Using a computer running a Windows interface, connect into the corporate Internet server.
Objective 4: Using a computer running a Windows interface, start the NETSCAPE browser.
Objective 5: Given a specific Web site address (e.g., ''URL'' [http://www.cgmp.com]), connect the NETSCAPE browser to a particular URL.
Objective 6: Given a particular topic of interest and the URL of ''http://www.yahoo.com,'' find three different Web sites related to the topic and visit all the sites within ten minutes.
Objective 7: Using a job aide, disconnect from the Internet and return to the Windows file manager.

mation systems, in which many activities are distributed to various people and sites and can be ''invisible'' to people.

- ''What's in it for me?'' Why should the participants in the program want to learn the material? What is their incentive? What are the expectations once they have completed the course?
- Ramifications. What can happen if something isn't done properly? What are the immediate and long-term consequences?

3. Selecting the Instructional Methods

With the objectives and the content known and sequenced, the methods for presenting the information to the learner can be identified. For each method, there are several techniques that can be used.

Instructional media are the tools for delivering the instruction; the media are chosen after the appropriate methods and techniques have been identified.

Table 6 presents suggested instructional methods for different learning domains.

For a particular method, there is a variety of techniques that can be used. For example, ''telling'' a learner information could make use of lecture, presentation, or a panel discussion. Alternatively, the same material could be covered using a case study, a technique that more completely involves the learner.

Table 7 identifies various instructional methods and specific techniques.

If instructors, facilitators, or mentors are to be used, they should be identified, as least preliminarily. If this isn't done at this point, incorrect assumptions about instructor availability and qualifications could cause later problems and delays.

One of the most critical aspects of the design phase is selecting instructional

Table 6 Learning Domains and Suggested Instructional Methods

Learning domain	Suggested methods
Information	*Tell* information to the learner. *Show* information. Have learner *read* information. Have learner *practice* using the information.
Intellectual skills	
Identifying differences	*Demonstrate* the differences with various examples. If situational differences, *discuss* the differences. Have learners *practice* making the distinctions between examples.
Concepts, rules, principles	*Show* the concept, rule, principle. *Tell* the concept, etc. *Demonstrate* the concept, etc. Have learners *read* about the concept, etc. Have learners *practice* using the concept, etc.
Procedures	*Demonstrate* the procedure. *Show* the procedure being done. Have learners *read* the procedure. Have learners *practice* using the procedure.
Motor skills	*Demonstrate* the motor skill. *Simulate* the motor skill. *Show* the motor skill. Have learners *practice* the motor skill.
Attitudes	*Show* someone behaving with the proper attitude. *Discuss* attitudes and behavior. Have the learners *simulate* using the proper attitude.

Source: Training for the Healthcare Manufacturing Industries. James L. Vesper (1993). Used with permission by Interpharm Press.

methods and techniques so they meet the requirements of the learners. This is where one must consider the special needs of adult learners discussed above.

As much as possible, try to select instructional methods and techniques that involve multiple senses of the participants (e.g., hearing, seeing, touching). This promotes learning and retention. Also, have people be active participants in the learning process. Having the learners work on real-life problems will not only help convey the information, but reinforce the relevance of what they are learning.

Another consideration when selecting methods (and media) is to try to get as close as possible to how the information or skills will actually be used in the workplace. For example, if a forklift driver is expected to read and respond to a data display mounted on the forklift's control panel as he or she is driving the vehicle, at least part of the training efforts should be on a working or simulated

Table 7 Comparison of Instructional Methods

Instructional method	Examples of specific techniques	Senses stimulated	Active involvment of learner (relative)	Ways to optimize
		Vision **H**earing **T**actile **K**inesthetic **A**ffective		
Tell (live)	lecture presentation panel discussion	H, A	low	Increase audience involvement. Combine with visuals.
Sound	play a recording generate	H, A	low	Increase audience involvement. Combine with live action, visuals.
Show	words/symbols diagrams still images moving images models	V, A	low	Combine with live action. If topic involves motion/changes, using moving images. Combine written words, symbols with diagrams, images.
Read	textbooks self-study books checklists	V, A	medium	Combine with diagrams, images.

Discuss	question/answers group discussions case studies	H, V, A	high	Combine with live action, visuals written words.
Tutor	instructor/learner learner/learner technology/assisted	H, V, A	high	Use small-sized groups for maximum instruction. Combine with reading, visuals.
Demonstration	real life	H, V, (T?, K?)	medium	Use actual equipment/environment if possible.
Play/simulation	role playing games simulations case studies	H V, A, T, K	high	Combine with practice. Use actual equipment/environment if possible.
Practice	hands on practice with feedback case studies	H, V, T, K, A	high	Provide coaching.

Includes work of Allen (1967), Reiser and Gagné (1983), Romiszowski (1988).
Source: Training for the Healthcare Manufacturing Industries, James L. Vesper, (1993). Used with permission by Interpharm Press.

forklift. Doing this significantly improves the transfer of the learning from the training session to the workplace.

Selection of the methods must be learner-driven. Unfortunately, choices are frequently made by what is easiest for the instructor or systems developers. For instance, it is much easier, faster, and cheaper to simply present a lecture or give the users an instruction manual to read. Unfortunately, this does not make for effective learning that will be readily transferred back to the job.

4. Selecting the Appropriate Media

The content, instructional methods, and techniques are delivered to the learner using instructional media. Media can range from a ten-cent printed pamphlet to a $15 million computer-controlled simulator; in a given situation, either of those options could be the preferred one.

When it comes to selecting the instructional media, there are usually several solutions that can potentially be used. Some are definitely better than others; sometimes, from a strictly instructional standpoint, it doesn't really matter. Some media are more effective vehicles than others for delivering particular instructional methods. Also, depending on the audience factors (location, numbers of people, time available) and how frequently the course is to be delivered, some media are more cost-effective than others.

A well-designed instructional program will make use of different media in complementary ways. This creates a more interesting instructional environment and builds on the strengths of the various media used. For example, a scenario could be established with a brief videotaped segment and then the participants could discuss the approach they would take in addressing it.

When selecting potential instructional media, the initial consideration is its effectiveness in delivering the content. Then other factors, such as audience, instructor availability, and cost, are used to refine the selection.

Cost is one of the more important factors in selecting instructional media; however, both initial and longer-term costs must be considered. Showing a videotape the first time is its most expensive use; after that, the costs per use and per student decrease dramatically. This pattern holds true for other media with high development and production costs, such as multimedia technology or computer simulations.

On the other hand, courses using "live" instructors or content experts cost more over the life of the course. Instructor time, travel, and availability all present recurring costs. Also, scheduling and administrative costs for assembling groups of people with their time away from the job and traveling need to be considered. In most organizations, these are hidden costs that are rarely examined, yet they are definitely there.

Interactive multimedia instructional courses are being used more and more. They can be costly to initially produce, but when used properly, they can be more effective and efficient than leader-led programs and significantly reduce the overall costs of delivering the instruction (11–13).

Simulations are another powerful teaching tool. While games are, technically speaking, more of a pure fun way to learn something, simulations have a much stronger grounding in reality. They are extremely useful as a tool for learners to discover the best way to respond to a given situation because they see the outcomes very clearly. If the verb in the objective is similar to "respond," "react," "investigate," or "monitor," a simulation could be valuable to include. Simulations do not necessarily need to be elaborate. The closer to reality you can make it, the higher the level of transfer back to the job you can expect. However, by focusing on the learning objective in a creative way, you may be able to create a learning situation with high impact.

It may be possible to incorporate scenarios initially used in the testing and validation of an information system or piece of equipment into a simulation.

On-the-job training (OJT) is a vehicle for delivering instruction that has a high potential for hands-on involvement. Unfortunately, OJT sometimes has takes a more passive turn. When done improperly, the British nickname for OJT, "sitting next to Nellie," becomes descriptive; learners simply watch while the experts do the task.

OJT should include mentors who are willing and trained to provide guidance and coaching to the learner. Also, there should be objectives that serve as a guide to what is expected of the learner. Some firms use OJT outlines that provide the sequence that topics and tasks should be taught as well as questions that the mentor is to ask the learner so the learner understands the "why" as well as the "how-to."

With the increased use of electronic performance support (EPS) systems (14,15), there are now ways of giving learners "electronic coaching" while they are using an information system or automated piece of equipment. Well-designed EPS systems that have context-sensitive help or that include online demonstrations of how to perform certain tasks can reduce the initial training. Then, when people have particular needs, support is immediately available. Performance support systems, whether they be electronic or paper-based, must be considered in the context of how they will be used. If reaction time and response are critical—say, the initial, immediate response to a disaster—there may not be time to use them.

As the instructional methods, techniques, and delivery media are selected, try to use a mixture of approaches. A variety will not only keep the training more interesting and give the learner a richer perspective on the topic, but more of the individual learning styles that we have as adults will be touched.

5. *Plan the Evaluation Strategy*

The instructional plan should also include a section on how the success of the training program is to be measured. Success should be examined on several different levels—from the learner's point of view as well as from the organization's. Success should be defined, along with the type of support given to learners who do not initially succeed. Thoughtful consideration must also be given to those not capable of performing the new skills and tasks.

The topic of evaluation and assessment is a minefield of potential problems; federal and local labor laws, union contracts, Americans with Disabilities Act, company culture, and employee relations are all forces that must be considered.

In the United States, FDA investigators are beginning to ask firms for information on how successful their training programs are. The investigators would like to see test scores, performance checklists, or deviations related to inadequate training that provide evidence of the program's adequacy.

Several features of a program that would be defendable from various positions include the following:

- An assessment program based on objectives identified using a well-documented, accepted process
- A competency-based or mastery type of program in which all personnel need to perform to a given standard
- An organizational and management attitude of trying to help people succeed

Chapter 14 discusses assessment of learning in more detail.

6. *Approval*

There should be a formal approval process of the instructional plan before it is implemented. Management from all affected areas should review and sign off on it, indicating its agreement with how the plan will be executed in the development and implementation phases.

VI. DEVELOPING THE INSTRUCTIONAL PROGRAM

The instructional plan that was completed in the design phase is a blueprint that is followed in developing the instructional program and materials.

Tasks in the development phase include the following:

Prepare a detailed outline	Add more details to the content as needed.
Sketch or storyboard the visuals and other materials	Prepare rough models of the visuals. This is especially important if video or multimedia instructional technology is used.
Develop evaluation tools	Produce checklists, tests, questionnaires, and so on based on the evaluation strategy that was selected.

Produce the lessons, visuals, and other materials	Develop the detailed content, activities, materials, video, simulations, and so on according to the instructional plan.
Plan the implementation	Develop the logistical plan and schedule for the final course(s).
Prepare the instructor's manual	If a facilitator, instructor, or mentor is used, prepare the materials that will support his or her work. If a computer-based program is used, develop materials that will help key personnel monitor and assist in its use.
Conduct a pilot course	Present the course to a specially selected group of learners; obtain and use feedback to improve the course.

Developing and producing the actual course is a period of creativity and excitement, but also a point at which things can get out of control rather quickly, especially if the project is a large one. Missed deadlines can ripple through, delaying other parts of the development process. Changes to the actual system that people are being trained to operate or use can have significant ramifications to the instructional content.

An important element in a new technology project is the change management process. Changes that are "simple" from the software or equipment perspective may require changes or additions to the training curriculum. Any proposed change should include a review by training professionals.

The look and feel of the training materials, whether they are print-based, videotape, or interactive multimedia programs have an important role in how they are received. If the materials have a quality look about them, it will reinforce the importance and value of the program. If they are amateurish, poorly produced, or insulting to the user, people will get that message as well. People are all affected to some degree by aesthetics; use it to your advantage.

Defining styles, formats, and other expectations is important to do at the beginning of the development phase, particularly if an outside firm is being used to produce the materials. Templates and style guides will take time to develop, but, especially if the project is large, will save many hours later on. Also, having development standards will help achieve a consistent identity and "look" to the program.

During the development of the lessons and activities, it is also important to consider how the participants will emotionally respond. Using humor can be a way to break down barriers to learning and have people remember important points. Activities that include the opportunity for learners to feel frustration, impatience, and confusion can also be useful to reinforce certain messages, such as what can happen if something is done improperly. Don't be afraid to carefully tap the emotions of the learners.

Opportunities to practice can be useful to include in a training course. If they are to be used, integrate them into the lessons; several shorter practice sessions are more effective than one longer one.

Ideas, sample materials, activity instructions, and job aides should be reviewed and tried by a variety of people before being printed. If a simulation or other activity is used, simple, understandable instructions, along with the goal of the exercise, need to be clearly thought out and written.

Planning the implementation of the instructional program needs to be a broad-based effort. People should not be surprised that it is coming or have last-minute resistance to it. As mentioned in Chapter 4, information should be given in advance to prepare all people in the organization about the impending changes and the training that will accompany them.

An essential part of the development process is conducting a pilot program when the program is formally given to a selected group of people. This is similar to a ''beta'' test. A good design and the pretesting of the materials should give the pilot a high probability of success; however, it is not uncommon to modify 20 to 30 percent of the course. Therefore, when developing materials for the pilot, the possibility for change should be considered. Spending large amounts for printed materials, slides, or videotapes that are costly to change will cause management to take a ''we'll make due'' attitude.

The audience for the pilot should consist of the actual learners. Having management present can lead to changes that may not be justified from a user or instructional basis. If managers want to see the program, it is better if they act as observers while target audience members participate.

It is very useful to have a neutral observer watch the pilot and comment on non-content-related issues. One course developer always invites a psychologist to observe. During a recent pilot that was not going well, the psychologist identified part of the problem on the attitudes of the participants; they were extremely angry with organizational issues not related to the pilot course. This comment helped the developer to better understand the negative evaluations from the people attending the course.

For complex instructor-led or multimedia courses, subsequent pilot sessions may be needed to assess the modifications made.

When the course is ready to be used, it should be formally approved. Firms should have an SOP that describes how this is done and who approves the course. Some regulatory investigators expect that any course that has an impact on good manufacturing be approved by the quality unit (i.e., quality control or quality assurance).

VII. IMPLEMENTATION

With the courses approved for use, the implementation phase of the process can begin. The curriculum and implementation schedule developed in the design phase are the driving forces of this.

Implementation can include preparing the instructors who will be training people. Train-the-trainer workshops for classroom and OJT trainers are important. Frequently these individuals are certified that they can effectively teach by the course developers and other master trainers.

Record keeping plays an important role during implementation. First, creating a master file of the important documents, such as the instructional plan, detailed course outlines, instructor and learner materials, and approval sheets should be kept for future reference. These documents should be ''readily accessible'' in the event of a quality audit or regulatory inspection. Also, most validation protocols refer to these documents or even require that a copy of the training materials be kept with the validation records.

Another element of record keeping is tracking those who have attended the course(s). Information about the numbers of people needing to attend, attending, and completing the training program is useful for management as it provides resources and priority to the training efforts. Also, this information is expected by the FDA. (Further detail on this topic is found in Chapter 13.)

VIII. EVALUATION AND MAINTENANCE

As the instructional plan is executed and learners complete the various courses defined in the curriculum, feedback about the course and the learning that has taken place will be collected as described in the evaluation strategy of the instructional plan. This information can be used to improve the courses.

If classroom or OJT training methods are used, it is important to periodically monitor the work of the instructors to be sure they are delivering the course consistent with the way the course was designed and produced. In one particular situation, training was not effective because the OJT instructors were not following their instructor's guide.

Chapter 14 describes various evaluation and assessment tools.

Besides user comments and performance data, other factors that can affect the content of the program are operational and procedural changes to the system itself.

There must be a strong connection that links the organization's change management system to the area responsible for maintaining the training materials. Periodically, SOPs and training materials need to be formally reviewed against actual practice to see if ''drift'' has occurred. This can be most apparent in OJT, when personal practices and shortcuts can affect how people are performing the tasks on a daily basis.

IX. CONCLUSION

Because of the rapidly changing state of the art and competitive pressures, firms are investing more and more in technologically based solutions. In the pharmaceutical industry today more than ever before, the investments are being made prudently and carefully with an eye on both short- and longer-term costs and paybacks. A key element in acheiving the payback is providing workers with the information, education, and training they need to use the technological innovations safely and efficiently. Applying the instructional systems design methodology to produce instructional interventions will have a significant, positive impact on the organization and its people.

REFERENCES

1. Skills needed, *Wall St. J.*: 1 (Nov. 9, 1993).
2. R. L. Mager and P. Pipes, *Analyzing Performance Problems*, 2nd ed, Lake, Belmont, California, 1984.
3. D. M. Smith, Training—the other automation investment, *INTECH*: 32–35 (Dec. 1991).
4. D. M. Gayeske, L. E. Wood, and J. M. Ford, Getting inside an expert's brain, *Train. Dev. 46*(8): 55–62 (Aug. 1992).
5. J. M. Carroll and R. L. Mack, Learning to use a word processor: By doing, by thinking, and by knowing, *Human Factors in Computer Systems*, J. C. Thomas and M. L. Schneider (eds.), Ablex, Norwood, New Jersey, 1984.
6. M. S. Knowles, *The Making of an Adult Educator: An Autobiographical Journey*, Jossey-Bass, San Francisco, 1989.
7. C. Rogers, *Freedom to Learn*, Merrill, Columbus, Ohio, 1969.
8. W. Hannum and C. Hansen, *Instructional Systems Development in Large Corporations*, Educational Technology Publications, Englewood Cliffs, New Jersey, 1989.
9. R. F. Mager, *Preparing Instructional Objectives,* rev. 2nd ed., Lake, Belmont, California, 1984.
10. R. M. Gagné, *Principles of Instructional Design*, Holt, Rinehart, and Winston, New York, 1985.
11. G. L. Adams, Why interactive? *Multimed. Videodisc Mon.*: 20–25 (March 1992).
12. A. C. Kay, Computers, networks, and education, *Sci. Am. 265*(3): 138–148 (Sept. 1991).
13. *Interactive Multimedia: Return on Investment Analysis for Learning and Communication*, Macromedia, San Francisco, 1992.
14. G. J. Gery, *Electronic Performance Support Systems*, Weingarten, Boston, 1991.
15. C. Ladd, Should performance support be in your computer? *Train. Dev. 47*(8): 23–26 (Aug. 1993).

13

Documenting Education and Training

James L. Vesper

LearningPlus, Rochester, New York

I. INTRODUCTION

Once the training program has been implemented and people are becoming proficient in using the new technology, there is one more element that must be considered: documentation. Records of who needs to be trained, what courses people need to complete, and evidence that a person has completed a given course are necessary to answer business and regulatory questions.

From a business perspective, having records of training that is required and training that has been completed helps in personnel and workload scheduling.

Having a systematic method of tracking people through their training regime is consistent with good management practice and quality system expectations. Periodic reports to management on the status of the training activities can give them an impetus to realign resources as necessary.

Regulators such as the U.S. Food and Drug Administration (FDA) examine training records to determine if the firm has a rational training program and if people have the training, education, and experience necessary to perform their assigned tasks safely and effectively. Additionally, if training was prescribed to correct a deviation, investigators will want to see if the training took place and had the intended effect.

There are other regulatory and certification bodies that are interested in training records. These include such U.S. agencies as the Occupational Safety and Health Administration (OSHA), the Environmental Protection Agency (EPA), and the Nuclear Regulatory Commission (NRC). Also, certification bodies for the ISO9000 quality program expect a documented training program and related records. Firms that must comply with agency mandates should review current expectations.

For business decisions and regulatory investigations, records related to training must be *readily available*—a Current Good Manufacturing Practice (cGMP) regulatory term that can be subjectively interpreted. In practice, it means that if you need to know something (for business reasons or to answer an FDA question), you can get the information within fifteen to sixty minutes.

Having readily available records also means having the information arranged systematically. Some firms do this on paper; a small biotechnology company can tell a visitor within five minutes the training required for anyone in his or her organization. Other firms, large and small, are using personal or mainframe computers to manage their training data. Whether on paper or via electronic systems, firms need to have more than one person who can access the information when it is needed.

This chapter discusses the data that should be kept as part of a training program and some special considerations about using electronic data systems.

II. RECORDS THAT SHOULD BE AVAILABLE

Based upon current practices found in some of the better pharmaceutical firms and recent requests by U.S. FDA investigators, there are several different types of information that pharmaceutical and medical device firms are expected to have.

A. Training Program Records

1. Training Policy/Standard Operating Procedures

These documents define the organization's training program, as well as

- Who should be trained
- Who is trained on what
- Who develops courses
- Who reviews and approves the courses
- Who is responsible for assuring personnel attend courses as required

Periodic reviews (including what is examined, who performs them, and when they are done) of the training program and courses should also be described.

If a firm uses assessment (such as qualification and certification), this should be described as well as what happens if someone fails.

The period for retaining the various training records should be described in the training Standard Operating Procedure (SOP) or refer to the appropriate records retention SOP.

Some organizations have a corporate procedure written in general terms, with each department having its own specific SOPs that apply.

Since the training program SOP is GMP-related, it should be approved by the firm's quality unit (e.g., QA [Quality Assurance]) prior to implementation.

2. *Course Outlines and Approvals*

Detailed outlines about the content and instructional methods used should be kept for reference. These can assist course developers in the future and provide a baseline of what information was covered. Records showing that the course material was reviewed and approved by content experts and management should also be retained.

3. *Needs Analysis Information*

Documents related to the needs analysis should be kept for future reference and to show the rationale for decisions made related to course content.

4. *Course Review and Change Control Records*

If changes are made in the source content information, there should be a formal examination to determine if the changes have any impact on the training program. Not all changes require that people be retrained. Sometimes, simply informing the affected personnel is adequate. Other times, training and assessment should be done. Firms should evaluate the change and determine the appropriate action(s) to take; this should be documented.

B. Job-training Requirements

1. *Curriculum*

The curriculum is the learning plan for a particular job position or set of similar positions. It would include the following:

- The training course titles required for the position
- The recommended sequence
- The time frames (if any) for completion

2. *Qualification/Certification Requirements*

If there are certain assessment requirements that result in qualification or certification for a position, they should be described.

3. *Equivalence*

If there are other courses, events, or experiences that would substitute for courses listed in the curriculum, the approach to be used for substituting them should be described. For example, a firm may allow its personnel to attend either internally offered courses or courses available through an outside, professional association covering the same objectives.

C. Documentation of Participation

1. Attendee Signature List

This is the most typical training record firms have to show that someone attended a course on a given day. Usually this consists of

- The course title and number (if any)
- Duration of the course
- Date
- Instructor name and signature
- Participant name, ID number, and signature

Obviously, the signature list only documents those attesting that they have attended the course; it says nothing about what was learned by the participants.

The method for collecting such information, such as a standardized form, should be described in an SOP. The SOP should authorize the instructor to ''invalidate'' an attendee; for example, if the attendee leaves early or arrives only for a moment in order to sign in.

2. Retention of Lists

There is a variety of ways that firms use and retain the paper-based attendance lists. Some firms make copies of the list and place one in the training folder of each attendee; the original is placed in a central training file. Other firms note in the employee's file that he or she attended a course on a particular date; the signature is kept in a central file of courses arranged chronologically. Whatever is done must be according to the SOP that describes the practice.

3. Transcription of Attendance Lists

Some firms transcribe information from attendance lists into a database. This process should be described by an SOP and include a verification step. What happens to the original sign-in sheet varies; some firms formally discard it after the entry has been verified, but most firms retain it in some form, including the archives, in microform, or as a scanned electronic image. Since FDA investigators take various positions on the retention of the original paper, this might be something to discuss with local regulatory authorities.

D. Attendance at Outside Programs and Conferences

Externally offered programs at a vendor, training organization, or conference can provide personnel with useful information that contributes to the person's performance on the job. These events should be documented. This can be handled in a variety of ways, such as a copy of the program's outline and a certificate of attendance or a trip report filed in the person's training file. Many electronic systems have the capability of recording externally offered programs.

E. Assessment Results

If any assessment data are collected that can be related to an individual, special care must be taken to ensure that they are properly used. If there is any possibility that the data might be used in a way that would affect a person's salary, rating, or position, the assessment program could face additional scrutiny.

It is highly recommended that when assessment results are retained, they be kept separate from other personnel information and be accessible only to authorized personnel.

Retention of assessment data should be described by an SOP. It should be available to answer questions such as the following:

- How do you know your training program is effective?
- How do you know that a particular person is qualified to perform a task?
- How do you know that a particular person is performing a task as required?

III. METHODS OF RECORD KEEPING

Pharmaceutical companies use a variety of paper-based and electronic methods for keeping training-related documentation. Current GMP regulations have no specific requirements of how to keep records; each firm must address the issue in a way that makes sense to it. Clearly, however, there is a role for both paper-based and electronic record-keeping methods.

A. Paper-Based Records

Certain documents, such as training course outlines and needs assessments, will be most easily kept on paper. Having files or notebooks for each course containing the course outline, approvals, periodic reviews, and so forth is an effective way of keeping the information together. Some firms keep an electronic copy (e.g., a diskette) archived along with the other materials.

For participation records, one paper-based method was described earlier; whatever is done needs to meet the readily available requirement.

B. Computer-Based Record-Keeping Systems

More and more firms have a significant part of their training records stored electronically because of the amount of data that must be kept as well as the advantages of being able to get a variety of reports for trainers, staff, and management.

Electronic systems that are being used are a variety of home-grown, customized, and off-the-shelf software packages. Depending on the number of personnel to be tracked, how the training database relates to other electronic sources of information, and how many people/sites need access, electronic systems could be Macintosh or PC-based, perhaps in a client-server relationship. Application programs such as FILEMAKER or Microsoft ACCESS, or database applications such as D-BASE4 could be used to develop them.

1. *Building Your Own Record-Keeping System*

Many firms initially consider building their own system, because, at least for general record-keeping purposes, and in concept, it isn't that complicated. Difficulties occur, however, when users want their internally built system to have the same performance and capabilities that packaged systems have, such as scheduling or sending out announcements. Another potential problem that some firms have is that their own systems do not have the control, security, and documentation that is needed. At least one company has learned the lesson the hard way; the programmer left after ''finishing'' the program, and maintenance fell to someone else who didn't understand some of the ''clever,'' undocumented features the initial programmer had included into the system.

Building a system should be considered, but both the initial and long-term costs must be weighed when making the decision.

2. *Packaged Programs*

There are a growing number of record-keeping packages that independent developers are marketing to the pharmaceutical and medical device industries. The applications packages run the spectrum of very simple to highly complex. When looking for a packaged program for tracking training, there are some particular points to consider, including the following:

- Connections to current company databases. Usually firms have employee databases with names, job titles, departments, and so on that are needed for training record-keeping systems. The packaged program should be able to read or share this information.
- Updating personnel information. Does this need to happen manually or can it be done on a scheduled, automated basis?
- Use on networks. Some record-keeping systems are incompatible with the local area networks some firms use.
- Change control. Does the vendor of the system practice change control that will simplify upgrades and fixes?
- Validation. Not all developers understand and practice validation as expected in the pharmaceutical industry. Some training record-keeping system developers think of validation only in the sense of fixing problems

observed during beta testing. Firms should ask to see the validation protocols and acceptance reports.

- Determine who will ''feed'' and maintain the system. Some firms have one or two people in a central area who enter training records into their system, while others have the function decentralized into all departments.
- Training required to use and operate the system. Some record-keeping systems have much steeper learning curves than others, making decentralization of data entry more difficult.
- Consider alternative data entry methods. If computer-based training is used, some systems will accept information sent directly from the PC. Also, dataloggers that work with worker ID cards may be an alternate way of having data enter the system.
- Use in administration. The more complicated systems have the capability of scheduling rooms, sending out E-mail messages, generating certificates, and so forth. Would you be using these capabilities if they were available?

3. *Validation of Training Record Systems*

A frequently asked question is, ''Do we need to validate our system?'' (whether purchased or internally developed). The short answer is yes.

A longer answer is, Why would you want to entrust valuable business and regulatory information to a system without documented and proven storage, backup, security, and processing capabilities? From business and regulatory points of view, validation is something that proves that the system works, that there is a plan for backups and change control, that there is adequate security, and that there is written documentation describing the design and operation of the software. Also, the validation would include a protocol that describes the testing to be conducted, specifies the acceptance criteria, and provides the results. It is important for the organization to keep the data, shouldn't there be some evidence that the data will be input and maintained in a way that assures their integrity? A carefully planned and executed validation should do this.

IV. CONCLUSION

Having readily available documentation and records of employee training is the finishing piece in a systematic strategy for training personnel. Such a system doesn't need to be overly complex or costly; it does need to meet the requirements of the organization and the expecations of regulatory inspectors. If a record-keeping system is well thought out and meets organizational needs, chances are it will also be found satisfactory by regulatory agencies as well.

14

Evaluation and Certification

James L. Vesper

LearningPlus, Rochester, New York

I. INTRODUCTION

One of the essential differences between instruction and other forms of communication is that instruction includes a mechanism to determine if the student is learning.

A classroom instructor informally assesses learner comprehension by asking questions and looking for signs of confusion and boredom on the faces of the students. More formally, tests or activities are used to measure learning.

There is also a difference between evaluation used in the traditional academic world and that used by business. In school, students are evaluated to see if they have a minimal (i.e., ''passing'') score to allow the student to proceed to the next level. Schools also rank the individual to others (the ''curve'') or to a fixed scale (an *A* is 93–100; a *B* is 85–92, etc.). In industry, however, the intent of assessment is usually to qualify a person for a particular assignment, predict how well the learner will perform in a job, or determine if the learner ''transferred'' the learning to the job.

Management more than ever before, wants evidence that the training program in which it is investing is making a difference (1). This is yet another type of effectiveness evaluation.

This chapter examines the broader picture of measuring the effectiveness of training and the ''certification'' of people who have been trained.

II. TYPES OF EVALUATIONS

There is a variety of reasons why an organization evaluates training, such as the following:

- To measure how well an audience likes a particular training course
- To assess what a participant has learned
- To determine if the learner has transferred what was learned back to the job
- To determine the level of proficiency that a person has doing a particular skill
- To evaluate the impact that training has on the department or organization
- To determine the improvements needed in both the courses and the overall training program

A. Four Levels of Evaluations

An approach for evaluating training that is widely used in industry was initially developed by Kirkpatrick (2). This model includes four levels of evaluations:

- Level I—trainee reaction
- Level II—trainee learning
- Level III—trainee performance
- Level IV—business results

The levels are not exclusive; each provides a different perspective on the instructional efforts.

Not all levels are used for every lesson, course, or training intervention. Because of the time and costs involved, some firms only do level III evaluations in situations in which performance is critical. Other firms choose to initiate level IV evaluations on programs that are widely used throughout the organization.

B. Level I: Trainee Reaction

This is the most common form of evaluation that is done, because it is the simplest. Usually a questionnaire is provided to participants to collect comments and reactions to the course they just completed. The data that come from a level I evaluation is useful in determining how satisfied the learners were with the instructional experience. Instructors and course developers use this information to refine a course; training managers use the data to evaluate learner reaction to particular instructors or instructional methods.

Level I evaluations are sometimes dismissed as ''smile sheets'' because they are frequently designed to elicit positive comments from the learners about the course. When they are provided for this purpose, they have no real benefit.

When using a level I evaluation, ask questions that will help improve the course, its content, and the way it is delivered. Questions concerning the pace, the emphasis on particular topics, any comparison to other courses, and the instructor's delivery are valuable. In addition, ask fill-in questions such as the following:

- What did you like most about the course?
- What did you like least about the course?
- What information did you receive that you will use immediately in your job?
- What other topics should have been included?

Level I evaluations are usually done at the end of a course, although sometimes a slightly different version is also given several weeks after the course when the learners have returned to their jobs.

C. Level II: Trainee Learning

Multiple choice, essay, computer simulations, and immediate demonstrations of performance are examples of level II evaluations. The goal is to see what the participants have learned during the course. This can be done with pen-and-paper tests or by having the person perform the task or skill he or she has learned. Level II evaluations are also used to predict how well someone will transfer the learning back to the job.

Selecting the level II method to best assess what the trainee learned depends upon the "learning domain" of what was taught. The domain should be evident from the objective that was written in the design phase. There are several different domains.

- Information (e.g., listing the specifications for a high-purity water system)
- Intellectual skills (e.g., developing a new validation protocol)
- Motor skills (e.g., assembling a piece of equipment)
- Attitudes (e.g., behaving in a certain way in a given situation)

Some types of tests are preferred over others for a given learning domain, as discussed below.

To make a valid prediction of transfer, the testing situation should be as close as possible to how the person will actually use what has been learned.

For information domains, multiple choice, short answer, essay, or oral tests are appropriate. The goal is for the person to write or tell what he or she has learned. Some of the tests listed above are more difficult than others. For instance, we all remember from school that it is (usually) easier to recognize a definition from a list than to have to write one in a blank space. This reflects several different levels of "knowing" something. Simple recall of facts is on the lowest level, while arranging and ordering facts is on a higher level. Higher yet is applying knowledge to analyze a situation and solve problems.

For intellectual skills, multiple choice, short answer, essay, or oral tests work, as well as simulations or demonstrations of performance. An example of this is having the learner write a short computer program.

Motor skills are best evaluated by demonstrations of performance or simulations. Written tests should *not* be used because they do not examine all of the skill aspects. For example, a learner may be able to match the characters to the correct keys on a keyboard, but that says nothing about the person's typing skills. Checklists and trained observers are useful in gathering consistent information.

Attitudes are harder to evaluate. Short answer, essay, oral, or anecdotal methods (e.g., when facing a situation, I would . . .) can be used.

Level II testing is done at the end of the training session. In special cases, such as when determining retention, testing is repeated weeks or months later.

D. Level III: Trainee Performance

"But are they using what they have learned back on their job?" is the question that level III assessment answers. This is a more complicated type of evaluation, because there are other factors besides training that contribute to a person's using what he or she learned.

Quality auditors and regulatory inspectors in essence conduct a level III assessment when they do inspections. They determine, by observing activities and examining documents, if people are performing their jobs according to standard operating procedures (SOPs) and good manufacturing practice (GMP).

Methods of assessing trainee performance include direct observation (such as watching a lab analyst enter data into a laboratory information management [LIMS] system), and interviews with supervisors (e.g., anecdotal information about the delivery of raw materials from an automated warehouse).

Performance on the job also can be used to rate how well a person performs. Performance indicators, such as errors per hundred keystrokes, time required to solve a "standard" problem, and so forth can be used to differentiate levels of the performers.

From the examples mentioned above, it is obvious that there is a variety of other factors that can influence performance. When there is a failure of performance in the workplace, these factors, as shown in Fig. 1, must be carefully examined before placing the blame on ineffective training.

A level III evaluation is best made three to six months after the training has been completed (3).

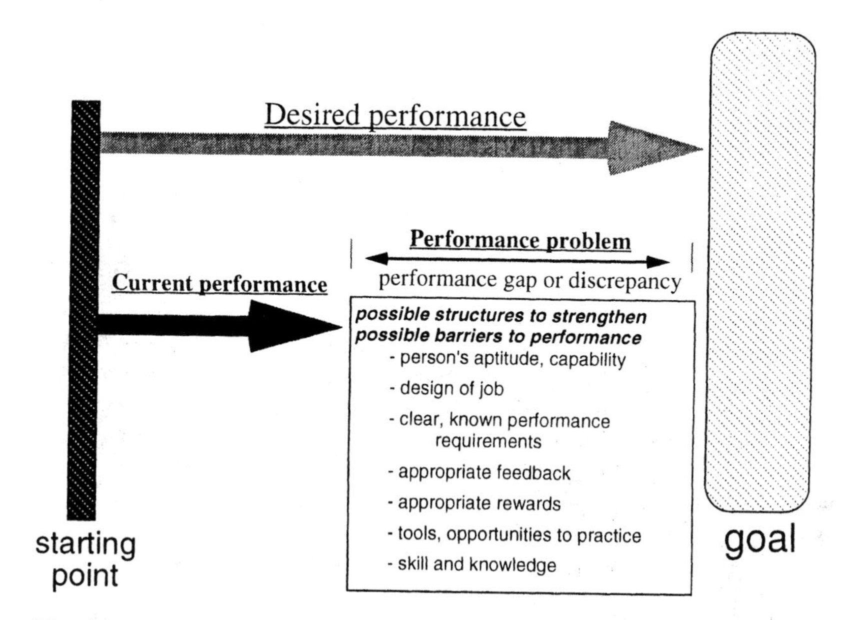

Fig. 1 Model that categorizes types of performance problems.

E. Level IV: Organizational Results

One of the claims typically made regarding worker training and education is that it is an "investment" in people that will benefit the organization. A level IV assessment is used to determine what, if any, the benefits are to the organization.

A level IV evaluation looks at indicators that are important to the organization. Examples related to new information systems might include the following:

- The length of time required for documents (SOPs, specifications, etc.) to be generated, approved, and distributed
- The number of out-of-date SOPs found at workstations
- The average time to process a lot
- Work-in-process
- The number of deviations in a given period of time
- Inventory levels required to fill orders at a 95 percent service level

As was seen in level III evaluations, there are a number of factors besides training that will influence the results. If less-than-expected results are seen, a thorough performance analysis should be conducted to determine the cause. Level IV evaluations do not give proof that the training was effective; rather, they give evidence.

III. DEVELOPING AN EVALUATION STRATEGY

During the design phase (discussed in Chapter 12) an instructional plan is prepared that includes a description of the evaluation strategy. A comprehensive strategy would use a combination of the levels mentioned above.

One critical decision that must be made concerns the assessment of people after they complete training. Many of the questions touch on organizational and human resources philosophies and practices of the firm. For firms in which assessment is new, these issues must be thoughtfully addressed.

For example, what does worker assessment really mean? Will it affect the pay or promotion of the individual? If so, the evaluation tools must be carefully developed with someone who has expertise in testing and labor law. The tests must be valid (i.e., the test questions must reflect the learning objectives they were meant to measure) and reliable (i.e., provide consistent and accurate information about the knowledge or performance being evaluated [4]). Failure to do this can put a firm at risk for litigation from individuals and labor unions (if present).

Another organizational consideration would be what happens if the learner fails an evaluation. Will the person be removed from the job or could the person continue to work but be paired with a person who has passed the evaluation? What would a regulatory official say if upon reviewing the training records he or she determines that a person who has failed the training is working on a critical task?

There may be situations in which the person cannot perform the required tasks because he or she does not have the skills or ability to do so. In these cases, there must be a process of working with the person to preserve his or her individual dignity no matter how the situation is resolved.

Still another question is, What is ''success?'' What is a passing score? Some firms require that an individual complete a test with 70 or 80 percent of the possible answers correct. Others require mastery, or 100 percent correct responses.

In some situations, using a percentage scale is fine; for instance, related to general knowledge and facts. However, at other times, everyone should be performing a task identically. This is important in a GMP setting, in which people are required to follow SOPs as written. Technically, if someone does not follow a procedure exactly, they have caused a ''deviation'' that is to be documented and investigated. Current GMP regulations do not accept 80 percent compliance; therefore, when it comes to skills and tasks, evaluating for mastery is the most defendable position. (Note: if certain alternate pathways are permitted, the SOP should be written to allow for them.)

In mastery or competancy-based programs, training, mentoring, practice, and coaching are used so the learner is able to demonstrate that he or she has mastered the particular skill or task. This is usually seen in jobs that involve a high degree of motor skill, such as operations, maintenance and crafts, and analytical chemists. However, there is no reason why people who use perception or intellectual skills cannot be included as well.

Defining mastery in a particular situation is based on the objectives that were written in the design phase.

IV. CONDUCTING A LEVEL I EVALUATION

Questionnaires are typically used to collect comments from participants of a training course. These can be one- or two-page paper documents or electronic forms at the end of a computer-based training application.

During the piloting or first several uses of a particular course, the evaluation may be longer (three to five pages) in order to collect more data that will be used to fine-tune the instruction. As the course becomes more refined, condensing the form to a simpler version is desirable.

Learners should be told at the beginning of a course that they will be asked for their comments. Building time into the end of the course will improve the quality of the comments. Some organizations require the participants to exchange their completed evaluation form for the individual's certificate of completing the course.

Evaluation questions should be developed with a purpose. What information are you expecting to receive? How will the response be used?

Experience has shown that giving participants a form to fill out and return after the session results in a very poor response rate.

Table 1 is an example of a one-page evaluation form.

V. CONDUCTING A LEVEL II OR III EVALUATION

A key to the success of both level II and level III evaluations is the quality of the objectives that were developed during the design phase. Objectives need to be behaviorally based; that is, learners need to do something (the PERFORMANCE) that can be observed and evaluated. Additionally, the objective usually includes the CONDITIONS and CRITERION (or standard) used to determine if the person has performed to the desired level. The better written the objectives are, the easier it will be to do a level II or III evaluation.

A useful tool that can be used if performance is being examined in either a

Table 1 Workshop Evaluation Sheet: Basics of Computer Validation

Your feedback and comments play an important role in helping the instructors meet your needs for high quality instruction. We would appreciate your taking a few minutes to evaluate the workshop, the instructors and the materials.

For each of the statements below, use the following scale. Rate each statement according to your level of agreement by circling the appropriate response. Use the back of the sheet for additional comments.

SD	D	N	A	SA
Strongly Disagree	**Disagree**	**Neutral**	**Agree**	**Strongly Agree**

SD	**D**	**N**	**A**	**SA**	1. This workshop was a useful way for me to learn basic information about computer validation.
SD	**D**	**N**	**A**	**SA**	2. The sections in the workshop were well organized and presented in a logical manner.
SD	**D**	**N**	**A**	**SA**	3. The pace of the instruction was about right for me.
SD	**D**	**N**	**A**	**SA**	4. As near as I can tell, the content of the workshop was technically accurate and complete.
SD	**D**	**N**	**A**	**SA**	5. The workshop covered the aspects of the subject that were most important to me.
SD	**D**	**N**	**A**	**SA**	6. The workshop contained information I can take and apply back at my job.
SD	**D**	**N**	**A**	**SA**	7. I felt the instructor had knowledge, expertise, and competence in the field.
SD	**D**	**N**	**A**	**SA**	8. I would recommend this workshop to others.
SD	**D**	**N**	**A**	**SA**	9. This workshop met my expectations.
SD	**D**	**N**	**A**	**SA**	10. I feel I have learned enough to begin applying the concepts and tools covered by the materials in my job.

Additional Comments

1. TWO things I am going to take back and apply to my work are:
2. Overall, I would rate this workshop as (please circle your response below):

   excellent good ok fair poor

3. Compared to other training programs and workshops I have attended, I would rate this as (please circle your response below):

   excellent good ok fair poor

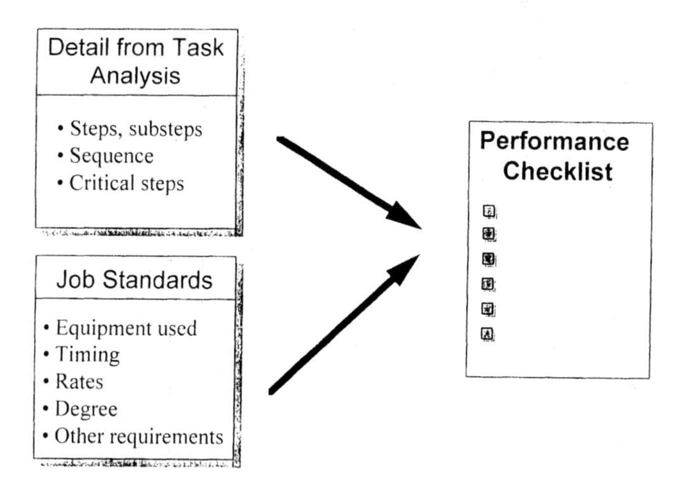

Fig. 2 Information used in preparing performance checklists.

level II or level III evaluation is a performance checklist. Checklists reduce the subjectivity as well as standardize what is examined. They can cover a particular task as defined by one or more SOPs or by a task analysis. Checklists may also include other performance requirements or expectations, such as general GMP compliance or departmental documentation standards that performers must do. Figure 2 shows the general process for developing a performance checklist; Table 2 is an example of a checklist.

Checklists should be completed by the observer concurrently while watching the performance.

In some industries, a frequently used type of performance assessment involves looking at the final product the person produces, for instance, whether or not a video monitor displays the proper image. In the pharmaceutical and medical device industry, performance assessment needs to include the *process* used to produce the object or information. This reflects the GMP concept that *how* something is done (i.e., the process) is just as important as the product. (This type of assessment is also commonly done when the object itself obscures what the person did, such as welding the interior of a pipe.)

Several other elements are needed besides a performance checklist when assessing performance. There should be a procedure identifying who conducts the assessment as well as the qualifications necessary for the observer. Providing training and qualifying the observer is especially important in maintaining consistency if there is more than one observer.

Qualifying the observer would include some basic training in the use of the checklist, its organizational and legal ramifications, and then a practice session.

Table 2 Performance Checklist

Task: **Using Basic Internet World Wide Web Resources** Associate: ____________

Control No. 36341 Rev: 3.2 (10.23.95) Badge No.: ____________

Yes	No	Rev	Comment	Expected Performance	General Requirements
☐	☐	☐		1. User connects to the corporate Internet server. • clicks open CONNECTION icon • clicks INTERNET icon	• Any pc using Windows.
☐	☐	☐		2. User starts NETSCAPE browser. • if NETSCAPE not automatically invoked, user clicks on NETSCAPE icon	• If user-induced error occurs, user can properly respond without personal assistance and continue.
☐	☐	☐		3. User connects NETSCAPE browser to a specific WWW address (URL). • moves cursor to input location • types in URL (e.g., http://www.cgmp.com) • connection is made	• If lockup or unexpected event occurs, user can recover and continue. • Time limit to complete checklist: 15 minutes.
☐	☐	☐		4. User connects browser to: **http://www.yahoo.com** and finds 3 sites related to a particular topic.	
☐	☐	☐		5. User connects to 3 URLs by either: • writing down URL for later connection or • connecting to website using links	

☐	☐	☐	6. User can travel back and forth between sites using command icons.
☐	☐	☐	7. User exits NETSCAPE and returns to Window's File Manager window. • uses exit command from NETSCAPE pulldown menu • closes connection using exit command from INTERNET pulldown menu • clicks open File Manager menu

NOTE: any task not successfully completed should be marked NO and commented upon. When the topic is reviewed with the performer with the REV box checked and dated. Whether to begin another assessment at a later date or continue with the current assessment is after a failure is at the discretion of the certifier.

The performer successfully accomplished the task in the manner described above and in accordance with all of the general requirements.

Performer's signature, date

Certifier's signature, date

Table 3 Terms and Suggested Definitions Related to Training and Evaluation

Trainee or learner	A person who is participating in a training course or program.
‘‘Qualified’’	A person who has the documented educational background, experience, and training and has demonstrated that he or she can perform a task or skill at the conclusion of a training program or in a controlled setting.
‘‘Firm-certified’’	A person who has been evaluated and shown to be performing a skill or task according to a standad on the job. The person certifying the performer states that the performer meets the performance standards at the time of the certification.
‘‘Board-certified’’	A person who has been evaluated by an organziation outside the firm and meets its criteria.

Here, a small group of observers would watch (live or on videotape) a person performing a task. The observers then compare their completed checklists and focus on differences that each perceived, trying to arrive at a consensus. This should be repeated using several checklists and different tasks until there is confidence that all observers would arrive at the same conclusions. If new people are trained at a later date, a previous qualifer should be part of the group to maintain consistency.

There is no universal (or GMP) definition of what to call people who have been evaluated at the different levels, however useful it may be for the firm. Whatever definitions are used should be consistent with the firm’s policies and practices. Table 3 provides several terms and examples of how to define them.

Having qualified employees who have demonstrated in a controlled setting that they can meet the objectives has several benefits to the firm. It provides evidence—and confidence—that the person should be able to

- Perform the task or activity safely, without endangering him- or herself, co-workers, the community, the environment, or the equipment and facility
- Perform the task or activity consistently
- Perform the task or activity to standards that will allow optimal operation of the system
- Perform the task or activity in accordance with applicable company policies and procedures
- Perform according to the expectations of regulatory agencies, such as the FDA
- Produce objects and information that meet the requirements

In addition, having been qualified and ''checked out'' in a safe setting will give the performer added confidence that he or she can do the job. This reduces anxiety on the part of the individual.

In a similar way, having personnel assessed and certified that they are performing on the job according to the appropriate standards can give the firm additional benefits, such as confidence that

- The training has been transferred to the work environment
- The information system, SOPs, work instructions, and so on are being used as intended
- In the event of a regulatory inspection or quality audit, people will be doing their jobs properly
- Items needed to support the performance are in place and working
- The products (e.g., drug products, information) are being made properly

Can a person be certified without first being qualified? Who can enter data into a LIMS system, someone who is qualified or only someone certified? This would be defined in an SOP.

A very fast way that can put a firm out of compliance is by writing tight, aggressive SOPs for training and certification that it cannot live with. Best intentions need to be tempered with reasonableness and reality.

VI. IMPLEMENTING A QUALIFICATION OR CERTIFICATION PROGRAM

In Chapter 4 we mentioned the anxieties that implementing a new technology or information system can cause to those who will be using it. Anxieties also occur when starting or expanding a qualification/certification program. Many of us had the same fears when we went to get tested for a driver's license. Will we pass the written test? What if the inspector administering the test doesn't like us? What if we can't parallel park on the first try? How will we explain to our friends at school that we failed? What if . . . ?

An essential element for a qualification/certification program is communication with personnel who need to feel comfortable that it is going to be done fairly and that all possible efforts will be made to help them succeed. The program must truly be a ''win–win'' venture for both the firm and the people.

As in other training, people need to see ''what's in it for me''; that is, what benefits they will get from being qualified and/or certified. A well-developed system should include a combination of benefits.

Some firms are now using a compensation system in which people are paid in part for what they know and what they can do. The thinking is that the more skills and tasks the person can competently perform, the more valuable he or she is to the organization and the higher his or her pay should be.

Beyond pay incentives, there is a variety of other creative ways to answer the what's in it for me question. Some of possibilities depend on the culture of the organization and the workforce. A key point to remember is that not all people are driven by the same reward systems.

- *Recognition*—publicly acknowledging that someone has attained a certain level. This can be done with photographs on a bulletin board, stickers on the employee's badge, or special baseball caps.
- *Visibility with senior management*—having a coffee break or lunch with a respected member of management.
- *Special outings or gatherings*—attending a special conference or getting together with other peers for a lunch.
- *Status*—being among the first to use a new piece of equipment or the beta version of a program and providing comments that will be used to improve it.
- *Potential mobility*—understanding that the training and experiences make them more valuable in the firm (or industry) should they ever want to change positions.

VII. CONDUCTING A LEVEL IV EVALUATION

Objectives were critical in evaluating the learners; specific, measurable *goals* are essential in assessing the effectiveness of the training program to the organization.

For a new technology or system, education and training are used to support its implementation. When education and training is not done (or not properly done) for a system that requires it, the system could fail or will not be optimally used; the system will not have the expected payback. One measure, then, to the organization is the success of the new system. Is it meeting the realistic expectations used to justify it?

(This points to the situation that sometimes happens when systems and technologies are ''sold'' with expectations that are not realistic. Failure to meet the unrealistic goals should not be shouldered by those using the system.)

Evaluating organization results not only require a specific identification of what is to be assessed, but also an initial baseline assessment that is made before the changes are implemented. These ''before'' results will be compared to results some months ''after'' the change.

Another level IV approach is to examine two similar groups at the same time. For example, if a firm has two identical sites and is installing a manufacturing execution system at one of them, it may be able to use the other site as the baseline.

VII. CONCLUSION

For the evaluation of the training efforts to be most successful, it should be done from a point of view aimed at continual improvement—improvement of the training programs, the learners, and jobs, and the organization itself. If assessment is positioned and actually carried out in this spirit, people will respond positively and the training investment will pay back substantial dividends.

REFERENCES

1. B. Geber, Does your training make a difference? *Training*: 27–34 March 1995.
2. D. L. Kirkpatrick, *Evaluating Training Programs: The Four Levels*, Derrett-Koehler, San Francisco; 1994.
3. D. G. Robinson and J. Robinson, *Training for Impact*, Jossey–Bass, San Francisco; 1989.
4. E. A. Davidove and P. A. Schroeder, Demonstrating the ROI of training, *Train. Dev.* **46** (8):70–71 (1992).

15

GMP Regulations and Computer Validation

Teri Stokes

GXP International, Acton, Massachusetts

I. INTRODUCTION

This chapter discusses the key ideas found in good practice regulations from various world authorities and looks to describe a common perspective on good practice for computerized systems. The use of computerized systems in drug manufacturing has become a way of life today. Computers not only control the process and product flow, they also control the data flow and often the work flow of the whole manufacturing organization.

Regulators recognized the importance of the shift of production control from manual operations to automated activities in the early 1980s. In February 1983 the U.S. Food and Drug Administration (FDA) responded to this trend with the publication of a guide for its inspectors titled *Guide to Inspection of Computerized Systems in Drug Processing* (1). This document became known by the color of its cover—the "blue book"—and continues to be used by inspectors today.

By the early 1990s other authorities and the FDA itself began to elaborate on computer system compliance with various annexes and appendices to good manufacturing practice (GMP) directives. In November 1990 the FDA published an inspector guide that applied the medical device GMPs to computerized devices and manufacturing processes (2). In January 1992 the European Commission published its guide to GMP which included an annex 11 on computerized systems (3), and in April 1993 the Japanese Ministry of Health & Welfare, the Koseisho, began enforcing its "Guideline on Control of Computerized Systems in Drug Manufacturing" (4).

Parallel to all the GMP focus on computer systems, various authorities published good laboratory practice (GLP) guidance for computer systems in the laboratory. While GLP has a strict application to animal testing facilities, quality control laboratories at production sites can find useful information in such directives to support general good practice for laboratory computer systems.

One of the most recent and most useful GLP computer directives is a joint effort by Europe, North America, and Japan as part of the Organization for Economic Cooperation and Development (OECD). The OECD GLP consensus for computerized systems (5) was published in 1995 and provides guidance in a number of areas. It gives clear, concise descriptions of the validation roles and responsibilities of laboratory personnel, including management. It also provides a list of ten mandatory standard operating procedures (SOPs) for computerized systems.

All of these regulatory documents have content that can be categorized within the following three themes:

- Management control
- System reliability
- Auditable quality

It is from the perspective of these three themes that we now examine the international directives for computerized systems in GMP-regulated environments. This chapter uses the term computerized system to include a software application and its platform system composed of the hardware, operating system, software tools, database, and network components required for the software application to function as intended. It uses the term electronic device for input/output (I/O) systems of limited function such as bar code readers and individual programmable logic controllers (PLCs).

II. THE BLUE BOOK (FDA 1983)

A. Management Control

The blue book was the first attempt by any regulatory authority to provide guidance to its inspectors about computer use in drug manufacturing. It was written at a time during which most people who were not computer professionals had little understanding of computer technology and the personal computer revolution had not yet reached the home market. The FDA used this document to bring its investigators into the new world of computerized production. The document provided a basic tutorial on the types of hardware and software found in manufacturing facilities, the general approach to the validation of hardware and software, and a glossary of common terms.

With this document, the FDA recognized the increasing use of computers by the pharmaceutical industry and wanted its investigators to identify and check "those computer controlled processes which are most critical to drug product quality" (1, p. 1). The blue book suggested starting with a broad overview of all the systems used in order to determine exactly what processes and functions were under computer control and had automated monitoring alarms. For each significant computerized system, it suggested a close review of the hardware and software.

The blue book advises inspectors to look for evidence of management control of both hardware and software systems used in the production process. It expects a firm to be able to produce documents that show an overview of all the hardware and software systems used in the production of a drug and to be able to identify those systems that are most critical to product quality. For the critical systems, full validation documentation is expected to be available for review to support the claim that the systems function as intended in the drug manufacturing process.

The document requires management control in the form of written and approved SOPs. A careful reading of the blue book shows that the topics listed in Fig. 1 are expected to be addressed by SOPs.

Management is expected to assess the quality of its system suppliers and to maintain some record of a supplier's quality testing of systems prior to purchase. Vendor certification of a system is not enough, and the FDA expects management to perform its own validation activities on systems in their final production environment.

1. Definition of the operational limits for critical systems
2. Defined process for accepting hardware and software systems
3. Documented testing practices
4. Maintenance procedures for hardware and software systems
5. Revalidation procedures for ongoing conditions and change situations
6. Security practices for protecting system programs and data
7. Performance of system overrides and manual overrides for computer-controlled processes
8. Documented change control mechanism for changes in equipment, software, and the exercise of manual or system initiated process control overrides
9. Backup operations for systems and data records
10. Alarm response procedures for correcting production problems
11. Manual production operations to be followed in case of system shutdown
12. Recovery from unplanned system shutdown

Fig. 1 U.S. FDA blue book: SOP topics.

B. System Reliability

1. Hardware Systems

The blue book goes into some detail to explain to investigators the types of hardware and software that might be encountered in production facilities, and it gives examples of the types of situations in which such hardware and software could have an impact on product quality. With the advance of computerized systems since 1983, some of the blue book examples may seem simplistic today, but they do provide a basic tutorial on how to go about thinking of the impact of automation and system reliability on product quality.

The types of hardware discussed include input devices (thermocouples, flow meter, load cells, pH meters, pressure gauges, control panels, and operator keyboards), output devices [valves, switches, motors, solenoids, cathode ray tubes (CRTs), printers, and alarms], signal converters (analog to digital, digital to analog), the central processing unit (CPU), peripheral devices (CRTs, printers, keyboards, disk drives, modems, and tape drives), and distributed systems, including networks.

Five key points for potential risk to hardware system reliability are presented. These are location, signal conversion, I/O device operation, command overrides, and maintenance. The first point discusses the location of CPUs and peripheral devices and identifies three potential problems due to location. A warning is given to avoid the following:

1. Environmental extremes of temperature, humidity, static, dust, power feed line voltage fluctuations, and electromagnetic interference
2. Excessive distances between the CPU and peripheral devices, where electromagnetic interference from electrical power lines, motors, or fluorescent lighting fixtures could occur
3. Input devices that are out of visual range of the drug-processing equipment so that operator acceptance might be low

The second point expresses the importance of proper analog/digital signal conversion to prevent interface problems. The third point stresses the system's need for accuracy in the performance of I/O devices and the need to have sensors systematically calibrated and checked for accurate signal outputs.

The fourth point talks about distributed systems and the importance of knowing how errors and command overrides at one computer are related to operations at another computer in the system. The blue book cautions that the limits on information and command flow within a distributed system should be clearly established by the drug firm. The sophistication of today's integrated distributed control systems (DCSs) makes charting such flows an enormous challenge. When validation of the system has not been built into the original design of the DCS, it can become an impossible task to fully document and validate systems with multiple levels of feedback loops.

The last key point discussed in the blue book for hardware systems' reliability is the need for an SOP on maintenance. It advises firms to use diagnostic software, to keep spare parts available, and to restrict system access to qualified service personnel for implementing the system maintenance program.

2. *Software Systems*

The blue book advises inspectors to identify critical computer programs used by the firm: "Of particular importance are those programs which control and document dosage form production and laboratory testing" (1, p. 8). For key programs, the items shown in Fig. 2 are expected to be identified.

The blue book discusses two key points for consideration with software systems—development and security. For software development, it advises inspectors to determine whether the software was "purchased as 'canned' from outside vendors, developed within the firm, prepared on a customized basis by a software producer, or some combination of these sources" (1, p. 10). Inspectors seek documented evidence that the acceptance process for the software provides full assurance that programs with complex algorithms that control or monitor a significant process will perform as intended. For programs developed by the drug firm itself, the blue book suggests that an examination of the source code may even be performed.

1. Program Language: high level language or application name.
2. Program Name: name associated with function of the software, e.g., production initiation, batch history transfer, alarms.
3. Function: what is the purpose of the program.
4. Input: inputs to the program, such as thermocouple signals, timer, or analytical test results.
5. Output: what outputs the program generates, e.g., mechanical action (valve actuation) or recorded data (generation of batch records).
6. Fixed Setpoint: the desired value of a process variable which cannot be changed by the operator during execution.
7. Variable Setpoint: the desired value of a process variable which may change from run to run and must usually be entered by the operator.
8. Edits: program written to reject or alter certain input or output information which does not conform to some pre-determined criteria or does not fall within certain pre-established limits.
9. Input Manipulation: how the program is set up to handle input data.
10. Program Over-rides: when an operator can override a sequence of program events or program edits.

Fig. 2 U.S. FDA blue book: software identification—descriptive elements.

For software security, inspectors are advised to ''determine how a firm prevents unauthorized program changes and how data are secure from alteration, inadvertent erasures, or loss'' (1, p. 10). An SOP for systems security is expected to cover both access to and change control privileges for software programs, data records, and storage devices such as tapes, disks, and magnetic strip cards. The use of keys, firmware, and magnetic cards is discussed as possible types of security measures to be reviewed for operator procedures and tamper potential.

3. Computerized Operations

The interaction and coordination of the many systems working together in computerized operations adds a new dimension to assuring system reliability in drug manufacturing. Alarm-activating problems in one part of a production control system may trigger the shutdown procedure for a system in another part of the process. Integration of human activities around alarm situations and shutdown/recovery procedures need to be defined and documented in order to avoid confusion and assure product quality is controlled. The blue book spells out FDA concerns for the following seven areas of computerized operations:

- Networks
- Manual backup systems
- Input/output checks
- Process documentation
- Monitoring of computerized operations
- Alarms
- Shutdown recovery

It advises that network security measures should be established and external companies interacting on the network should be identified. The types and locations of production I/O activities performed across network systems should be understood, and remote monitoring and controlling activities need to be documented. The use of networks has increased dramatically since 1983 and is often dynamic, with systems coming on- and off-line frequently. Today the use of automated network mapping techniques may be needed to keep up to date with network topology for mid-sized to large companies.

Inspectors are advised to determine to what degree company personnel monitor computerized operations, which functions are monitored, and how often. During an inspection, the blue book advises them to spot-check such computerized items as the following:

- *Calculations*—for alternate method verification
- *Input recording*—for sensor versus computer indications
- *Component quarantine control*—for actual warehouse location versus batch data

- *Timekeeping*—for clock accuracy in real-time control
- *Automated cleaning in place*—for assuring adequacy of cleaning and residue elimination
- *Tailings accountability*—for what limits, if any, the firm places on residual material (tailings) carried over between batches in continuous processing

The goal is to keep in as much control of product quality during computerized operations as during manual production. Human monitoring and intervention should be prescribed by SOP and documented at the time of action.

C. Auditable Quality

The ability to audit quality is based on providing documented evidence for actions planned and actions taken. Without a written plan, procedure, log, or report, an inspector has no objective way to give credit to a company for its computer validation activities. For hardware systems the blue book makes the following statement:

> The suitability of computer hardware for the tasks assigned to pharmaceutical production must be demonstrated through appropriate tests and challenges . . . The validation program need not be elaborate but should be sufficient to support a high degree of confidence that the system will consistently do what it is supposed to do (1, p. 6).

In order to inspect for confidence in hardware systems the FDA advises its inspectors to consider several questions.

1. Does the capacity of the hardware match its assigned function?
2. Have operational limits been identified and considered in establishing production procedures?
3. Have test conditions simulated "worst-case" production conditions?
4. Have hardware tests been repeated enough times to assure a reasonable measure of reproducibility and consistency?
5. Has the validation program been thoroughly documented?
6. Are systems in place to initiate revalidation when significant changes are made?

While much hardware validation can be performed by the computer vendor, the ultimate responsibility for suitability of equipment used in drug processing rests with the pharmaceutical manufacturer, according to the FDA.

When looking at the validation of software, the blue book comments that "It is vital that a firm have assurance that computer programs, especially those that control manufacturing processing, will consistently perform as they are supposed to within preestablished operational limits" (1, p. 1). Inspector review questions for checking software include the following:

1. Does the program match the assigned operational function?
2. Have test conditions simulated worst-case production limits?
3. Have tests been repeated enough times to assure consistent, reliable results?
4. Has the software validation been thoroughly documented?
5. Are systems in place to initiate revalidation when program changes are made?

While software vendors do much testing of their software, the ultimate responsibility for program suitability rests with the pharmaceutical manufacturer.

In general, for both hardware and software the blue book recommends that three separate test runs covering different operating conditions be performed to demonstrate consistent, repeatable performance. Validation documentation should include a validation protocol and test results that are specific and meaningful in relation to the attribute being tested. The individuals who reviewed and approved the validation should be identified in the documentation.

III. ANNEX 11 OF EU GMP GUIDE (1992)

A. Management Control

While the 1983 blue book has nineteen pages of inspector guidance followed by five pages of glossary, the 1993 European Union (EU) GMP guide annex 11 has nineteen paragraphs of directives to pharmaceutical companies. It is a concise discussion of all the key points from the blue book in a format that is suitable for reading by senior management without requiring technical terminology to explain the concepts. Annex 11 can build a bridge of understanding about computer validation between computer systems management and production management and computer systems management and senior management.

The EU GMP guide holds senior management responsible for ensuring that a medicinal product is manufactured so that it is fit for its intended use and does not place patients at risk due to inadequate safety, efficacy, or quality. Annex 11 of the guide makes it clear that introducing computerized systems into systems of manufacturing, including storage, distribution, and quality control, does not change the need to fulfill all other EU GMP regulators. A strong system of quality control under a comprehensive program of quality assurance is expected to apply to computerized systems as well as to other aspects of GMP production. The basic principle of annex 11 is stated as follows:

> Where a computerized system replaces a manual operation, there should be no resultant decrease in product quality or quality assurance (3, p. 139).

The blue book made no mention of life cycles, but annex 11 describes validation as being part of the complete life cycle of a computer system. It then describes the cycle as including the stages of planning, specification, programming, testing, commissioning, documentation, operation, monitoring, and modifying. Life cycle management for an operational system is a common theme with the Japanese GMP computer guideline, the FDA device GMP, and the OECD GLP consensus, to be discussed later.

Annex 11 is more specific than the blue book in assigning end user management with validation responsibilities for computerized operations. It discusses the need for training end user managers who have computerized systems operating within their areas of responsibility and states that ''it is essential that there is the closest cooperation between key personnel and those involved with computer systems'' (3, p. 139). It places responsibility on the user of software to take all reasonable steps to ensure that the software has been developed in accordance with a system of quality assurance. It is production management that has the final annex 11 responsibility for GMP compliance of software used, not computer systems management.

When management decides to outsource a computer service, annex 11 requires that a formal agreement be prepared to specify the responsibilities of the outside agency. It references Chapter 7 of the guide, which defines roles and responsibilities for the contract giver and the contract acceptor and discusses key elements to be included in the contract itself. Although this chapter is written to cover contract manufacture and analysis, its advice can easily be adapted to apply to computerized systems (3, pp. 59–61).

B. System Reliability

Sixteen of the nineteen paragraphs in annex 11 focus on system reliability. It considers a computerized system to be both hardware and software, and thus its use of the word *system* refers to the total package of hardware and software working together to perform an operation in the production environment. Annex 11 requires that a written detailed description of the system be made and kept up to date. It prescribes that the description should include the principles, objectives, security measures, and scope of the system, the main features used, and how it interacts with other systems and procedures.

A new element in annex 11 is an explicit request that the system include built-in checks of the correct entry and processing of data wherever appropriate. It also suggests the use of systems that record failed attempts at entry as well as other identification and security measures for authorizing system use, data access, data edits, and system changes. When critical data are entered manually, it says there should be a second check on the accuracy of the record made either by a second operator or by validated electronic means. It further recommends use of an ''audit trail'' function to record the identity of individuals entering, confirming, or making changes to critical data.

Annex 11 requires a change control procedure for alterations to a hardware system or to a computer program. It expects this defined procedure to provide for validating, checking, approving, and implementing the change. It cautions that the changes should only be implemented with the agreement of the person responsible for the relevant part of the system, e.g., end user of the function, and that the alteration should be recorded. Every significant modification should be validated and checked for its potential impact on stored data.

As with the blue book, annex 11 expects auditors to be able to get clear printed copies of electronically stored data for quality assurance checking purposes. Annex 11 is more specific, however, in its statement that data should be checked for accessibility, durability, and accuracy at a frequency appropriate to the storage medium used and that it should be secured by physical or electronic means against willful or accidental damage. At this point annex 11 references 4.9 of the guide, which advises that batch records electronically stored should be protected by backup transfer to magnetic tape, microfilm, paper, or other means (3, p. 34).

In addition to backing up data at regular intervals, annex 11 discusses making alternative arrangements for backup systems in cases in which operations need to continue in case of a system breakdown. As with the blue book, annex 11 requires a breakdown recovery procedure to be defined and then it goes further by requesting that the recovery procedure be validated or exercised so that it is proven to be adequate. It also states that a procedure should be established to record and analyze errors to enable corrective action to be taken. Monitoring trends in errors can provide diagnostic information before a breakdown occurs to support preventive maintenance activities.

C. Auditable Quality

For a system to be auditable to annex 11 standards, there must be some documented evidence for validation activities in each of the life cycle phases mentioned. Although the annex 11 text does not prescribe a list of recommended documents, experience has shown that auditors and inspectors usually look for the types of documents shown in Fig. 3 to support system life cycle activities.

Although annex 11 mentions retrospective as well as prospective validation, it is very clear about the need for prospective validation of new systems. In paragraph 7 it states, ''Before a system using a computer is brought into use, it should be thoroughly tested and confirmed as being capable of achieving the desired results. If a manual system is being replaced, the two should be run in parallel for a time, as part of this testing and validation'' (3, p. 140).

Both the blue book and annex 11 share the common goal of seeking validation evidence to show that computerized systems operate as intended to achieve the desired results. The blue book is a tutorial for inspectors and annex 11 is a guide for manufacturers, but the concise format of the annex makes it a useful tool for building awareness for validation concerns in senior management. The numbered structure of the nineteen paragraphs makes annex 11 a useful benchmark for auditors to use and an outline format for organizing and reporting their review of computer validation activities.

System Life Cycle	Documented Evidence
1. Planning	- user requirements, supplier proposal
2. Specification	- requirements specification, design description
3. Programming	- documented source code, programming standards, audit reports
4. Testing	- test plan, test scripts, testing logs, test summary report
5. Commissioning	- acceptance criteria, validation plan, validation report
6. Documentation	- system descriptions for hardware and software, user manuals
7. Operation	- training program, experience records, system and department SOPs, company policy
8. Monitoring	- maintenance logs, operations logs
9. Modifying revalidation	- change control procedure, change logs, testing records

Fig. 3 EU GMP guide annex 11: system life cycle and documented evidence.

IV. JAPANESE GMP GUIDELINE (1993)

A. Management Control

Ten years after the publication of the blue book, in April 1993, the Ministry of Health and Welfare (the Koseisho) in Japan activated its eleven-page ''Guideline to the Control of Computerized Systems in Drug Manufacturing.'' It is designed to provide guidance for the development and use of computer systems in process control, production control, and quality control, which ensure proper implementation of drug GMP and other regulations in drug manufacturing plants. The guideline specifies the following systems as being included within its scope:

- Systems for manufacturing process control and management, including recording batch data
- Systems for production control, such as storage and inventory of starting materials, intermediates, and final products
- Systems for documentation of manufacturing directions, testing protocols, or records
- Systems for quality control and recording of quality control (QC) data

The Japanese document is particularly interesting in that it also states which systems are outside the scope of its directives. Small, embedded systems with limited function and prescribed parameter settings are exempted from the guideline's directives. In addition, all systems already developed or under development as of April 1, 1993, are exempted from the guideline.

Another feature of the document is that almost every paragraph begins with words assigning responsibility to people in management. They start with ''the manufacturer shall,'' ''the manager shall,'' or ''the person in charge shall.'' The guideline's sections on system development, operation control, and documentation are all written with a focus on the responsibilities of management for the quality of computerized systems.

B. System Reliability

1. Development of the System

The largest part of the guideline is devoted to system development, and it begins by directing the manufacturer to designate an overall manager and person or persons in charge for each major step of development, from system design through to acceptance testing. It then prescribes a fully documented procedure for developing systems. For the design of hardware and software systems, the important controlling documents are listed in Fig. 4.

The guideline places considerable emphasis on system performance testing, and states that even for systems developed by outside suppliers, this type of testing ''shall be directly supervised, evaluated, and accordingly approved by the responsible person designated by the manufacturer concerned'' (4, section 3.6). It also describes suggested evaluation criteria for such testing, as follows:

- *Function*: Does it match provisions in the system engineering document?
- *Capability*: Is there an Assurance of system response as designed in the system engineering document?
- *Reliability*: Does the recovery function work properly?
- *Operation*: Is there appropriate operation of terminal devices, etc.?

2. System Installation

The guideline requires the preparation of an installation plan that describes a documented process for installation and testing of hardware and an operation test plan for the software program. The operation test plan includes all testing performed under practical production conditions for the evaluation of production and control performance to specifications. The use of external contractors is allowed, but as with performance testing, operation testing must be supervised, evaluated, and approved by a responsible person designated by the pharmaceutical manufacturer.

3. Operation Control

Ongoing support of systems after installation is a key concern for the Japanese guideline, and again it begins this section with having the manufacturer assign an overall manager who specifies the duties of another person or persons in charge

1. System Development Manual
   - with engineering standards, documentation standards, design change control procedures, exit criteria for each phase of the development process

2. Development Schedule
   - with development objectives, time schedule, staffing resources, selection criteria and equipment plan for hardware

3. System Engineering Document
   - with hardware composition, outline of system functions, tabulation of input/output data, file structure outline, countermeasures against system shutdown, security control functions, and title or name of the manager and person/s in charge. (This document to be prepared in compliance with the System Development Manual.)

4. Program Specification
   - with details of input/output data, data processing, and title or name of manager and person/s in charge. (This document to be prepared in compliance with the System Development Manual.)

5. Trial Test Plan for the Program
   - with test methods, a provision for test records, and evaluation criteria of test results. The Manager shall evaluate results of the trial test and thereafter approve it.

6. System Performance Test Plan
   - to confirm the system performance in compliance with its design specifications in non-production conditions this plan includes testing conditions, check items and test data to be used, test methods, test records, problem logs, evaluation criteria for results, testing schedule, and assignment of tasks during testing. The Manager evaluates and approves results.

Fig. 4 Koseisho GMP guideline: systems development control documents.

of specific operation steps. Then considerable detail is given for developing SOPs to address the topics shown in Fig. 5.

4. Documentation

The guideline requires management to store and maintain the documents and records developed for systems operating under its directives either as paper printouts or in electronic form. If electronic means are employed, a backup copy for documents and records is to be kept and their authenticity checked by the manager.

- Operation of Hardware and Software to SOPs and Training of Personnel
- Daily Inspection and Periodic Maintenance of Hardware and Software
- Accident Prevention, Alarms and Accident Recovery Measures
    - ⇒ System halt conditions and organization in case of accidents
    - ⇒ Procedures for recovery, cause finding studies and future prevention
    - ⇒ Evaluation of product impact from system accidents
    - ⇒ Procedures for necessary manual backup systems
    - ⇒ Training for backup manual systems
- Security Control for both physical and logical access to systems and data
    - ⇒ Control of passwords and identification codes
    - ⇒ Assigned privileges to enter, modify or delete data
    - ⇒ Limited access to hardware
    - ⇒ Backup copies of programs and data
- Change Control for System Alterations and Testing of System after Change
- Self Inspection and Monitoring Records

Fig. 5 Koseisho GMP guidelines: SOP topics.

Documents and records relevant to system development are to be retained for three years after the date that the system is taken off-line. Records relevant to system operation are to be retained for three years from the date of recording.

C. Auditable Quality

The Japanese GMP guideline provides for a thorough documentation trail from system development through installation and up to three years after retirement of the system. Such a trail gives inspectors and auditors a clear view of the history and performance of computerized systems, and the points of required management approval show exactly where responsibility has been designated for assuring GMP compliance. Auditing a system that complies with the Japanese GMP guideline should be very straightforward, as there will be a lot of documented evidence for system quality.

Like the EU annex 11, the Japanese GMP guideline is addressed to drug firms and not to inspectors. It is longer and more technically focused than the EU annex 11, and constantly refers to management's role in the compliance process. The Japanese GMP guideline discusses system development in much more detail than either annex 11 or the blue book. Its directives cover all phases of a system's life cycle without specifically naming any of the life cycle phases the way that annex 11 does.

All three documents stress security measures and backup/recovery procedures for both systems and data. They all emphasize the need for testing systems prior to production use and after significant modifications have been made to the software or hardware. The Japanese guideline, however, is the most specific in describing documented testing procedures across the various stages of development, installation, acceptance, operation, and maintenance of both hardware and software.

V. COMPUTERIZED MEDICAL DEVICE GMP (FDA 1990)

A. Management Control

Once more writing to instruct inspectors, the FDA published a draft document in November 1990 titled "Application of the Medical Device GMPs to Computerized Devices and Manufacturing Processes" (2). This document applies to medical device manufacturers who use automated systems for manufacturing, quality assurance, and/or record keeping. It also applies to firms making medical devices that are driven or controlled by software. The value of this document for general pharmaceutical manufacturers lies in its various discussions of ways and means to ensure system quality and its confirmation of key points from the blue book, EU annex 11, and the Japanese guideline.

The strongest and most constant theme of the computerized device GMP is the basic concept of documented evidence for management's total control of critical hardware and software. It expects management to ensure adequate quality assurance controls so that hardware and software systems perform as intended to produce safe and effective final product. The document expects management to have written policies and procedures that define roles, responsibilities, and actions to be taken for ensuring that GMP requirements are implemented and maintained for critical hardware and software components at supplier sites as well as inside the device manufacturer's own premises.

In order to maintain control, a written contract with well-defined specifications must be prepared for software and/or hardware purchased from external suppliers. This directive has its echo in paragraph 17 of the EU annex 11 for required formal agreements with outside computer service agencies. In the device GMP, the contract must also include provision for the ongoing monitoring of the supplier's quality assurance practices and their quality control records during the development of software and hardware. Methods for assessing the quality and acceptability of component software prior to production of the final device must also be documented (6, section 4.2).

Another area of management responsibility shared with the blue book, annex 11, and the Japanese guideline is that of personnel training, and the device GMP particularly discusses requirements for software developers. It states that individuals responsible for producing and evaluating software must have the necessary education, training, and experience to assure that software is properly prepared and maintained. They must know how to develop the software and how to properly test the program to minimize with an adequate degree of confidence the effect of latent faults. Individuals responsible for duplicating software and handling magnetic storage media (e.g., floppy disks, tapes, and Programmable Read Only Memory (PROM) chips), must also be trained to understand and follow the procedures and controls necessary to assure that software incorporated into the final medical device is not adversely affected and performs as intended (6, section 4.3).

B. System Reliability

1. Environmental Control

Section 4.4 of the computerized device GMP discusses environmental concerns whereby conditions could have an adverse impact on a device's fitness for use. It discusses in some detail the control of temperature, humidity, electrostatic discharge (ESD), dust, dirt, and electromagnetic interference (EMI) to protect hardware and software from erratic performance problems or permanent loss or damage. The degree of environmental control desired is to be determined by the device manufacturer. Specifications are then developed for the environment and maintained in the device master record, and a control system is implemented to assure that environmental specifications are not exceeded. Environmental control is periodically inspected for proper functioning, and the inspections are documented.

2. Software and Hardware Control

When software is a part of the final product, precautions must be taken to be sure that a master copy of the approved version is kept safely archived. Working master copies of the software must be periodically challenged and compared against the archived master to be sure that the working copy of the released version is a true copy of the master. Various utilities and approaches are available to do this checking, including check-sum calculations, directory comparisons, and printouts of code differences. Control of software revisions and updates should also be covered in a written maintenance procedure.

To establish confidence in the adequacy of computerized equipment, the hardware is calibrated and the software is challenged and validated to assure fitness for intended use. The computerized device GMP goes into considerable detail to discuss calibration and acceptance procedures for computerized measurement equipment and component acceptance and handling for computerized devices. Of general interest is its discussion of the following:

> Calibration of computer hardware is similar to calibration of any other electromechanical system. The sensor's measurement of temperature, voltage,

resistance, etc., is compared against the measurement of a known standard traceable to the National Institute of Standards and Technology or other acceptable standard. An important part of the calibration activity is to assure that measurements are properly transmitted across computer communication lines and properly interpreted by the computer system. Verification of properly transmitted measurements is accomplished by comparing the measured value that has been input into the computer system with the value of the traceable standards (6, section 4.6).

The document goes on to advise that an SOP should be written for handling modifications to hardware or system configuration, which may require system recalibration. It also states that software programs must be validated for automated production or quality assurance (QA) systems. For a discussion of verification and validation of software, the computerized GMP refers the reader to the FDA's reference manual titled *Software Development Activities* (7).

C. Auditable Quality

Readers who are familiar with the types of rigorous controls required for manufacturing medicinal products will find the remaining sections (4.9–4.16) of the computerized device GMP to provide a parallel process of documented control for the production, labeling, quality assurance, master record, history record, and complaint files of computerized devices. The paper trail for a computerized medical device must be in place, and must be just as accurate as the paper trail for a tablet or liquid medicinal product. Similarly, documented evidence for the quality of computerized systems used to produce the device must also be ready for review and audit.

For pharmaceutical manufacturers in general, section 4.9 of the computerized device GMP provides a concise discussion of some of the key points of the blue book. It discusses process validation and process control, as shown in Fig. 6 (2, section 4.9).

The computerized device GMP is quite consistent with the blue book, EU annex 11, and the Japanese GMP guideline in seeking to make critical hardware and software systems auditable. For further clarification, the list of definitions at the end of the document includes the following items:

- *Validation.* Establishing documented evidence that provides a high degree of assurance that a specific process will consistently produce a product meeting its predetermined specifications and quality attributes.
- *Verification.* The process of reviewing, inspecting, testing, checking, auditing, or otherwise establishing and documenting whether or not items, processes, services, or documents conform to specified requirements.
- *Worst Case.* A set of conditions encompassing upper and lower processing limits and circumstances, including those within SOPs, which

"When a manufacturing process is automated, the computerized system is validated to assure it performs as intended. In validating computerized equipment, parameters that the system is designed to measure, record, and/or control are evaluated by an independent method until it is demonstrated that the computer system will function properly in its intended environment.

When a manufacturing process is controlled by computer, functional evaluation of the control system may include, but is not limited to, the following activities:

- equipment (peripherals, etc.) and sensor checks using known inputs, which may consist of processing test or simulated data;
- alarm checks at, within, and beyond their operational limits; and,
- evaluation of operator override mechanisms for how they are used by operators and how they are documented.

In case of system failure, evaluations would include:

- how data is updated when in manual operation;
- what happens to data 'in process' when the system shuts down;
- what procedures are in place to handle shutdown; and,
- how product or information handled by the computerized process is affected."

Fig. 6 FDA device GMP: computerized process validation and process control.

pose the greatest chance of process or product failure when compared to ideal conditions. Such conditions do not necessarily induce product or process failure.

VI. OECD GLP Consensus (1995)

A. Management Control

The last regulatory document to be analyzed here is the most recent in this group and has been produced as a joint effort by the OECD, which includes Europe, North America, and Japan. Its focus is the application of GLP principles to all computerized systems used for the generation, measurement, or assessment of laboratory data intended for regulatory submission. When applying this definition to quality control laboratories, one could categorize the laboratory data as data that are intended for proving to authorities the safety, efficacy, and quality of manufactured product.

The approach presented by the GLP consensus document has three major themes that by now can be seen as consistent themes across all the GMP documents as well. Computerized systems are to be

- *Suitable for purpose*: Computerized systems should be of appropriate design, adequate capacity, and suitable for their intended purposes.
- *Controlled and maintained*: There should be appropriate procedures to control and maintain these systems, and the systems should be developed, validated, and operated in a way that is compliant to GLP principles.
- *Validated prior to use*: The demonstration that a computerized system is suitable for its intended purpose is of fundamental importance and is referred to as computer validation. The validation process provides a high degree of assurance that a computerized system meets its predetermined specifications. Validation should be undertaken by means of a formal validation plan and performed prior to operational use (5, p. 4).

The first section of the GLP consensus document defines responsibilities for management, study directors, personnel, and quality assurance. Its description of the responsibilities for management provides a concise review of the management concepts given in the blue book, EU annex 11, Japanese guideline, and device GMP. (See Fig. 7; 5, p. 5).

While all the other regulatory documents talked about management devel-

"1. Responsibilities

a) Management of a test facility has the overall responsibility for compliance with the GLP Principles. This responsibility includes the appointment and effective organization of an adequate number of appropriately qualified and experienced staff, as well as the obligation to ensure that the facilities, equipment and data handling procedures are of an adequate standard.
Management is responsible for ensuring that computerized systems are suitable for their intended purposes. It should establish computing policies and procedures to ensure that systems are developed, validated, operated, and maintained in accordance with the GLP Principles. Management should also ensure that these policies and procedures are understood and followed, and ensure that effective monitoring of such requirements occurs.
Management should also designate personnel with specific responsibility for the development, validation, operation, and maintenance of computerized systems. Such personnel should be suitably qualified, with relevant experience and appropriate training to perform their duties in accordance with GLP Principles."

Fig. 7 OECD GLP consensus: management responsibilities for computerized systems.

oping policies, the OECD GLP consensus has the most explicit listing of the policy areas that should be covered. It expects written management policies to address the whole life cycle of computerized systems (e.g. the acquisition, requirements, design, validation, testing, installation, operation, maintenance, staffing, control, auditing, monitoring, and retirement of computerized systems; 5, p. 12).

B. System Reliability

The consensus document defines a computerized system as ''a group of hardware components and associated software designed and assembled to perform a specific function or group of functions'' (5, p. 7). It is as specific as the device GMP in discussing environmental issues for systems such as extremes of temperature and humidity, dust, electromagnetic interference, proximity to high-voltage cables, and the need for reliable power supply. Documented maintenance activities and disaster recovery procedures are other consensus priorities shared across all regulations.

In its section on security, the OECD consensus requires documented measures for the following:

- *Physical security*: Restricting physical access to hardware, peripheral, and communications equipment and storage media
- *Logical security*: Preventing unauthorized access to computerized systems, applications, and data
- *Data integrity*: Training all personnel in system procedures for data security and using system features to support security and data integrity (e.g., access failure rates, file verification routines, and exception reporting)
- *Backup*: Making backup copies of all software and data to allow for recovery from such system failures as disk corruption

In the validation section of the consensus document, the goal is stated that ''Computerized systems must be suitable for their intended purpose'' (5, p. 11). In discussing ways and means to ensure suitability, the OECD consensus considers four major topics—system acceptance, retrospective evaluation, change control, and system support.

System acceptance: For new systems, the OECD consensus looks for all the same acceptance activities as the Japanese GMP guideline. The system is to be developed in a preplanned, documented, and controlled manner and preferably to recognized technical standards. The system is to have formal testing and acceptance prior to use and all documentation is to be retained.

Retrospective evaluation: For systems currently in use, the OECD consensus expects suitability to be assessed by retrospective evaluation. The first step in retrospective evaluation is to gather all historical records related to the computerized system. After reviewing the records, a written summary is produced. This summary should specify what validation evidence is available and what needs to be done in the future to ensure validation of the computerized system.

Change control: Change control procedures need to be in place to protect the system's validation status and to ensure data integrity. Once a computerized system is operational, responsible persons need to be identified to assess the extent of changes to the system and the need for revalidation activities and to approve the documentation associated with the change and retesting.

System support: Once a system has been validated and put into operational use, the OECD consensus recommends that support mechanisms be put in place to ensure that it is functioning and being used correctly. These may periodically involve system management, training, maintenance, technical support, auditing, and/or performance assessment to ensure meeting stated performance criteria (e.g., reliability, responsiveness, and capacity).

Procedures for:

1. Operation of computerized systems (hardware/software), and the responsibilities of personnel involved.
2. Security measures used to detect and prevent unauthorized access and program changes.
3. Authorization for program changes and the recording of changes.
4. Authorization for changes to equipment (hardware/software) including testing before use if appropriate.
5. Periodic testing for correct functioning of the complete system or its component parts and the recording of these tests.
6. Maintenance of computerized systems and any associated equipment.
7. Software development and acceptance testing and the recording of all acceptance testing.
8. Backup of all stored data and contingency plans in the event of a breakdown.
9. Archiving and retrieval of all documents, software, and computer data.
10. Monitoring and auditing of computerized systems.

Fig. 8 OECD GLP consensus: basic set of SOPs.

C. Auditable Quality

Section 8 of the OECD GLP consensus provides a guide to the minimum documentation needed for development, validation, operation, and maintenance of computerized systems. Application software programs are expected to have detailed descriptions similar to that of the blue book, and some countries require source code to be retrievable if needed. The consensus document expects that much of the documentation will be in the form of SOPs. Quality can then be audited by reviewing documented evidence for activities performed to SOP requirements. A basic set of ten topics for SOPs is listed in Fig. 8 (5, p. 13).

The OECD consensus notes that electronic data are to be stored with the same levels of access control, indexing, and timely retrieval as other types of data. Managing long-term access to electronic data when systems have to be retired may require producing hard copy printouts or transfer to another system to maintain continued readability of the data. Other data supporting the validation of a system should be maintained as long as study records (batch records) associated with that system are kept for use.

VII. CONCLUSION

All five regulatory documents studied in this chapter agree on the following major concepts:

- Systems must be shown to be suitable for their intended purposes.
- Systems must be controlled and maintained throughout their life cycle, from development through to retirement.
- Systems must be formally validated prior to use.
- Systems must be kept in a validated state through change control mechanisms for systems and data and various maintenance, backup, and recovery procedures.
- For audit purposes, system and data quality must be supported by documented evidence; if an activity is not documented, it did not happen.

Firms must be prepared with documented evidence to show that management is in control of computerized systems and computer controlled processes, resulting in system reliability and data integrity supporting the safety, efficacy, and quality of manufactured medicinal product. The ultimate responsibility for validated computerized systems rests with the manufacturer.

REFERENCES

1. FDA, *Guide to Inspection of Computerized Systems in Drug Processing*, U.S. Government Printing Office, Superintendent of Documents, Washington, D.C., 1983-381-166:2001, Feb. 1983, pp. 1–25.

2. FDA, *Medical Device Good Manufacturing Practices Manual*, 5th ed., U.S. Government Printing Office, Superintendent of Documents, Washington, D.C., FDA 91-4179, Aug. 1991, App. pp. 1–24.
3. European Commission, ''Guide to Good Manufacturing Practice for Medicinal Products—Annex 11: Computerized Systems,'' *The Rules Governing Medicinal Products in the European Union Volume IV*, Office for Official Publications of the European Communities, Luxemburg, Jan. 1992, pp. 139–142.
4. Koseisho, ''Guideline on Control of Computerized Systems in Drug Manufacturing,'' *Manual for Control of Computerized System in GMP*, Yakuji Nippo-sha, Tokyo 1993, ISBN4-8408-0278-5. pp. 23–32.
5. OECD, *GLP Consensus Document: The Application of the Principles of GLP to Computerized Systems*, Environment Monograph no. 116, Environment Directorate, OECD, Paris, 1995, pp. 3–15.
6. FDA, Ref. 2, computerized device GMP.
7. FDA, *Software Development Activities, Reference Materials and Training Aids for Investigators*, U.S. Government Printing Office, Superintendent of Documents, Washington, D.C., FDA 84-4191, July 1987.

16

Validation Concepts for Manufacturing Systems

Kenneth S. Kovacs

Bailey Controls Company, Wickliffe, Ohio

Joseph F. deSpautz

INCODE Corp., Herndon Virginia

I. INTRODUCTION

As process control systems become increasingly sophisticated, the ability to meet regulatory validation requirements becomes more complex. The objective of this chapter is to provide the reader with an introduction to validation concepts for manufacturing systems and an understanding of the following:

- GMP compliance issues
- Validation concepts and principles
- Computer-related systems validation concepts
- Typical elements necessary for a computer-related system validation project plan

It is ultimately the responsibility of each end user to plan and implement a validation that meets the intent of the good manufacturing practices (GMP). The exact method to accomplish validation is not prescribed by regulation. It is important to note that the Food and Drug Administration (FDA) will be interested more in the content and exact implementation of systems validation as opposed to the methodology of that validation. The problems found by investigators tend to be more in the nature of incomplete implementation of a chosen methodology.

A computer-related system validation program is outlined in this chapter to provide insight into a typical validation project plan. Detailed policies, procedures, protocols, and validation documentation are necessary for each step in the program to ensure the success of validation efforts. Since validation is based upon specific applications and operating environments, there are no warrantees or guarantees implied in the use of the information presented here.

II. REGULATORY ISSUES

The FDA is empowered by the Food, Drug, and Cosmetic Act to enforce the federal regulations defined in Title 21 of the Code of Federal Regulations (21 CFR). Current good manufacturing practices (CGMPs) are defined within the CFR; for example, 21 CFR 211 ''CGMP's for Finished Pharmaceuticals,'' and 21 CFR 820 ''Good Manufacturing Practice Regulations for Medical Devices.''

The FDA publishes guides to explain these regulations. Their guide entitled ''General Principles of Process Validation'' states that process validation is a requirement of the CGMPs (1). The manufacturer of a drug or medical device is responsible for validation of both the process and their facilities and equipment. Process validation is defined by FDA as: ''Establishing documented evidence which provides a high degree of assurance that a specific process will consistently produce a product meeting its predetermined specifications and quality attributes'' (1).

Each company that manufactures products under federal CGMP regulations is responsible for validation within its own organizations; validation provides documented evidence that the control system hardware and software function as designed and will continue to function as intended reliably and consistently.

In order to obtain the pertinent information needed for process validation, a validation impact study should be undertaken to analyze all process equipment, controls, and distributed computer control systems for their GMP implications in the quality and manufacture of applicable products. A thorough knowledge of company products, manufacturing equipment and processes, procedures, operating environments, and computer system functionalities is required. The intent is to determine the scope of the validation effort by assessing the computer system's role in the process. If product quality can be affected, or if any GMP-related records are stored or generated by the computer system being reviewed, it should then be included in the scope of validation. Validation of computer-based process controls places specific demands on the user of these systems, therefore a *computer system validation plan* should be utilized for organizing the validation methodology of these types of control systems.

Federal regulations mandate compliance with these requirements. The importance of this is emphasized in 21 CFR 210.1 (b): ''Failure to comply with regulations renders a drug to be adulterated, and the drug, as well as the person who is responsible for the failure to comply shall be subject to regulatory action'' (2).

III. COMPUTER SYSTEM VALIDATION

The CFR specifically allows the use of computer systems within 21 CFR 211.68 (a), ''Automatic, Mechanical, and Electronic Equipment.'' Note the provisions: ''Automatic equipment, including computers, may be used provided they are routinely calibrated, inspected or checked according to a written program designed to insure proper performance'' (2).

In 1983 the FDA issued the ''Guide to Inspection of Computerized Systems in Drug Processing'' as a reference and training aid for investigators. Although general guidelines and concepts are presented, *there are no specific regulations itemizing the details for computer system validation*. Because of this, professional societies have helped to provide clarification and interpretations of CGMP validation stipulations. The Pharmaceutical Research and Manufacturers Association (PhARMA; formerly the PMA), the Parenteral Drug Association (PDA), and the International Society for Pharmaceutical Engineering (ISPE) all have active computer system validation committees to provide guidance in this area. Basically, as with process validation, computer system validation can be viewed as: ''Establishing documented evidence which provides a high degree of assurance that a specific Computer-Related System will consistently operate in accordance with pre-define specifications'' (3).

In addition, the U.K. Pharmaceutical Industry Computer Systems Validation Forum launched guidelines in its ''Good Automated Manufacturing Practice (GAMP) in the Pharmaceutical Industry,'' which states: ''The guidelines are intended to add technical depth to the existing ISO 9000 series of standards that will streamline the prospective validation of new computer-related systems'' (4).

The principles and concepts presented here are intended to provide methodologies that encompass approaches to validation by the PDA, PhARMA, and GAMP guidelines.

IV. COMPUTER-RELATED SYSTEMS

As computer systems and their applications become more complex for companies throughout the world who market products in the United States, where the FDA has jurisdiction, there is a growing need for global definitions and methodologies associated with the validation of these systems.

It is important to understand current terminology used in the validation of computer-related systems. Referencing PDA Technical Report No. 18, the basic components of a ''computer system'' are the software and hardware. Equipment (such as that used in a GMP function for production or a laboratory) that is to be controlled, along with the pertinent operating procedures to define the function of the equipment, comprises the ''controlled function.'' A ''computerized system'' is the ''controlled function'' operating with the computer system.

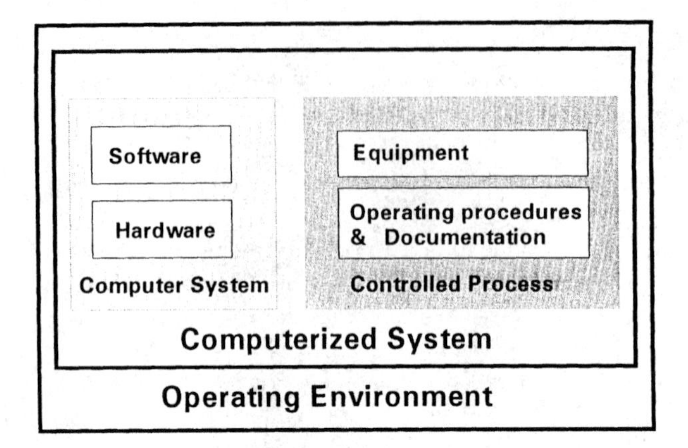

Fig. 1 Computer-related system (3).

When the computerized system performs its intended function while working in its operating environment, the result is a computer-related system. This is an important concept, because "it is the Computer-Related System that must be validated for use in a GMP function" (5). A graphical representation of the computer-related system can be seen in Fig. 1 (3).

The validation effort must include the operating environment of the system because of the factors that can affect the state of control of the computerized system. The physical operating conditions, operator inputs, input/output interfaces with other sources and systems, and plant utilities can play a major role in how effectively a computer system can operate the controlled function; "A Computer-Related System cannot be validated unless the process it is executing can be validated" (3).

V. VALIDATION LIFE CYCLE APPROACH

A computer-related system validation project plan is required for the validation program. This validation program is best addressed through a validation life cycle approach, which can be defined as: "An approach to computer system development that begins with identification of the user's requirements, continues through design, integration, qualification, validation, control, and maintenance, and ends only when commercial use of the system is discontinued" (6).

The PMA (PhARMA) life cycle approach to validation shows that the validation effort must begin early in the project. This is fundamental to the validation methodology presented in this book. Validation *cannot* be delayed until all components are integrated, since it is often impractical or impossible to adequately test software functions in an integrated system.

It should be noted that the validation of an existing computer system is no less exhaustive than the validation of a new computer system. It is crucial that the software component of the system be defined and verified. If this documentation is not available from the vendor, it must be created by the user. The user must provide a system specification for his or her own application, and all testing and resultant reviews must be performed against this specification.

Although previous use and historical documentation can support the validation of an existing computer system, *the FDA does not recognize validation through use*. Operating experience will seldom exercise all parts of the software; therefore, additional software testing will be needed. If operating experience is included in the validation, that experience must be analyzed and documented. In addition, the intended function of the system must be completely and objectively defined. Finally, the documentation of operating experience must be compared to the defined intended function. This final analysis for the validation of an existing computer system may prove more difficult to complete than performing the validation of a new system (Fig. 2).

VI. VALIDATING COMPUTER-RELATED SYSTEMS

As a suggested pragmatic methodology, the PDA's model can be used in a life cycle approach to the validation of computer-related systems through the application of specific steps in an organized process (3). These steps include the following:

- Planning validation activities
- Defining system requirements
- Selecting vendors
- Designing the computerized system
- Constructing the computerized system
- Integrating and installing
- Qualifying
- Evaluating the computer-related system in its environment

Using these steps as an outline will provide a basis for the validation project plan through a life cycle methodology. This methodology can be seen in a flow chart format in Fig. 3. By properly considering validation issues and documenting the details of each step of the project, pertinent regulatory requirements can be addressed in a timely manner.

VII. USING THE VALIDATED SYSTEM

A milestone is achieved after all documentation and reports, along with the computer-related system summary report needed to satisfy validation require-

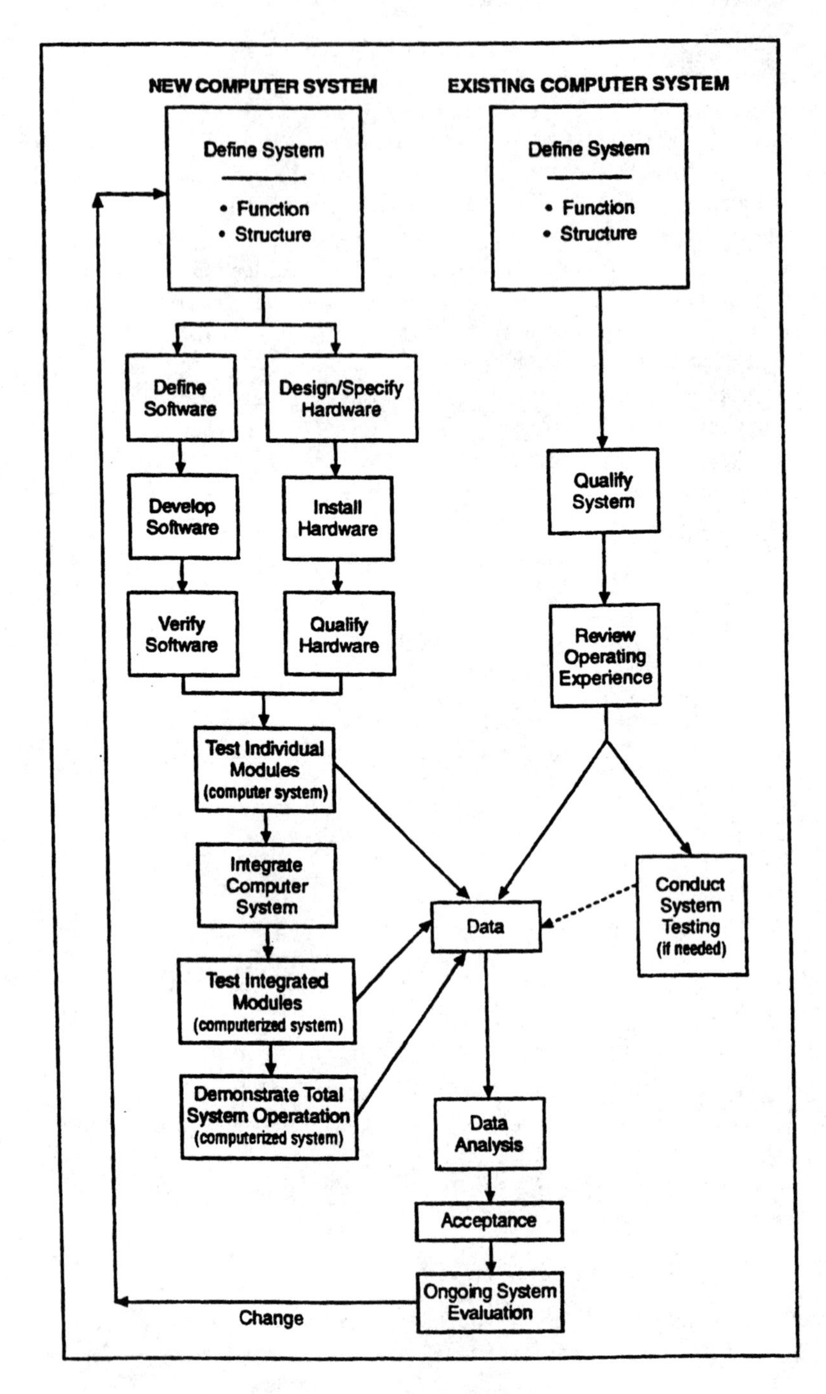

Fig. 2 PMA CSVC validation life cycle approach (6).

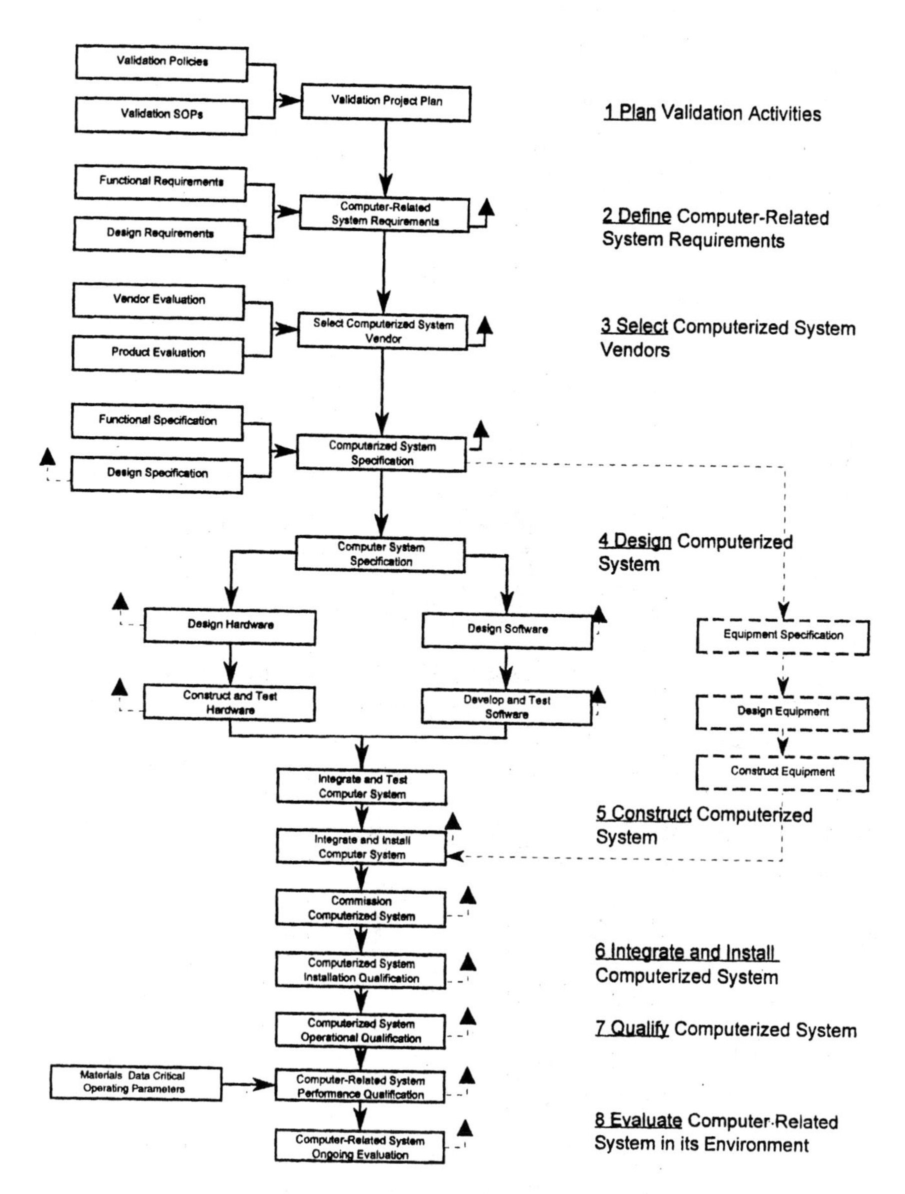

Fig. 3 Steps in validating computer-related systems (3).

ments, are formally reviewed and accepted. System reports, data files, and statistical capability studies generated by a validated system can provide the necessary "documented evidence" required for process validation. Properly utilized, a computer system with the applicable functionalities can greatly simplify documentation required for process validation.

VIII. TOTAL LIFE CYCLE COSTS

As with any project task, there are costs attributable to associated activities. The amount of funding required for executing the validation project plan should be included in the total life cycle costs for the computer-related system. Long-term cost benefits can be derived from integrating the validation process with project management activities during the early planning stages of the project. Only through proper planning and vendor selection can the long-term life cycle costs be identified and controlled.

Low-cost hardware with quickly developed applications software can be attractive when project funds are limited. In order to keep development costs low, these systems may not be developed with the methodologies required to ensure long-term system reliability and product quality. If this is the case, additional testing (along with possible design changes) will be required during start-up and qualification. It is during this phase of the project that the risk of introducing new errors into software systems is significantly increased. This "secondary development" can be extremely costly and detrimental to any project schedule. In addition, the ongoing costs for maintaining these systems can be high, since software problems may arise only through longer-term operations in production. This is the very time when problems cannot be tolerated because of the negative impact on manufactured product quality and GMPs.

Products manufactured in accordance with ISO 9001 (7) now provide end users with some assurances that a life cycle approach is integrated with the design, development, and delivery of a system. Documented procedures, specifications, and quality data ensure that delivered products meet established performance criteria. Start-up and qualification testing may not need to be as rigorous with systems produced under these conditions as with the previous case, since much of the lower-level product testing and documentation has been done by the vendor. The initial cost of this delivered system may be higher than the low-cost solution, but the long-term benefits will provide a more economical system over its life cycle.

Purchasing systems from a vendor that has an understanding of FDA issues and that is capable of supporting end user validation efforts to meet compliance requirements should provide the most economical long-term project solution. Although initial costs of the delivered system may be higher, long-term costs and detrimental effects to the system user's organization should be minimized. A close user–vendor relationship will ensure that the delivered system meets established specifications and that the system will continue to operate in accordance with ongoing validation criteria (8).

IX. A VALIDATION METHODOLOGY

By following the steps of the PDA's model previously outlined, a validation methodology can now be detailed. This section provides a description of the steps in this validation methodology.

A. Planning Validation Activities

Each company must have its own documented validation policies to follow for the execution of projects requiring validation. These policies should include formally written standard operating procedures (SOPs) and guidelines for validation activities, such as the following:

- Communication of management expectations
- Validation policy statements
- Validation SOPs
- Validation guideline documents
- Project management techniques
- Vendor assessment and audit criteria

A resultant document of the planning step is the validation project plan. This document defines the scope of the validation effort, how it will be accomplished, and who will be responsible for the protocols, test data, and approvals required to assure that each step in the validation project meets established objectives.

B. Definition of Computer-Related System Requirements

Functional requirements for the system must be prepared and approved. At this stage of the project, the system is best defined through functional requirements and high-level system-related design requirements. This document is referred to in Ref. 3 as the system requirements specification and is essential for a successful validation effort. It functionally defines *what* the system must do to satisfy the process, information, application, and technology requirements and becomes a foundation for all subsequent design documents. The system requirements specification should be included with submitted requests for proposals from vendors.

Elements of the system requirements specification are shown in Table 1 for process, information, software application, technology, and people-related requirements.

By following established company project management guidelines detailed in the "planning" step, process equipment and systems can be identified at this

Table 1 Elements of the System Requirements Specification

Description	Process	Info.	App.	Tech.	People
System purpose and description	✓	✓	✓	✓	✓
Description of the controlled function	✓				
Required system functions	✓	✓	✓	✓	
Performance requirements			✓	✓	✓
Physical requirements such as utilities	✓			✓	
Environmental considerations	✓			✓	✓
Recipe management	✓	✓	✓		✓
Input/output information		✓			✓
Security and alarm management	✓		✓		✓
Operator–machine interface requirements	✓		✓	✓	✓
Interfaces to other operations and systems		✓	✓		✓
Data processing strategies and algorithms			✓	✓	
System-generated reports	✓	✓			✓
Emergency operations and interlocks	✓			✓	✓
Disaster control and recovery	✓		✓	✓	✓
Operating mode criteria and interlocks			✓		✓
System documentation	✓	✓	✓	✓	✓
Specific project validation criteria	✓	✓	✓	✓	✓

time. The validation project plan should identify the systems to be included and the procedures to be followed during the validation project.

C. Selection of Computerized System Vendors

Potential computer system vendors and developers must be identified, requests for information issued, and evaluations completed. Based upon established company assessment criteria and vendor audits, a final list of qualified vendors, developers, and system integrators is then produced.

The ability of each vendor in meeting project objectives must be established and considered in choosing a system supplier. Along with purchasing specific hardware and software, end users are purchasing the vendor's ability to provide support for the validation and ongoing maintenance of the system.

In order to establish the competency of a vendor, specific qualifications should be verified through a site visit and an audit of its operations.

D. Design of the Computerized System

A detail design specification describing *how* the system will satisfy the defined system requirements is prepared during this step. Both functional and design specifications should be addressed at this time for all components: process, information, application, technology, and organization. This document, also known as the computerized system specification, should be generated and approved through the combined efforts of both the end user and the vendor providing the system. Once approved, the foundation computer system specifications should be revised in accordance with ''change control'' procedures to ensure all related documents such as program listings, operator manuals, and installation drawings are also modified to reflect changes.

A detail design specification that details how the system hardware and software operates and satisfies the system requirements will provide the cornerstone document required for validation. All system installation and operating performance parameters, along with acceptable values, will be detailed in this document. Properly written and detailed, the system specification will provide the basis for qualification protocols that are required later in the validation program.

Design specifications for the computer system hardware and software can now be generated by the selected vendor. To assure the quality of the system design, a formal program for engineering, developing, testing software and hardware should exist for any organization providing systems. A quality assurance program must be comprehensive to assure that predefined quality requirements are integrated with the application of all products and systems. Software engineering standards are published by the Institute of Electrical and Electronics Engineers (9), and should be an integral part of the software quality assurance system.

E. Construction of the Computerized System

Once the design phase is completed, construction and testing of system hardware can proceed, along with development and testing of system software. Vendor integration of the hardware and software produces an integrated computer system that should be thoroughly tested during this step.

Engineering methodologies are procedures driven to meet a product life cycle approach for developing hardware and software. The design and development process utilizes a series of distinct planning and production phases with clearly defined evaluations and reviews, all of which require adherence to documented quality standards.

This life cycle approach typically ensures the following:

- Functional system requirements are written.
- System specifications are written.
- A development plan is issued.
- Written test plans are completed, along with procedures, methods, and acceptance criteria.
- The system is designed, and tests and inspections are executed.

- Test results are documented.
- After software and hardware are integrated, additional testing is done and the results are documented.
- Acceptance testing is accomplished.

Thorough inspection and testing procedures by each vendor should ensure that the design is functional and that each step of the design process is monitored and controlled. At lower software levels (and modules), structural verifications should be performed. As software modules are put together, and also integrated with hardware, functional tests are then performed. Performance and functional tests are done on hardware. Formal supplier documentation of inspections and tests provides the user with the "documented evidence" that all systems and applications-specific software are capable of functioning as specified.

Configuration and structural verification is documented to ensure the integrity of product and applications software. Along with documented product hardware and assembly quality assurance tests and inspections, this provides the first level of documented evidence for system quality and design to specifications. A functional test plan detailing the hardware and software testing as well as the integrated system functional testing is also generated during this phase of the project.

A factory acceptance test (FAT) developed jointly by the vendor and end user can be a milestone in the validation project plan. Execution and documentation of the FAT test plan in accordance with the system specifications and procedures detailing the acceptance criteria provide a verification of design to specifications. This verification can be incorporated in the validation project as the "documented evidence" to satisfy the criteria for system release and subsequent shipment to the end user.

A formal process for verification to specifications ensures that products and systems released for delivery perform accurately, consistently, and reliably. Factory acceptance testing verifies that system hardware and software adheres to design criteria and that it satisfies the project design specifications. Detailed FAT test plans should be provided to clients for this critical step in the validation process. This verification to specifications includes the following:

- Review of functional requirements and high-level, system-related design requirements (system requirements specification)
- Engineering design to specifications
- Defined release criteria
- Factory acceptance testing and review
- Review of test results

The software quality assurance report (SQAR) ensures that the applied system released for delivery meets established user specifications.

Comprehensive documentation is essential for the installation, operation, and ongoing service of delivered systems and products. Proper documentation is mandatory for all validation programs. To meet the needs of user validation programs, application and product-specific documentation should be available for review, including the following:

- Quality assurance system: Formal documentation such as quality assurance policy and procedures manuals
- Product development: ISO 9001 documentation for engineering design, development, and testing
- Product manufacturing: Assembly procedures along with test plans, procedures, and results

Documentation that may be specified with the purchased system hardware and software typically includes wiring and interconnection diagrams, hardware layouts, bills of material, system tests and results, system configuration, and applications-specific user manuals. Installation qualification (IQ) and/or operational qualification (OQ) documents should be provided on a project-by-project basis for supplied products and systems. Product documentation includes configuration guides, programmer's manuals, instruction bulletins, and operator's manuals.

F. Integration and Installation of the Computerized System

Installation of the computer system and related controls and instrumentation follows a logical path in project management. All hardware must be installed according to approved engineering specifications and drawings. In this step, all inputs, outputs, communications, and other interconnections with process and production equipment to be controlled by the system are to be completed.

Vendor support can positively impact the validation schedule during this phase. All test plans and results performed at the vendor's location during the FAT should be available to the purchaser. Once installed on-site, the FAT can be used as the basis for a site acceptance test (SAT). Test results can be compared to the FAT to determine if the system was affected during shipping or installation. This step verifies the baseline from which all qualification work will proceed.

G. Qualification

After the installation and integration step, the qualification phase of the computerized system can begin: "Qualification is the procedure of collecting appropriate data that, when documented properly, provides a high level of assurance that a Computerized System will operate in accordance with the System Specification" (3).

In this step, written and approved qualification protocols for verifying and testing the installation, operations, and performance of the computer-related system are provided and executed in accordance with the validation project plan.

> The System Specification is the cornerstone to the qualification effort. A clear specification will yield detailed acceptance criteria for specific functional testing. Qualification of complex Computer-Related Systems may require breaking down the system to define sub-systems. Each sub-system can then be qualified separately. After completing the qualification of the sub-systems, the qualification of the integrated complex system will be an easier task to accomplish. The specific approach to be used in the qualification of the Computer-Related System should be described in the Validation Plan and the appropriate validation SOP's (3).

Appropriate testing protocols can be generated from the system specification to ensure that functional requirements satisfy the acceptance criteria. For expediency, work performed during the SAT can be documented concurrently with the execution of both the IQ and OQ protocols.

Three types of qualification verification and testing systems should typically be performed to assure that the system is installed properly, that it operates properly, and that it will produce a product having the desired attributes.

1. Installation qualification provides the documented verification that all important aspects of the computerized system hardware and software installation adheres to the system specification, manufacturer recommendations, and appropriate codes or regulations.
2. Operational qualification provides the documented verification that the computerized system performs in accordance with the system specification throughout all anticipated operating ranges.
3. Performance qualification (PQ) provides the documented verification that the computer-related system operates in accordance with the system specifications while performing its intended function in its operating environment. The PQ should include verification that the computer-related system consistently produces a product meeting its predetermined specifications and quality attributes.

Documentation provided to the purchaser by the system supplier should be comprehensive enough to generate the IQ and OQ documents needed for the computer-related system validation program. If the purchaser does not have the expertise required, it may be advantageous to have the vendor and/or a consultant generate the system qualification documents and execute the test protocols.

Qualification protocols are written and approved documents that are prepared in advance of testing and describe the objectives of the test and the preapproved test methods and acceptance criteria to be used. Protocols will specify who is responsible for conducting the tests, what specific method is to be used for each test, how data are to be collected and reported, and what review and evaluation procedures will be used to determine if the acceptance criteria are met. Acceptance criteria will be based on the system specification (10).

All test results and data obtained through the execution of the qualification protocols must be formally documented and approved in test reports. These test reports will include clearly displayed summary data. The use of tables, graphs, and charts is customary for this report. All results should be checked for accuracy and completeness. Test reports will compare test data against predefined acceptance criteria, and clearly state the basis for concluding that system performance is found acceptable. For a successful qualification phase, analysis of the accumulated information must formally confirm that the operation satisfies all requirements specifications (10).

H. Evaluation

With the computerized system installed in its environment and performing its intended function, the PQ protocols can be executed. Production materials and data must be input to the system and satisfy specifications while operating under approved procedures and critical parameters. Properly documented, this step will provide the verification that the computer-related system operates in accordance with system specifications. As part of this step, product analysis must be documented to verify that specifications and quality attributes of all products are satisfied consistently and reliably through the computer-related system.

Ongoing evaluation with written procedures and documentation must also be provided to ensure that programs are enacted to maintain the system in a validated state.

Formal ongoing programs with written procedures should be established to provide for such issues as the following:

- Training of personnel impacting on the system operation
- Contingency planning and disaster recovery
- Security access confirmation
- Maintenance and calibration
- System audits and reevaluations
- Provisions for remedial action and revalidation
- Periodic auditing of the system
- Change control procedures for the validated system

For ongoing support, services should be provided by the vendor that provides the follow-up field service to ensure all installed systems continue to operate within specifications. These services can include the following:

- Assistance at local, regional, and national levels
- Global organization offering worldwide support

- Flexible maintenance agreements
- Customer training for all products and systems
- Parts repair and exchange services
- Qualified representation to consult with regulatory personnel
- Access to review source code as required by the FDA
- Bulletin board service for system news
- Telephone technical support

REFERENCES

1. ''General Principles of Process Validation,'' Food and Drug Administration, Center for Drug Evaluation and Research (CDER), Rockville, Maryland, May 1987.
2. *Code of Federal Regulations*, U.S. Food and Drug Administration, Rockville, Maryland, Title 21 (21 CFR).
3. ''PDA Technical Report No. 18, Validation of Computer-Related Systems,'' PDA, 1995 Supplement, Volume 49, Number S1, Bethesda, Maryland.
4. M. Rosser, Draft guidelines on good automated manufacturing practice: An extract, *Pharm. Tech.* (April 1994).
5. C. A. Kemper, Vendor support required in control system validation, presented at the PDA International Congress, Basel, Switzerland, 1993.
6. Pharmaceutical Manufacturers Association (PMA), Computer System Validation Committee (CSVC), Validation concepts for computer systems used in the manufacture of drug products, *Pharm. Tech.* (May 1986).
7. ISO 9001: Quality systems—model for quality assurance in design development, production, installation and servicing, International Organization for Standardization, Geneva, Switzerland (March 1994).
8. K. S. Kovacs, *Validation Assurance and GMP Compliance*, Elsag Bailey Process Automation, Wickliffe, Ohio, 1995.
9. *Software Engineering Standards*, 3rd ed., the Institute of Electrical and Electronics Engineers, Piscataway, New Jersey, Aug. 1990 (ANSI/IEEE Std. 729-1983, ''Glossary of Software Engineering Terminology''; ANSI/IEEE Std. 730.1-1989, ''Software Quality Assurance Plans''; ANSI/IEEE Std. 828-1983, ''Software Configuration Management Plans''; ANSI/IEEE Std. 829-1983, ''Software Test Documentation''; ANSI/IEEE Std. 830-1984, ''Software Requirements Specifications''; ANSI/IEEE Std. 1008-1987, ''Software Unit Testing''; ANSI/IEEE Std. 1012-1986, ''Software Verification and Validation Plans''; ANSI/IEEE Std. 1016-1987, ''Software Design Descriptions''; ANSI/IEEE Std. 1028-1988, ''Standard for Software Reviews and Audits''; ANSI/IEEE Std. 1042-1987, ''Guide to Software Configuration Management''; ANSI/IEEE Std. 1058.1-1987, ''Standard for Software Project Management Plans''; ANSI/IEEE Std. 1063-1987, ''Standard for Software User Documentation'').
10. ''System Integration Methodology in Support of FDA Compliance,'' Bailey Controls Company, Wickliffe, Ohio, 1994.

17

Management's Role in Computer Validation: Policy and Procedures

Teri Stokes

GXP International, Acton, Massachusetts

I. INTRODUCTION

As seen in Chapter 14, one theme common to all good manufacturing practice (GMP) computer directives from regulatory authorities is that company management has the responsibility to be in control of computerized systems that are critical to the safety, efficacy, and quality of medicinal product. The GMP directives suggest that the mechanism for management to exert this control is through the development and implementation of policies and standard procedures. Writing policy is not enough, however, and inspectors look for evidence of how personnel are trained on policy and procedures for computerized systems and how compliance is monitored.

This chapter examines management's role in providing policy and procedures for computer validation. It looks at ways to develop a practical approach to computer validation that ensures system control and reliability to world standards in an organized fashion. In order to pass inspections and audits, a practical policy approach must address the issue of organized documentation for validation activities. A picture of the documented approach to computer validation discussed in this chapter is shown in Fig. 1.

II. BUSINESS CYCLES FOR COMPUTER VALIDATION

Pharmaceutical manufacturing companies participate in a business cycle oriented to produce quality product for sale at a profit that can sustain the firms through

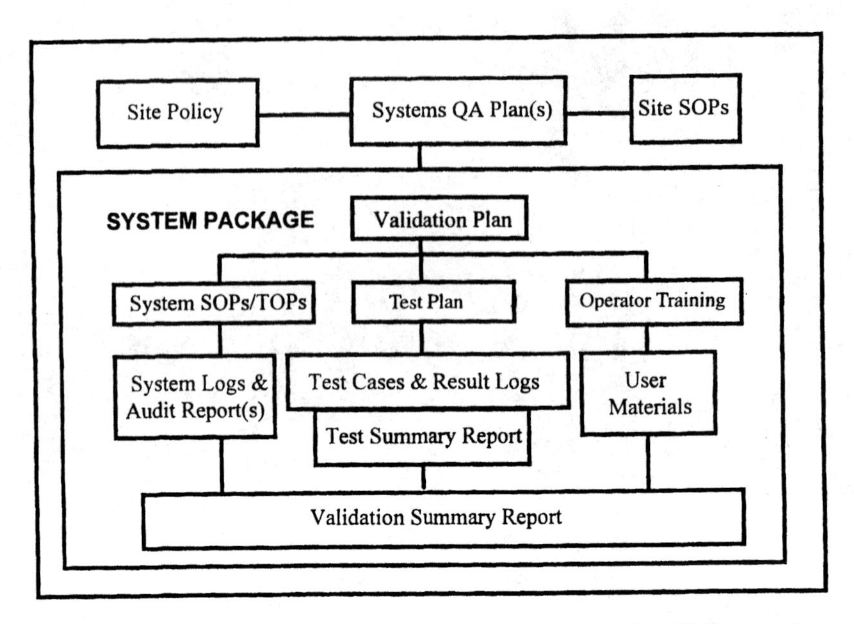

Fig. 1 Documented computer validation approach for site GMP compliance.

future endeavors. Regulatory authorities participate in an audit and inspection cycle designed to ensure quality product that is safe and effective for consumers. Medical reimbursement plans participate in a health care delivery cycle that seeks to use quality product at a low cost. Computer validation is a discipline that can contribute positively to each of these cycles.

At first glance, it may seem to management that computer validation work is both a cost overrun and a loss of profits for the company. Time pressures to get a newly automated line up and running can lead to requests to shortcut the documentation and testing procedures required for validation. Experience has shown, however, that giving in to such pressures can often result in costly, unexpected line interrupts after production begins and untested problems arise.

Developing a computer validation policy and implementing it with plans and procedures can ensure data integrity and system reliability. Data integrity and reliable systems are key components in making a quality product at reduced cost. Reliable systems reduce the cost of line interruptions, rework, and nonconforming product in the manufacturing cycle. Reduced cost of manufacture provides an opportunity to achieve profit goals at lower reimbursement prices; thus computer validation efforts should be seen not as a necessary evil but as a necessary good for profitable business practice in automated production.

Management, regulators, and consumers all share some common goals for drug manufacturing with computerized systems. They all want to have the following:

- Systems that produce a quality product because they perform their intended functions in a consistent and reliable manner throughout the full range of production conditions
- Product prices based upon cost-effective production that includes computerized systems with optimal uptime, ease of repair, and no damage to controlled processes or loss/corruption of critical data

Within the pharmaceutical manufacturing production cycle it is important for management to define the business priorities for computer validation work. People, time, and money are always in limited supply and it is management's job to provide direction for applying them to system validation projects in a manner that best achieves the objectives of safety, efficacy, quality of product, operator safety, and cost-effective operations.

III. MANAGEMENT'S ROLE IN COMPUTER VALIDATION

The role for senior management in computer validation is to set policy, establish procedures for implementing the policy, train personnel in policy and standard operating procedures (SOPs), and monitor compliance to the policy over time. When inspectors look for documented evidence of management commitment to validated systems, they look for signed and approved policy, SOPs, training records, and audit reports. Style, format, and content may vary from firm to firm, but the essentials of GMP regulations should be covered for the critical systems being used. Management's definition for what constitutes a GMP system in its operations should be clearly stated, and the rationale for prioritizing validation efforts should also be clearly stated. Examples of policy definition statements are shown in Fig. 2.

The definition of both a computerized system and an electronic device allows management to differentiate between the two in its validation procedures so that documentation and resource allocation can be proportionate to the size and scope of the GMP activity. This will let the SOP for device validation be more calibration-oriented and the documentation demands more focused than for larger systems.

A site validation policy can be written in a number of styles, depending on the corporate culture involved. Some common orientations are the following:

- *Data/process centric*—All validation tasks are initiated and driven by the regulatory status and ownership of the data being handled or the process being controlled by a computerized system.

- **GMP Data:** Any data used to prove to authorities the Safety, Efficacy, and/or Quality of regulated product.
- **GMP Electronic Device:** Any electronic device used to gather GMP data for upload to a GMP System or to control critical activities in a GMP process. A GMP Device is composed of two parts, software code written to perform a limited range of predetermined functions and hardware designed to perform the predetermined functions, e.g., programmable logic controller (PLC), portable bar code reader, analog/digital converter.
- **GMP Computerized System:** Any computerized system which handles GMP data or which controls a GMP-regulated process. A GMP System is composed of two parts, the software application and the platform system.
- **GMP Software Application:** Software code written to provide a specific set of functions used to handle GMP data or to perform/control a GMP-regulated task or process.
- **GMP Platform System:** The configuration of hardware and peripherals, operating system, utilities, database, and other software and network components required to allow the GMP Software Application to perform as intended.
- **Validation Priority:** First priority for validation resources will be placed on computerized systems and devices whose failure to perform would have a direct impact on the Safety of medicinal product or the Safety of the system operator. Second priority for validation resources will be placed on systems and devices having an impact on product Efficacy. Third priority will be for systems and devices having an impact on other Quality attributes of medicinal product.

Fig. 2 Site policy—definition examples.

- *User centric*—All validation tasks are initiated and driven by end user management, which uses systems to perform regulated work.
- *System centric*—All validation tasks are initiated and driven by the information systems department based upon the types of hardware and software systems provided for regulated operations.
- *ISO centric*—All validation tasks are initiated and driven by a policy that is part of the ISO 9000 manual of a company and maintained by the quality department.

Whatever the focus chosen, it is important that computer validation be recognized as a team effort that requires the active support of multiple disciplines, including (but not limited to) application users and system providers.

Senior management is in the best position to establish the organization's focus for computer validation and for resolving resource and interdepartmental issues that may arise during early efforts. Large manufacturing sites usually have

⇒ Senior Management Introduction - Signed rationale for Site Policy
1. Business Objectives for Systems GMP Compliance
2. Technical Objectives for Systems GMP Compliance
3. System Acquisition & Supplier Relations Policy
4. Policy for System Development on Site
5. GMP System Acceptance Process
6. System Life Cycle Management - Change Control through Retirement
7. Training Programs for System Use and Validation
8. System Audit and Inspection Policy
9. Documentation Requirements for System Validation
10. Roles & Responsibilities for System Validation Team Activities

⇒ Appendices - Terms & Definitions, Document Templates, SOP Listing

Fig. 3 Site policy outline topics.

a mix of manual and automated operations, with older and newer facilities operating in very different states of computerization. A site policy should reflect all states of computer use. (For more detail on policy content see Stokes reference 1.)

To develop a site policy, senior management should assemble a working site team that represents all types of computerized environments involved in their manufacturing. Drivers of computer validation policy from a technical perspective would come from plant engineering for automated control devices and systems, the computer department for materials and resource planning (MRP) systems, and quality control for laboratory systems. The business point of view would be driven by plant managers and by shift managers for various types of operations and logistics concerns. Regulatory concerns are usually represented by the quality assurance role.

Experience has shown that a facilitated workshop approach to developing content for validation documents is both time-effective and cost-effective. The outline for typical chapter or section topics forming a site policy is shown in Fig. 3.

The site team working group develops a consensus for content about each topic in the policy outline using a consistent format approach.

- Management summary
- Defined terms associated with the topic
- Bullet list of validation tasks with associated roles and responsibilities

The management summary is a brief policy statement (one to two paragraphs) of a site consensus on the topic. This is developed by adapting corporate policy, GMP regulations, and local business practices to site-specific needs. The site team working group also identifies and defines any terms related to the topic that need clarification. Policy language must be clearly understood by all people at the site as well as by external inspectors; that is, computer support people must be able to understand the regulatory and business issues and all others must be able to understand the computer issues. The computer validation policy should be in English for international inspectors and should also be available in the local language of the site to facilitate the understanding needed for implementing compliance.

The process of developing content for management summary and defined terms provides a good opportunity for the site team to decide the various validation tasks associated with each topic. Once tasks are identified, the roles and responsibilities can be assigned. Using a bullet list approach for validation tasks, roles, and responsibilities provides a concise way to communicate multiple ideas in a reduced amount of text.

For the final site policy document, the terms and definitions are stripped out of the sections and consolidated into a glossary in an appendix. The roles and responsibilities can then be organized into a coherent last section on validation roles and responsibilities. The final consolidation allows a site team to look for redundancies and conflicts of purpose in various activities and to resolve any such issues.

A steering committee of the site's senior management board then reviews and approves the site computer validation policy. Usually the policy is presented

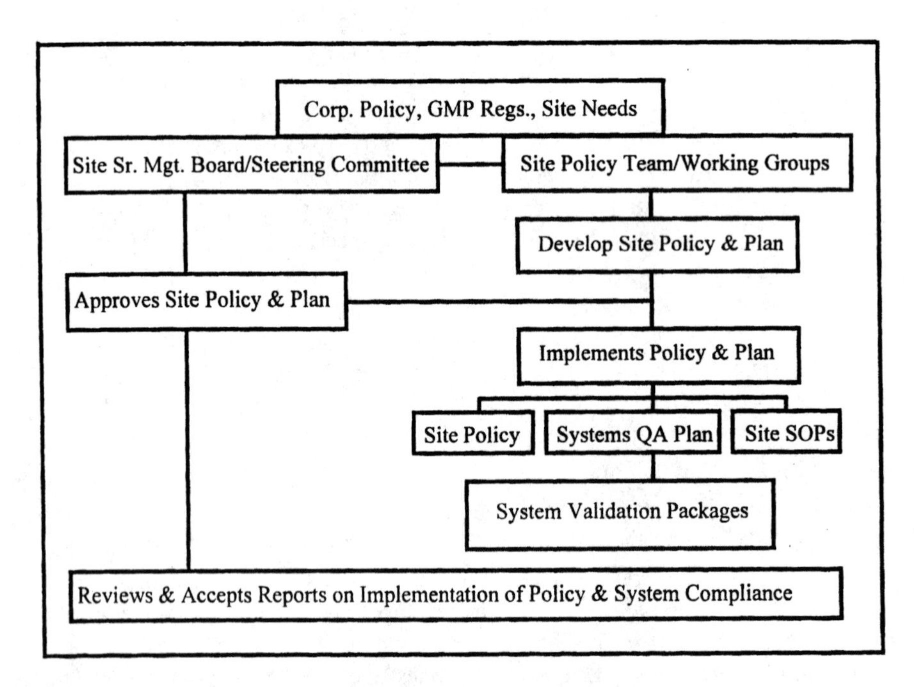

Fig. 4 Site process for computer validation compliance.

along with an implementation plan to test its practical usefulness on a short list of selected systems. Management then applies its priorities to the short list to direct validation resources in line with site business objectives. Periodic reports back to the steering committee provide ongoing monitoring information to senior management, and written minutes of such meetings provide documented evidence of management's commitment to monitoring compliance for GMP computerized systems. (See the site validation process in Fig. 4.)

IV. IMPLEMENTING COMPUTER VALIDATION POLICY

Management's role in supporting policy implementation is to configure organizational support that allows resources to be applied to system validation tasks as part of normal business operations. Elaborate superstructures for computer validation should not be necessary when everyone associated with a computerized system understands his or her role in keeping it reliably operational and in compliance. Organizational supports usually include GMP and system training, SOPs for site practices, technical operating procedures (TOPs) for system-specific actions, and policy guidelines for validation roles and responsibilities with templates for validation documents.

- *Training*: Validation concepts for computerized systems need to be cross-trained among quality assurance, information systems, and end user organizations until they become as much a part of people's thinking as GMP procedures are today for the production process itself. Training for the proper use and care of the computerized system itself must also be provided and formally documented.
- *Standard procedures*: SOPs can be used at various levels of the organization to define consistent ways for performing system operations and validation tasks. At the corporate level SOPs can define how to work with suppliers. At the site level SOPs can define validation priorities and how validation tasks are to be assigned and performed at a particular manufacturing site. At the system level SOPs can address the specific safety and alarm concerns of an individual application. For platform system support and maintenance it is often helpful to meet changing technical demands by using TOPS, which are managed by change control at the system level instead of through the more formal process normally in place for SOPs.
- *Guidelines*: Policy needs to be supplemented with other guides that explain life cycle practices for various types of systems within the context of site manufacturing practice. In particular, the interactions during maintenance and change control for all parties concerned with a computerized system should be thought through, and a documented process should be established. Standards need to be written for documenting and writing code for any GMP software developed on site. Individual roles and re-

sponsibilities during inspections and audits of key systems should have guidance.

When first implementing a new validation site policy, experience has shown that it is useful to identify one new system for a prospective validation effort and one currently used system for a retrospective evaluation effort. These should be systems of moderate size that are considered critical to operations and that are on management's priority list for validation focus. It is a mistake to waste resources on a low-priority system or one that will be retired in six to twelve months. To get validation focus into the mainstream of people's thinking, the systems chosen should also be mainstream to site operations.

Once the first system is identified, a system team composed of individuals associated with the operation of that computerized system should be formed in accordance with the site policy. Developing the system validation package is a team effort. Role titles may vary from policy to policy, and the size and scope of teams may vary, depending on the size and scope of the computerized system, but in general a system validation team is formed from the generic roles shown in Fig. 5.

Usually the system owner forms and leads the system team through the pro-

System Sponsor: Manager responsible for the GMP process and data tasks using the computerized system

System Owner: Person charged by Sponsor with daily responsibility for having a computerized system ready for GMP use

System Support: Internal support person responsible for technical performance of software application and platform system

System Supplier(s): Internal/external software application and platform system suppliers, system maintenance and consulting services

System User(s): User/Operators representing various constituencies using a system

System Quality Control: Individual responsible for testing and/or calibrating the system

Site Quality Assurance: Individual who audits system validation activities to Site Policy, GMP regulations, and system plan, but is not involved with quality control testing of the system

Fig. 5 System validation team—GMP computerized system.

cess of developing a system validation package to provide documented evidence of the compliance of the system to GMP requirements. Guidance about the roles and responsibilities of the different team members for developing the system package is provided in the site policy and site SOPs. All team members share the common goal of ensuring that the system performs its intended functions in a reliable and consistent manner and that documented evidence to support such performance is available for audit and inspection purposes. The items of evidence contained in a system validation package for a GMP software application and/or its platform system are shown in Fig. 6.

Usually the system sponsor funds the validation effort and reviews and signs approval of the system validation plan and the validation summary report. When several different organizational units use the same GMP system, a user council may be the system sponsor and its chairperson would serve as the designated sponsor on behalf of all the user groups. Any validation costs would then be shared across the sponsoring user council. System sponsors are expected to keep validation efforts in line with the company's business objectives (e.g., validation efforts are focused on systems critical to product and process safety and efficacy concerns and testing is performed on functions critical to those same issues).

The development of a system validation package takes time, money, and human and physical resources. While the execution of some test cases may require product materials and production resources, not every computerized system in a large manufacturing facility can have a full package of its own. Hard decisions must be made, and an organized approach must be used to identify those

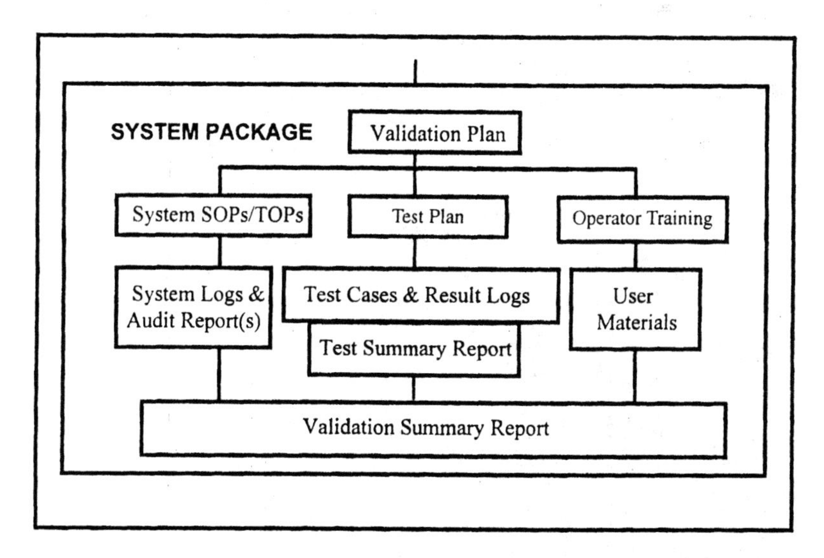

Fig. 6 Application/platform system validation package.

systems that are most critical to GMP concerns. One method for organizing such an approach is to develop a systems quality assurance plan (SQAP) for major functional units on the site (quality control (QC) laboratories, plant A, warehouse B), for types of systems (programmable logic controller (PLC)s, handheld devices, spreadsheet applications), or for large projects (new sitewide MRP or distributed control system (DCS) controlled facility; see Fig. 7).

The value of an SQAP is that it translates the site policy into action areas with a clear statement by management of how computerized systems will be checked for GMP performance. This document describes the inclusions, exclusions, and limitations for validation activities in a particular domain. Its section on purpose and scope states just what kind of systems merit full validation packages and how other systems will be checked for performance. The SQAP document provides an opportunity to look across all the computerized systems within its domain and to apply GMP regulations and site policy across the board in a systematic fashion. This is also the ideal place to document what will not be done and why it will not be done.

The Institute of Electrical and Electronics Engineers, Inc. (IEEE) Standard 730–1989 for Software Quality Assurance Plans is a good one to use as a basis for adaptation to a broader use as a Systems QA Plan. The standard gives an outline format for an SQAP and provides a discussion of points to consider for each of the items included in the outline. The discussion applies directly to application software and can be easily adapted to include platform systems. The IEEE outline for a software quality assurance plan is the following (2):

1. Purpose and scope
2. Reference documents
3. Management—organization, tasks, and responsibilities
4. Documentation requirements

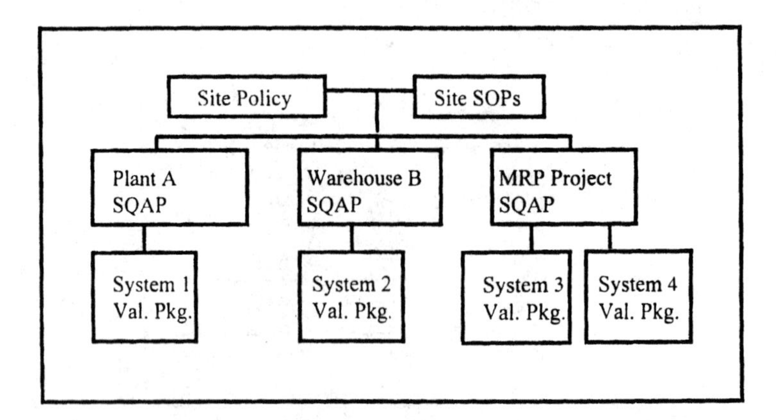

Fig. 7 Site policy and SQAP structure for system validation.

5. Standards, practices, conventions, and metrics
6. Reviews and audits
7. Test
8. Problem reporting and corrective action
9. Tools, techniques, and methodologies
10. Code control
11. Media control
12. Supplier control
13. Records collection, maintenance, and retention
14. Training
15. Risk management

Many items in the system validation package can be developed using various IEEE standards as guides and supports. The U.S. Food and Drug Administration itself made heavy reference to the IEEE standards when compiling a software development training book for its inspectors (3). The standards are designed to be complete enough for use with all systems up to the very largest. For GMP purposes, one must read the standards with the idea of scaling them to fit the scope of the system(s) under consideration.

Working computer validation projects on an international scale can sometimes lead to time-consuming discussions about whose format should be used for documentation in the system package. Experience has shown that a good way to remove such wasted effort is to start with the IEEE document formats whenever possible and adapt from there. The IEEE is an international standards body based in the United States with active membership and full recognition around the world. The primary focus for its standards activity is ensuring good-quality practices in general for information technology. It can be a neutral source of useful computer validation ideas for companies to use to defuse territorial discussions.

The IEEE standards are most reasonably purchased in the latest edition of the *IEEE Standards Collection* on software engineering. The following standards have been found very useful as a basis for formats for system package documentation (4):

1. Validation plan and validation summary report
   a. IEEE std. 1012-1987: Standard for Software Verification & Validation
   b. IEEE std. 1059-1993: Guide for Software Verification & Validation Plans
2. Test plan, test cases and result logs, and test summary report
   a. IEEE std. 829-1983: Standard for Software Test Documentation
   b. IEEE std. 1008-1987: Standard for Software Unit Testing
3. Audit reports
   a. IEEE Std. 1028-1988: Standard for Software Reviews & Audits

It is not the goal of computer validation to create mountains of paper, yet the documented evidence produced by validation activities does become significant. It is important to provide system validation teams with standard formats for all system package documents so that no time is lost in trying to figure out what to do. A consistent look to documents across systems and departments at a site will instill confidence in auditors and inspectors that management is in control of the validation process and then by default appears to be in control of the systems being validated.

One site SOP for validation practices should discuss an organized way to number, track, and store documents produced in the system package. The identifier number for a test plan should, for example, correlate to the identification of its associated validation plan and software application or platform system. Test case and test summary report identifier numbers should relate back to the associated test plan. Having an organized process for storing and accessing validation documentation also makes it easier to support audit and inspection requests to see evidence of compliance.

V. PEOPLE AND COMPUTER VALIDATION

People tend to rise to the occasion of validating a new system as part of the excitement of installing something new but find it hard to sustain interest in keeping up with validation of the system over time. Part of the problem is the perception that validation is a one-time major experience instead of a daily journey of quality tasks throughout the life of a system. It is important to design the application or platform system SOP/TOPs with ongoing routines that put application checking, system calibration, and on-the-job training into the normal workflow of system use.

People have special expectations around computerized systems that control critical production processes and batch-handling tasks. The essential expectation is that such systems should never break and if they do break that they should be fixed and put back on line immediately. The GMP procedures for documented change control, documented programming of code, and careful testing of any changes to critical application software may be seen as impediments to business profits rather than a guarantor of reliable future performance.

Production people may apply pressure to systems people to "fix it and do the testing and paperwork later." Here is where GMP training on computerized systems for both sides can prove helpful to people. Manufacturing folks can learn something about the unpredictable consequences of changes to code and systems people can learn about GMP requirements and the impact of system failures on product safety, efficacy, and quality.

Taking a computer validation site policy out to the people through an ongoing training program can provide the opportunity for people from all disciplines to learn together and see GMP for computerized systems as a shared responsibility. It is important for systems people to learn the real-world implications of a system breakdown and for production people to understand that computers are not magic and that software applications and platform systems need care and protection to be kept fit to perform their intended tasks.

The lessons of a computer validation GMP training program are reinforced for people who participate on a system validation team. The involvement of user representatives on such teams can be seen as continuing education in validation concepts and recorded on an individual's personnel record as relevant GMP experience. Since the system team operates throughout the life of the critical system, its members can take pride in maintaining "their" system in a validated state through both routine and change situations. Daily compliance can be less irksome when you yourself have participated in developing or adapting some of the system SOPs/TOPs.

In a similar fashion, operational managers who have to implement site policy do so with a different view if they have been involved in developing the policy. The site team approach of multiple disciplines coming together in work groups to decide content for the site policy sections provides an opportunity for people to express their practical issues and concerns and then get onboard with the final policy content. People on the site team train themselves further in the concepts of GMP for computerized systems and their experience should be noted on resumé records as relevant GMP experience.

A site policy should be a living contract that management has with itself for achieving the goals of reliable systems, management control, and auditable quality. Once the site team has produced an approved site policy, it should continue to operate as a task force to do the following:

- Review the policy on an annual basis and update it as needed
- Share learning with colleagues back in their respective domains at the site
- Serve as a support for any site groups trying to implement the policy.

The site team should be a reservoir of talent for policy implementation as well as a good arbitrator of practical concerns and a source for monitoring and measuring the success of GMP system compliance.

People will watch the site team carefully. The competency and level of management assigned to it will define its prestige and power and send a message to the site for how seriously senior management believes in GMP systems compliance. For this reason, at least one and preferably two of the senior board members should actively participate on the site team. Such participation shows the importance of systems compliance to senior management and provides a direct link into the operational knowledge shared among the group.

VI. CONCLUSION

Many people assume incorrectly that computer validation is primarily a testing exercise. The site policy approach and validation system package discussed in this chapter clearly show otherwise and reflect the directives of international GMP regulations reviewed in Chapter 14. Three common themes were seen across all international documents for computerized systems—management control, system reliability, and auditable quality.

The approach described in this chapter addresses all three themes with people, process, and documentation.

Management control

- People: senior management steering committee and site policy team
- Process: policy development, training, and monitoring
- Documented evidence: site policy, SQAP, site SOPs, operator training, system SOP/TOPs, monitoring reports

System reliability

- People: system validation team
- Process: system package development and life cycle management
- Documented evidence: validation plan, test plan, test cases and results logs, test summary report, validation summary report

Auditable quality

- People: quality assurance person
- Process: periodic reviews and audits for compliance
- Documented evidence: audit reports, system package

REFERENCES

1. T. Stokes, R. C. Branning, K. Chapman, H. Hambloch, and A. J. Trill, *Good Computer Validation Practices: Common Sense Implementation*, Interpharm Press, Buffalo Grove, Illinois, 1994, pp. 35–46.
2. IEEE, IEEE standard for software quality assurance plans, std. 1030-1989, *IEEE Standards Collection: Software Engineering*, the Institute for Electrical and Electronic Engineers, Piscataway, New Jersey, 1994.
3. FDA, *Software Development Activities, Reference Materials and Training Aids for Investigators*, U.S. Government Printing Office, Superintendent of Documents, FDA 84-4191, Washington, D.C., July 1987.
4. IEEE, *IEEE Standards Collection: Software Engineering*, the Institute for Electrical and Electronic Engineers, Piscataway, New Jersey, 1994.

18

Electronic Records, Electronic Signatures, and FDA Regulation Final Rule

Teri Stokes

GXP International, Acton, Massachusetts

I. INTRODUCTION

Published in the *Federal Register* on March 20, 1997, and effective as of August 20, 1997, the long-awaited final rule for electronic records and electronic signatures has been defined and approved and is now ready for implementation. The final rule provides criteria under which the U.S. Food and Drug Administration (US FDA) "will consider electronic records to be equivalent to paper records and electronic signatures equivalent to traditional handwritten signatures" (1, p. 13430).

The scope of this final rule applies to any paper records required by statute or agency regulations and allows electronic records to be used in lieu of paper records. Electronic signatures that comply with this ruling will be considered equivalent to full handwritten signatures, initials, and other general signings required by agency regulations. Such a final rule opens the path for more extensive use of automation and lights-out manufacturing technology by the pharmaceutical industry.

II. ELECTRONIC RECORDS—FINAL RULE DEFINITIONS

In order to understand the ruling, a number of terms had to be defined by the FDA. These are shown in Fig. 1 (1, p. 13465), and form a major part of the general

FDA Electronic Rule Definitions

- ***Biometrics*** - means a method of verifying an individual's identity based on measurement of the individual's physical feature(s) or repeatable action(s) where those features and/or actions are both unique to that individual and measurable.
- ***Closed system*** - means an environment in which system access is controlled by persons who are responsible for the content of electronic records that are on that system.
- ***Digital signature*** - means an electronic signature based upon cryptographic methods of originator authentication, computed by using a set of rules and a set of parameters such that the identity of the signer and the integrity of the data can be verified.
- ***Electronic record*** - means any combination of text, graphic, data, audio, pictorial, or other information representation in digital form that is created, modified, maintained, archived, retrieved, or distributed by a computer system.
- ***Electronic signature*** - means a computer data compilation of any symbol or series of symbols executed, adopted, or authorized by an individual to be the legally binding equivalent of the individual's handwritten signature.
- ***Handwritten signature*** - means the scripted name or legal mark of an individual handwritten by that individual and executed or adopted with the present intention to authenticate a writing in a permanent form. The act of signing with a writing or marking instrument such as a pen or stylus is preserved. The scripted name or legal mark, while conventionally applied to paper, may also be applied to other devices that capture the name or mark.
- ***Open system*** - means an environment in which system access is not controlled by persons who are responsible for the content of electronic records that are on the system.

Fig. 1 CFR 21 11.3—FDA definitions.

provisions section of the ruling. Most pharmaceutical manufacturing systems will be considered in the category of closed systems, in which the company responsible for good manufacturing practice (GMP) compliance of data and systems also has control of all access to its GMP systems. In these cases, subpart B—Electronic Records 21 CFR 11.10 Controls (for closed systems)—would apply.

> Persons who use closed systems to create, modify, maintain, or transmit electronic records shall employ procedures and controls designed to ensure

> the authenticity, integrity, and, when appropriate, the confidentiality of electronic records, and to ensure that the signer cannot readily repudiate the signed record as not genuine (1, p. 13465).

In the case of the contract manufacture of GMP product outside the drug firm's own premises, or with the extensive use of electronic data interchange (EDI) with many suppliers, an open system would be in use. Then section 21 CFR section 11.30 Controls (for open systems) would apply.

> Persons who use open system to create, modify, maintain, or transmit electronic records shall employ procedures and controls designed to ensure the authenticity, integrity, and, as appropriate, the confidentiality of electronic records from the point of their creation to the point of their receipt. Such procedures and controls shall include those identified in 21 CFR 11.10, as appropriate, and additional measures such as document encryption and use of appropriate digital signature standards to ensure, as necessary under the circumstances, record authenticity, integrity, and confidentiality (1, pp. 13465–13466).

III. ELECTRONIC PROCEDURES AND CONTROLS—21 CFR 11.10

This final rule provides one set of procedures and controls to be applied to both closed and open systems when electronic records and/or electronic signatures are to be used for any regulatory purpose—GMP, good laboratory practice (GLP), good clinical practice (GCP), or various electronic submissions to the agency, such as electronic new drug applications (e-NDAs). The eleven paragraphs describing procedures and controls in 21 CFR 11.10 are shown in Fig. 2 (1, p. 13465). They give a concise view of what the FDA considers to be good practice in computer validation for all regulated systems and they show common themes in counterpoint to the nineteen paragraphs of the European Union (EU) GMP guide annex 11 on computerized systems discussed in Chapter 14. Management control, system reliability, and auditable quality continue to be major themes for all legislative rulings.

IV. ELECTRONIC SIGNATURES

The FDA has long been concerned about the cost of biometric measurement technology for use as electronic signatures. Retinal scans, fingerprint reading, and voice patterns have been used by military and nuclear security systems for many years, but have been considered to be too expensive for common manufacturing uses. The FDA was reluctant to consider electronic signatures until less expensive alternatives could also be deployed with confidence.

The FDA's electronic ruling states that nonbiometric methods may be used

21 CFR Subpart B - Electronic Records - 11.10 Controls
Such procedures and controls shall include the following: a) Validation of systems to ensure accuracy, reliability, consistent intended performance, and the ability to discern invalid or altered records. b) The ability to generate accurate and complete copies of all records in both human readable and electronic form suitable for inspection, review, and copying by the agency. c) Protection of records to enable their accurate and ready retrieval throughout the records retention period. d) Limiting system access to authorized individuals. e) Use of secure, computer-generated, time-stamped audit trails to independently record the date and time of operator entries and actions that create, modify, or delegate electronic records. Record changes shall not obscure previously recorded information. Such audit trail documentation shall be retained for a period of at least as long as that required for the subject electronic records and shall be available for agency review and copying. f) Use of operational checks to enforce permitted sequencing of steps and events as appropriate. g) Use of authority checks to ensure that only authorized individuals can use the system, electronically sign a record, access the operation or computer system input or output device, alter the record, or perform the operation at hand. h) Use of device (e.g., terminal) checks to determine, as appropriate, the validity of the source of data input or operational instruction. i) Determination that persons who develop, maintain, or use electronic record/electronic signature systems have the education, training, and experience to perform their assigned tasks. j) The establishment of, and adherence to, written policies that hold individuals accountable and responsible for actions initiated under their electronic signatures, in order to deter record and signature falsification. k) Use of appropriate controls over systems documentation including: 1) Adequate controls over distribution of, access to, and use of documentation for system operation and maintenance. 2) Revisions and change control procedures to maintain an audit trail that documents time-sequenced development and modification of systems.

Fig. 2 Procedures and controls for closed and open systems using electronic records.

for electronic signatures as long as they meet certain criteria. Electronic signatures that are not based upon biometrics shall

1. Employ at least two distinct identification components such as an identification code and password

2. Be used only by their genuine owners
3. Be administered and executed to ensure that attempted use of an individual's electronic signature by anyone other than its genuine owner requires collaboration of two or more individuals (1, p. 13466)

The general requirements for an electronic signature, whether biometric or nonbiometric, are given in 21 CFR subpart C section 11.100. Each electronic signature is to be unique to one individual and cannot be reused by or reassigned to anyone else. An organization must verify the identity of an individual before it establishes, assigns, certifies, or otherwise sanctions an individual's electronic signature. Persons using electronic signatures must, prior to or at the time of such use, certify to the agency that the electronic signatures in their system, used on or after August 20, 1997, are intended to be the legally binding equivalent of handwritten signatures.

Electronic signatures and handwritten signatures executed to electronic records must be linked to their respective records to ensure that the signatures cannot be excised, copied, or otherwise transferred to falsify an electronic record by ordinary means, such as "cut and paste" technology. Signed electronic records must contain information associated with the signature that clearly indicates all of the following:

1. The printed name of the signer
2. The date and time when the signature was executed
3. The meaning associated with the signature, such as review, approval, responsibility, or authorship

The three items of signature information listed above are also subject to the same controls as for electronic records and must be included as part of any human-readable form of the electronic record (such as electronic display or printout; 1, p. 13466).

V. CONTROLS FOR IDENTIFICATION CODES/PASSWORDS

The FDA's electronic final rule requires that controls be used to ensure the security and integrity of electronic signatures based upon identification codes in combination with passwords. The recommended control measures are just a listing of the usual good practice activities that computer professionals have been using, when password security was taken seriously. Such controls include the following:

1. Maintain the uniqueness of each combined identification code and password, so that no two individuals have the same combination.
2. Ensure that identification code and password content are periodically

checked, recalled, or revised in order to cover such events as password aging.

3. Follow a loss management SOP to electronically deauthorize lost, stolen, missing, or otherwise compromised tokens, cards, and other devices that carry or generate identification code or password information. Follow SOP to issue temporary or permanent replacements using suitable strong controls.
4. Use program safeguards to prevent unauthorized use of passwords and/or identification codes and to detect and report any attempts at their unauthorized use in an immediate and urgent manner to system security personnel, and, as appropriate, to organizational management.
5. Perform initial and periodic testing of devices, such as tokens and cards, that carry or generate identification code or password information to ensure that they function properly and have not been altered in an unauthorized manner.

VI. CONCLUSION

This most recent ruling of the US FDA on electronic records and electronic signatures continues to elaborate on the major themes of other computer validation regulations as discussed in Chapter 14. The primary goal of all authorities and of good business itself is to maintain the integrity of the electronic data required for the safety, efficacy, and quality of regulated product. When paper records become electronic records and handwritten signatures become electronic signatures, regulatory authorities expect management to remain in control of the situation, the systems to be reliable, and the integrity of the records and signatures to have auditable quality.

Companies invest huge sums of capital in their information technology systems, and the return on that investment is achieved in an auditable way through computer validation good practices such as those discussed in Chapter 16. This chapter provides another view of the procedures and controls that are useful to ensuring management control, reliable systems, and auditable quality for electronic information in pharmaceutical processing.

REFERENCE

1. U.S. Food and Drug Administration, 21 CFR part 11—electronic records; electronic signatures; final rule, *Federal Register*, vol. 62, no. 54, U.S. Government Printing Office, Washington, D.C., Thursday, March 27, 1997, pp. 13430–13467.

19

Applied Computer Validation Plan for Manufacturing Execution Systems

Frederick R. Bickel

Kineticon Group, Inc., Loveland, Colorado

Richard E. Blanchette

Green Mountain Technology Inc., Boulder, Colorado

I. INTRODUCTION

Many pharmaceutical and process-oriented companies are installing a manufacturing execution system (MES) to improve efficiencies, reduce cycle times, and facilitate manufacturing control processes. The primary areas in which the MES is implemented are in material preparation (in which raw materials and intermediates are weighed and prepared for use in the manufacture of specific products), processing (in which raw materials and intermediates are converted to products), and packaging (in which the final product presentation is assembled.) Since any of these functions potentially impact the identity, strength, quality, and purity of the products, these functions are regulated by good manufacturing practices (GMP) requirements defined in the Code of Federal Regulations (CFR), title 21, chapter I, parts 210 and 211. These GMP regulations require that the system used to control and support product manufacturing functions be validated. Herein is described an approach to the implementation and validation of a computer-based control system.

II. PURPOSE

One purpose of the validation plan is to define the scope of the system validation effort required for the MES project. A second purpose is to establish the approach to be used to address validation requirements in order to ensure compliance of the completed system to FDA and internal guidelines. This validation plan defines why the validation is occurring, describes the validation methodology, outlines the required steps, specifies associated deliverables, and assigns responsibility. All of these activities should be based on a company-approved validation master plan.

III. TERMS AND DEFINITIONS

A few terms are used in this article that may be used with different meanings and connotations. Rather than risk any misunderstanding, these terms are defined. Other terms can be substituted.

Validation master plan. The validation master plan is the highest-level description of the validation approach. This is sometimes referred to as the validation policy, validation Standard Operating Procedures (SOP), or corporate validation plan.

Validation methodology. The validation methodology is the functional level description. This is sometimes referred to as the project validation plan, master validation plan (project level), or the validation system.

Validation protocols. The validation protocols are the lower-level description of the validation approach. These are sometimes referred to as test plans or test cases.

IV. VALIDATION MASTER PLAN

Much has been written, both from the regulatory agencies and from industry, concerning the need for a validation master plan. This plan identifies the activities to be undertaken that will ultimately compose the company's validation documentation package. Specifically, this plan establishes not only the format but also the content for the testing undertaken and for the approval of the data and conclusions. The validation master plan sets the standard for the validation approach.

Following the validation master plan, specific protocols and test cases are developed as outlined in the validation methodology. One approach to the validation of computer systems that has been applied is described.

V. OBJECTIVES

In order to validate the essential and critical features of a system, the goals and objectives must be clearly understood. Companies must formally define and document the intended operation of the MES by

Verifying that the system performs in a reliable and reproducible manner through functional, performance, and qualification testing of all system components and subsystems, as defined in the functional requirements
Creating/updating SOPs and manuals to reflect the actual installation and configuration
Creating a file of evidence that will demonstrate managerial control of the system for regulatory review.

VI. SYSTEM OVERVIEW

A. Software Description

The software chosen for the shop floor control component of the MES should be completely understood and described. This description includes the operating system and any adjunct programming (packaged or developed) that will be associated with the final implementation. The vendor must demonstrate a sound knowledge of the area addressed by its software or gather expertise from representatives in the field.

B. System Environment

The system environment must be well documented. The documentation should include the technical architecture, such as a client/server architecture (computers or terminals connected to a host computer), as well as the system architecture, such as the relationship of various software components. A description of any connections and/or drivers needed for the implementation should be described in detail. For example, the connections to scales and bar code printers used in weighing procedures and system logic and processing steps that will be controlled by that workstation should be spelled out. Data flows and ownership of data must be documented. If data are to be accumulated in a remote database (e.g., Oracle or DB2/2), this must be documented.

C. Functional Requirements

The processes to be controlled or supported should be described from the perspective of what functions they are designed to perform. For example, material preparation could begin with the staging activities and end with the delivery of weighed, labeled material to a granulation staging area. The detailed functionality could include preparing a picklist automatically, recording and verifying each material weighing, preparing and printing bar coded labels, and performing required system updates. Requirements for communication with other systems and resulting design solutions might also be determined at this time. The systems that could require some form of information exchange need to be identified (e.g.,

Manufacturing Resource Planning (MRP), inventory management, receiving, scheduling, document management, maintenance management, Laboratory Information Management System (LIMS), distribution, and finance). Initial implementations may be limited and may not interface with other systems.

VII. SCOPE OF VALIDATION

The computer-based system validation effort for a project will primarily focus on the functions described in the functional requirements. Any interfaces between systems will also be validated to ensure that data integrity and accuracy are maintained. Any nonvalidated, computer-based systems that pass data to the control system must have processes in place to ensure the integrity of the data. Similarly, the validation effort should ensure the integrity of data passed from the MES to other systems. Ensuring the proper use of data within the nonvalidated system remains outside the scope of the validation. The scope boundaries are at the MES (control system) interfaces to other nonvalidated business systems.

VIII. VALIDATION METHODOLOGY

A. Introduction

It is recommended that the validation methodology follow a system development life cycle as described by the Pharmaceutical Manufacturers Association (PMA). A number of life cycle approaches have been described and can be adapted to fit individual companies. It is important to adopt an approach that addresses ensuring the control of your processes and information. The life cycle approach described herein includes the following phases:

1. Project planning
2. Requirements
3. Design and development
4. Procedures development
5. Testing
6. Final approval
7. Ongoing evaluation

All phases need not be performed sequentially. A number of activities from the first four phases can be performed in the same time periods. In particular, key project team members will gain exposure early in the implementation to better understand opportunities made possible through process automation with an MES installation. The increased knowledge from this exposure will facilitate clear refinement of functional requirements and development of precise system specifications to meet those requirements. Early refinement of the project plan based on new knowledge and the ability of team members to make an informed assessment are both extremely useful in reducing costs. Appropriate rigor should be applied throughout the project to ensure the production of high-quality project outputs that meet validation requirements. The system must not be used in the production of finished product during development activities or until adequate validation has occurred.

B. Project Planning Phase

The project planning phase describes the approach to be used for implementation and validation, and will define the project and its boundaries. A project plan will be produced during the planning phase that will both detail project tasks and assign responsibilities, set timelines, and establish deliverables for each task. All required validation tasks defined in the validation plan should be included as part of the MES project plan. This planning will help in establishing and managing the project's scope and both user and management expectations. This will facilitate timely project completion and the realization of expected value.

C. Validation Deliverables

1. Scope and objectives document: Provides project background, scope, specific objectives, and resources to complete the project
2. Validation plan: Provides the scope and method for validating the system

D. Requirements Phase

The requirements phase will specifically define system needs for every system component: software, hardware, environment, and procedures. Activities will include defining functional requirements for the hardware platform, response time, and business process needs of all kinds. Work in this phase provides a foundation from which decisions can be made for specifying the right combination of hardware and software for the system. These requirements are normally defined in a functional requirements document. The functional requirements document should include a section on MES overview and requirements addressing requirements common to multiple functions across the shop floor. The functional requirements document for a specific project phase will define specific requirements for that process.

E. Vendor Audit

A software supplier's development process must be evaluated to determine whether it uses appropriate industry practices and can demonstrate acceptable control of its software. The standard approach for this determination is a vendor audit. A company team with expertise in auditing, quality assurance, and information services should visit the supplier to evaluate its practices and conformance to its standards. A report should be written recommending use, qualified use, or nonuse of the vendor software.

F. Validation Deliverables

1. Functional requirements: Details the system needs from a business perspective for all system components
2. Vendor evaluation: Summarizes the results of evaluating the supplier's software development practices and recommends software use, qualified use, or nonuse.

G. Design and Development Phase

The design and development phase will provide a definition and specification of actual hardware and software needed to provide the functionality specified in the functional requirements document. In order to build quality into the system and identify problems early, design and unit test reviews should be performed and documented as part of any development. Where custom procedures must be developed or custom interfaces with other systems are required, additional design and code reviews should be performed to ensure functional integrity and conformance to development standards. Some additional integration testing may be required.

H. Validation Deliverables

1. System specification: Details how the requirements will be met with specific screen, report, and software configuration, new application code, and associated hardware
2. Development testing documentation: Shows the quality checks during the development and documentation design phase
3. Programmed/configured software and hardware components: This is the system state (the actual software) resulting from programming and configuring the system as specified in the system specification

I. Procedures Development Phase

The procedures development phase creates the user and system management procedures for operating and managing the system. User procedures should be defined and written during the design and development phase, they should be available for qualification testing, and they must be approved before the final system may be approved. System management procedures should address the system administration and other SOPs that describe specific system management needs. Any new SOPs should be written.

J. Validation Deliverables

1. Operating (user) procedures
   a. Documents day-to-day operations for the user from sign-on to sign-off
2. System management procedures
   a. Security: physical and software security
   b. Backup and recovery: identifies timing and step-by-step procedures to backup and recovery
   c. Archiving: defines timing and procedures for removing but keeping historical data
   d. Disaster recovery: defines step-by-step procedures and verification of recovery in the event of a server, server room, or site disaster
   e. Change control: describes the process needed for system changes, both hardware and software
   f. Training: describes the content of training, who should receive the training, and how functional competence should be documented
   g. System administration: Documents day-to-day procedures for performing system administrative functions
   h. Revalidation: documents procedures for performing ongoing quality checks for either a standard system check, a new software release, a major system functional improvement, or complete revalidation of the system

K. Testing Phase

The testing phase starts after system development and associated testing is complete, and utilizes draft or approved SOPs where appropriate. A test plan will be developed to detail the qualification testing activities. This test plan will include a definition of what specific environments will be used for each type of qualification test, what set of specifications will be tested by each set of protocols, and who will perform the testing and verification. The test plan will also define how test results will be recorded and how exceptions to expected results will be tracked to a satisfactory resolution.

Generally, system development work and associated prequalification testing will occur on a development system. Other development work that must be performed outside the core software (such as system interfaces), should be performed in a development environment. For final qualification testing, the software should be installed on the hardware and in the locations in which it will operate after final system acceptance. The preapproved installation qualification (IQ), operational qualification (OQ), and performance qualification (PQ) protocols will then be executed as defined in the test plan.

Once final system acceptance has been achieved, required system changes will be addressed differently. Development work and associated testing should occur in the development environment. Qualification testing will start with an initial IQ and subsequent OQ in the development environment. Upon successful completion of these tests, the system will be relocated to the production environment and the PQ will be performed. This approach will allow continued use of the currently approved system until the updated system is ready for PQ activities.

L. Installation Qualification Protocol

The installation qualification protocols check that the installed hardware (as defined in the system specification) is installed properly and that the proper software was installed correctly. The current configuration should be documented. The IQ may reference technical documentation provided by the vendor. Any deviations or omissions from the manuals should be documented. After installation and/or data conversion, verification procedures should be performed ensuring proper installation, including communications and data integrity.

M. Operational Qualification Protocol

The OQ protocols describe the steps and any necessary setup instructions to test the system against the system specification. This testing should focus on functional characteristics of the system, and include testing error conditions as well as conditions within normal acceptable ranges. Response times should also be tested as appropriate. The OQ identifies the expected and actual results, with the actual results being documented with screen prints, reports, or other definitive proof. Each test will define a single step or a process—the emphasis being on the correct result and its corresponding documentation to meet the specification. Any exceptions to the expected results should be logged and investigated by responsible personnel, and appropriate actions should be taken. Sufficient testing should be performed to assure that actions taken on exceptions are appropriate. When the protocols are finished a report could be created.

The OQ should be designed to take advantage of the any modular design of the MES software, if possible, and the testing already performed by the supplier or integrator. By recognizing and understanding the modularity, the OQ can be written to minimize redundant testing. After making an assessment of this testing and documentation, the OQ should be written to minimize overlap with previous testing that was adequately performed. Any application code developed for the site implementation will require more exhaustive testing than the supplier's application code.

N. Performance Qualification Protocol

The PQ protocol should demonstrate proper system operation during normal operating conditions. Any exceptions must be investigated and reconciled.

O. Validation Deliverables

1. Test plan: defines the approach to be used in qualification testing.
2. Installation qualification: provides documented evidence that the hardware and software have been installed properly. The IQ protocol must be approved before execution.
3. Operational qualification: provides documented evidence that the system operates properly throughout its defined ranges. The OQ protocol must be approved before execution.
4. Performance qualification: provides documented evidence that the system operates properly under normal operating conditions. The PQ protocol must be approved before execution.
5. Validation reports: summarizes the results of the IQ, OQ, and PQs.

P. Final Approval Phase

The final approval phase packages the project documentation and the validation deliverables for review. Quality assurance or a designated validation group normally leads a review of these documents, and after any questions or issues are satisfactorily addressed, final validation certification will be provided. Involvement of the appropriate personnel and periodic reviews should result in a timely review and approval of all documents.

Q. Validation Deliverables

1. User documentation package: contains all user procedures/SOPs.
2. System documentation package: Contains all system procedures/SOPs.
3. Training documentation: includes appropriate training materials and documentation showing that operators have been trained.
4. Validation package, including final validation certification: contains all validation documents.

R. Ongoing Evaluation Phase

The purpose of the ongoing evaluation phase is to maintain control of the system while allowing for a continuous improvement process. The MES system should be maintained in a validated state through the change control process, and required revalidation should be defined and applied per the validation master plan. Revalidation can occur as either a validation for a new software release or a standard system check. The standard system check should reference existing validation documents, while the new release validation will emphasize validation of the new features and their interrelationships. Appropriate effort must be placed into the testing of the specific upgrades and the related PQ to verify proper system functioning and data integrity.

S. Validation Deliverables

1. Change control documents: documents showing control of the change process, including approval, as defined in the change control process
2. Revalidation documents: documents required to demonstrate that the system has been revalidated as defined in the revalidation plan

IX. OPERATIONAL AND VALIDATION RESPONSIBILITIES

Overall, the production operations department should be ultimately responsible for the implementation and validation of the MES system. Support and assistance should be provided by the information systems department. One approach to this type of implementation has been the deployment of diverse teams with specific areas of expertise. This approach brings together the shop floor operational personnel and the management staff, as well as the supporting groups, such as quality assurance, information systems, and validation. Each department has a significant role in making these projects successful. Particular functions within the teams include the following:

1. System operations
2. System administration
   a. Application security
   b. New user setup
   c. Old user removal
   d. Management report generation
   e. Archiving old data
   f. Backup and recovery/archiving
3. User support
4. Training
5. Revalidation of application
6. Application of change control process
7. Disaster recovery
8. Revalidation of hardware

A. MES Project Team

The skill sets required for the MES project may be met with assigned individuals from each area or by allowing specific individuals to assume multiple roles. The following skills comprise the core of the MES project team:

Skill	*Responsibilities*
Project manager	Responsible for ensuring overall project completion, guiding project direction, ensuring proper communication and participation of managing vendors and consultants, and executing project tasks.
Information systems analyst	Responsible for ensuring technical system integrity, ensuring integration with other systems, and providing ongoing system support after implementation. Responsible for installing and configuring the system.
Industrial engineer (IE)	Responsible for providing IE perspective to requirements and application/solutions.
Documentation specialist	Responsible for defining batch record and report contents, determining document management requirements and solutions.
Operations	Responsible for defining processing requirements, reviewing design solutions, reviewing and approving project outputs, ensuring availability of manufacturing personnel, and operating the shop floor portion of the MES on an ongoing basis.
Automation specialist	Responsible for system interfacing.
Compliance specialist	Responsible for ensuring project outputs and the completed system meet compliance requirements on regulatory issues, approving validation deliverables.
Validation	Responsible for ensuring validation requirements are met, providing resources to write qualification protocols, approving and managing validation deliverables.
Vendor/consultants	Responsible for providing hardware/software and specific expertise not available, ensuring availability of additional consulting as needed.

Other personnel may be involved in project activities. Specific task responsibilities will be defined in the project plan. Project oversight will be provided by a project steering committee composed of senior management, typically from operations, quality assurance, and finance and administration.

B. Validation Document Approval

The creation of a checklist, including approvals required to ensure that all tasks are completed, is useful to support this approach. An example matrix showing departmental responsibilities for the creation and approval of each validation document is included in Table 1.

Each signature will certify that the document being signed has been reviewed by the signer, and that the contents achieve the purpose of the document, are functionally and technically sound, and conform to cGMP and company requirements. Multiple approvals may be needed.

Table 1 Departmental Responsibility Matrix

Phase and task	Operations	QA	IS	Validation
Project planning phase				
1. Scope and objectives	R,A	A	A	A
2. Validation plan	R,A	A	A	A
Requirements phase				
1. Functional requirements	R,A	A	A	A
2. Vendor evaluation		R,A	A	A
Design and development phase				
1. System specification	A	A	R,A	A
2. Development testing documentation	A	A	R,A	A
3. Programmed/configured software and hardware	A	A	R,A	A
Procedures development phase				
1. Operating (user) procedures	R,A	A		A
2. System management procedures		A	R,A	A
Testing phase				
1. Test plan	A	A	R,A	A
2. Installation qualification	A	A	R,A[b]	R,A[a]
3. Operational qualification	R,A[b]	A	A	R,A[a]
4. Performance qualification	R,A[b]	A	A	R,A[a]
5. Validation reports	A	A	A	R,A
Final approval phase				
1. User documentation package	R,A	A		A
2. System documentation package		A	R,A	A
3. Training documentation	R,A	A	A	A
4. Validation package	A	A	A	R,A
Ongoing evaluation phase				
1. Change control documentation	A	A	A	R,A
2. Revalidation documents		A		R,A

Note: Only primary responsibilities are identified. Activities may require key participation from multiple departments.
R = Responsible for activity completion.
A = Approver of activity deliverables.
[a]Primary responsibility for writing protocol.
[b]Primary responsibility for executing protocol.

20

One Keyboard Pounder's Views on Validation

Joseph A. Hercamp

Eli Lilly & Company, Indianapolis, Indiana

Let's face it. Validation is about "document envy." Who's got one? Whose is biggest? I've read a mountain of validation documents from the Federal Food, Drug, and Cosmetic Act to our own validation guidelines and numerous articles and white papers presented by people trying to cope with this issue. From all of this, I can identify two functions that keep America's best and brightest occupied: keep your products on the market and keep your management out of jail! Now, admittedly these are not fringe area objectives, but they do not satisfy the mandates of the government, private industry, or consumers.

Simply stated, validation should be based on values. When this is the case, a company's best talent uses data to make cost-effective, rational decisions about the best way to manufacture products. If it's not, the result is a cumbersome, adversarial system of fatigued compliance that's in no one's best interest.

Probably the right amount of validation documentation is somewhere between the amount your company did before its first "483" and less than it has done in the years since. The natural reaction to a 483 is to validate everything! As has been pointed out in numerous articles written on the subject, the quality of software and documentation generally benefits from a well-thought-out validation plan, but when validation is being done as a knee-jerk reaction to an audit, chances are the values part goes out the window and volume becomes a measure of quality.

In this chapter, I will try to cover the following points:

1. Why things are the way they are (there is enough blame to go around)
2. Why validation doesn't work the way you might think it does
3. Why technical people hate doing this stuff
4. Why now is the right time to change the way validation is done
5. An alternative approach to traditional process control software validation
6. Two examples of how I implemented the suggested approach
7. Summary—in case you don't really want to read this whole thing

I. WHY THINGS ARE THE WAY THEY ARE (THERE IS ENOUGH BLAME TO GO AROUND)

The government wants to assure the public that it can expect and rely on a safe and wholesome food supply and access to safe and effective drugs and medical devices. No one would disagree with this end. After all, we are all consumers. But the government has a problem. The FDA inspects and oversees almost 95,000 establishments producing food, drugs, medical devices, and animal health products. Many of these businesses are highly technical. FDA inspectors are expected to go to these companies and perform audits based on limited knowledge and limited time. In order to get an idea of how well the company is making its products, the inspector examines things that tend to run in parallel. Good paperwork means good software. There is some validity to this approach. Good paperwork probably does mean that good practices were followed in the development process. But we don't manufacture products in a file drawer. Real-time computing is affected by conditions that may or may not exist the day the initial testing was done. The indirect approach, therefore, can provide only limited assurance that the system is operating as it is intended. More on this later.

The government has as attitude problem. In a speech delivered on March 16, 1995, President Clinton remarked, "The Food and Drug Administration has made American drugs and medical devices the envy of the world and in demand all over the world." (Excuse me? I don't mind sharing the credit, but that's like going to a sporting event to see the referees!) Mr. Clinton is overinflating the role of the overseer. The FDA has an important role as overseer, but the government agencies are not the only ones watching what's going on. The public does not have the technical expertise or inclination to examine complex scientific data. This is where the FDA can add value. Market forces will provide the common sense. For example, last year Monsanto introduced an FDA-approved drug to be given to cows to boost milk production. Several grocery chains asked their suppliers not to ship milk from cows on the drug. The grocery chains believed the drug was safe but were worried about consumer reaction. So who is the overseer, the FDA or CNN? In today's world, a company's reputation is absolutely of paramount importance. No manufacturer can afford to have news stories about negligent manufacturing practices. Even in cases in which the manufacturer is not at fault, serious market damage can occur because of bad publicity. The real reason American drugs and medical devices are the envy of the world is the free enterprise system. As a consumer, I want products that are manufactured by reputable companies with the honest, best efforts of experts. I do not want that expertise overburdened with busywork that does not reflect their expert judgment and keeps them from applying their time in the best way.

There is more that can be done by those of us in private industry for the cause of good validation practices. We should always be asking ourselves, "How is this document adding value to the products of my customers?" Too often the validation documents produced are only for the auditors. It is ironic that the documentation strategy we use for computer validation uses a "paper" mentality. We would be better served by a system that is "smart"; that is, a monitoring functionality that notifies an expert when something requiring his attention has occurred. This is a departure from the traditional documentation scheme and it is up to private industry to make this kind of innovation. Staying with a paper system just because we have become proficient at generating paper documents will limit the effectiveness of the manufacturing expertise in private industry and underutilize the technology that allows for innovation in manufacturing.

II. WHY VALIDATION DOESN'T WORK THE WAY YOU MIGHT THINK IT DOES

The problem with the paper approach is that it ignores the facts! There are fundamental differences between the general purpose software world, in which the traditional validation scheme works fine, and real-time manufacturing. In the general purpose software world, software is written for the widest possible customer base. Therefore, special cases are usually avoided and it's left up to the user to pick the right application for the job. Also, there are usually few outside connections other than networks running specific protocols. The environment that the "shrink-wrap" software runs in is fixed. Feedback from thousands of users supply much of the "validation." Corrections and enhancements are made to the software in response to competition and to this customer feedback. In a pharmaceutical operation, the software is one-of-a-kind, written specifically for one situation. It connects to thousands of measurement and control devices. The dependencies of thousands of variables are extremely complex and may change, based on the real-time environment. In addition, there are not thousands of customers with feedback on system performance. While the initial testing of software is very useful, from a validation standpoint, data gathered as a process runs are more useful. Consistent data from one run to the next is a good indicator that the computer system is doing what it is supposed to do. A significant portion of the deficiencies in real-time software will only show up in the real-time environment.

Private industry wants to make safe and effective products at the lowest cost and market the products as widely as possible. An adversarial system encourages companies to develop validation protocols geared toward passing audits instead of producing the best manufacturing practices based on useful data, which was the idea in the first place. If it's paperwork that's needed to keep business going, then paperwork is what you'll get! But for special one-of-a-kind software developed by experts and supported by experts, is all this documentation necessary? (I am reminded of the packing materials that come with computer components that are stamped with the warning "DO NOT EAT." Darwinism will take care of the packing eaters in the first generation! Packing eaters do not read labels!) Much of the documentation produced will only be used during an audit or by a novice who is trying to familiarize himself with the software. By the time the novice has learned enough to be effective, the novice is no longer a novice! So we're back to the audit being the only time much of the documentation is used. Am I making this stuff up?

III. WHY TECHNICAL PEOPLE HATE DOING THIS STUFF

Once I asked my eight-year-old daughter why she didn't like playing goalie on her soccer team. She answered, "Because it's boring and it's hard!" I would add, "and you get kicked a lot and they score anyway!" So what's that got to do with validation? If you give someone enough latitude, no matter what you do, they can find something inconsistent in the complex paperwork describing the operation of a pharmaceutical plant. Most people that I have worked with would much rather be on the offensive side of solving problems and making improvements rather than trying to prove that no problems exist. It runs counter to personal and professional values.

We have a business belief statement that says, "I will use data and statistical thinking to make decisions that improve my business." When I am faced with solving a problem or making an improvement, I need DATA! I have never used a validation document in the normal course of my work. This is a very telling fact.

Another business belief statement says, "I will act with HONESTY and INTEGRITY and will treat people with RESPECT." Does this include while talking to auditors? An adversary system's main focus is to keep your mouth shut and hope that the auditor doesn't find out as much as you know! It doesn't matter what happens as long as you have some piece of paper somewhere that says it's not your fault! Can you think of a single technical expert who doesn't know of something that could show up in an audit? Would your answer be affected if you were currently being audited?

On the human nature side, most people will expend extra effort in order to avoid doing any amount of "boring" work. This characteristic can be used as an asset. Coercing people to produce documents that no one reads is fighting human nature. The inclination to do more than is useful can become the basis for better validation documents.

IV. WHY NOW IS THE RIGHT TIME TO CHANGE THE WAY VALIDATION IS DONE

If there was ever a time when people in both the public and private sectors were in a mood for change, this is it! In private industry, competition dictates that every expenditure must have a business driver. Companies have gone back to their core businesses and are examining all aspects of the business. Technology today can do a better job than merely making a paper system faster. The resources spent on validation can be used more effectively if the technology is used correctly. Validation should not just result in documents used during audits, but should be a part of the development process itself. The specific cases detailed later illustrate how tools used for checking out the program initially are used to provide continuous, comprehensive DATA to monitor system performance without adding unnecessary workload.

Political pressure and budget constraints are causing the government generally and the FDA in particular to examine regulations. In the report on the National Performance Review (April 1995), several significant reforms are outlined that change the way businesses are regulated. In the area of medical device manufacturing, it is reported that nearly 125 categories of low-risk medical devices will be exempted from premarket review. In the area of biologics manufacturing, a new FDA policy will permit the use of small-scale and pilot facilities during the development of biologics. In the area of insulin and antibiotic manufacturing, sections 506 and 507 of the Food, Drug, and Cosmetic Act may be repealed and section 505 used for the regulation of both insulin and antibiotic drug products. This would remove the special requirements that were imposed because of the limitations of technology in the 1940s. In the area of environmental assessment, virtually all drug product approvals will be excluded from the requirement for submitting environmental assessment or environmental impact statements.

New technology is being used within the FDA itself to improve service and cut operating costs. There is a system known as OASIS (operational and administrative system for import support) that the FDA is implementing to process imported products. Phase I was implemented nationwide in 1994. The system operates in conjuction with the Customs Service, with which import brokers are already online. Routine approvals that took days with the old paper system now can be processed and moved into commercial channels within minutes. According to the April 1995 National Performance Review, "In February 1995, 67 percent of all shipments processed in FDA's electronic system received final clearance within minutes.''

According to the same report, the FDA has proposed a regulation to permit regulated companies to use electronic records and signatures in place of paper. With the climate for change in both private industry and the government, this is the right time to change the focus and technology used for validation in our industry.

V. AN ALTERNATIVE APPROACH TO TRADITIONAL PROCESS CONTROL SOFTWARE VALIDATION

How do we usually handle jobs that are boring and hard? Let the computer do it! It makes sense to let the computers do the audits. The information needed for audits as well as to actually solve real problems is already in a computer somewhere. The data for traditional tests and those affected by real-time environmental conditions are both already being tracked for optimization reasons. Innovative tools can be developed for diagnostics and validation. Furthermore, the tools that are used to diagnose problems should be the same tools used for validation. This way, the company expertise is being used to cost-effectively make product; time is not being filled by unproductive activities. The data to verify that the products are being manufactured properly are constantly being generated. Manufacturing processes have predictable outcomes. What if we started by writing a program that checked to see if the desired result was obtained? Then, the job would be done when the testing program no longer found any errors! As changes are made, the data continue to be collected. Of course, if examination of the test data shows a deficiency in the tests, these adjustments can be made. In any case, the data will represent the expert's best efforts to manufacture products as correctly and cost-effectively as possible. This is not all fantasy! The examples described in the next section illustrate how this has been implemented for two different situations.

VI. TWO EXAMPLES OF HOW I IMPLEMENTED THE SUGGESTED APPROACH

A. Example 1

The first example describes how a program evolved from the initial idea of simplifying the testing procedure and making it more accurate to the development of a continuous, comprehensive monitoring program that notifies the appropriate person when an error is detected. And if that isn't enough, it was done with existing software. No additional purchases were made to accomplish this. It is simply a better way to use technology.

As a part of our data integration initiative, software adapters were written to transfer data from legacy systems to the common data exchange (CDE) based on triggered events. The details of the program are not important here. The simplified diagram below illustrates the basic function of the adapter, which is to move data from the legacy system to the CDE. The ultimate destination of the data is an Oracle database (see Fig. 1.)

A traditional approach for testing this type of application might be: for each event for which data are to be transferred, repeat the following five steps:

1. Look up the data associated with the event in the legacy system.
2. Calculate the statistical values to be sent to the CDE.
3. Find the output file in the output directory of the adapter.
4. Compare the results in the output file with those manually calculated.
5. Sign a piece of paper to document that the event has been checked.

Given the fact that there were hundreds of these events to check, I really didn't want to go through the above steps a few hundred times. I'm one of the people mentioned above who would rather expend extra effort doing something that I like doing than doing a moderate amount of boring work.

So I wrote a program that would extract the data for each event and another one to extract the same data from the Oracle database. One important attribute of this pair of programs is that not only was the adapter functionality checked out, the entire data path was checked out. As a matter of fact, all the components and configurations must be correct in order for the correct data to wind up in Oracle. Errors in components other than the adapter were identified as a result of these programs. After these two programs were written, lots of files were produced for the data in the data historian and in Oracle.

What a pain! Not only did I not want to extract data manually and do manual calculations, I didn't want to correlate the files for the two systems. So I changed the programs so that the data from both systems for a given event were written to the same file. This solved the correlation problem. Now I could compare the data by looking at one piece of paper for each event.

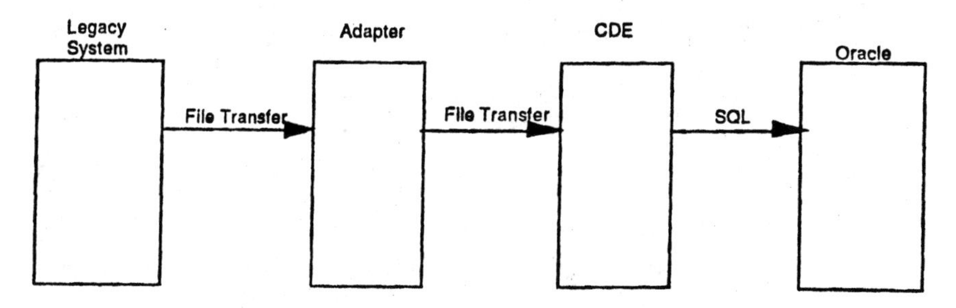

Fig. 1 Simplified diagram to illustrate the basic function of the adapter.

What a pain! Not only did I not want to extract data manually and do manual calculations or correlate the files, I didn't want to compare the data either! So I wrote another program to compare the data and produce a report. I could now read a report that marked all the "good" data and the data with errors.

What a pain! Not only did I not want to . . . , I didn't want to read the report either. So I wrote another program that reads the report and sends me a mail message telling me the correct conditions and the error conditions.

Well, you might have guessed it—I don't even want to read the mail message unless I have to, so the program that sends the mail message was changed so that the subject line of the mail message will be the word "OK" or "DISCREPANCY" . . . . So then all I had to do was read the directory of my mail messages. If OK appears in the subject of the message, I just file the report and go on to other activities. If the word discrepancy appears, I know I need to read the message and follow the lead. The nice thing about it is that all the backup information has been prepared and formatted in the mail message. The validation program is what I use for diagnostics!

The mail directory looks like this when everything goes well.

```
---------------------------------------------------------------------

NEWMAIL
    # From                   Date          Subject

    1 BHIHIST::KK24769        16-DEC-1994  HISTORIAN - ORACLE OK
    2 (Deleted)

LMail>
---------------------------------------------------------------------
```

This is what the mail directory looks like when an error has been detected.

```
---------------------------------------------------------------------
                                                        MAIL
    # From                   Date          Subject

   51 BHIHIST::KK24769        15-DEC-1994  HISTORIAN - ORACLE DISCREPANCY

Press RETURN for more...

      LMail>
---------------------------------------------------------------------
```

There is one rule that results in the above error message. The word ERROR appears in the report file. In other words, any error will be reported electronically to the responsible person. It's getting harder to lie these days!

If the mail message indicates an error, I now have a choice. I can either read the mail message or go to the report file directly and see what errors have occurred. Actually, the body of the mail message *is* the report. Again, the diagnostic tool is the same as the validation/notification tool. Following are a few lines from the report file. (These are the same lines that appear in the body of the mail message.) Here we can examine three types of errors.

```
-----------------------------------------------------------------------------

flt2555cip       30-NOV-1994 22:54:29.00                  Start Time OK
flt2555cip       01-DEC-1994 00:06:11.00                    End Time OK

col3388elute     30-NOV-1994 20:59:13.00                  Start Time OK
col3388elute     01-DEC-1994 00:31:12.00                    End Time OK
col3388elute     COL3388ELUTE FC3388A-H_TWAV-APVCUR           Value ERROR
col3388elute     COL3388ELUTE FC3388APO-H TWAV-AMVCUR         Value OK
col3388elute     COL3388ELUTE PC3388A-H_TWAV-APVCUR           Value OK
col3388elute     COL3388ELUTE TC3388A-H_TWAV-APVCUR           Value OK
-----------------------------------------------------------------------------
```

The first couple of lines show a successful event that supplies only the start and end times to the Oracle database. The second group of lines shows an error that occurred as a result of the data compression tolerance and capture rate of the variable. The details are not important for the purpose of this discussion. The point here is that a difference was detected between what the data historian recorded and what someone will see when he or she extract the data from the Oracle database. A person was notified by electronic mail that human analysis is required for this piece of data.

The next few lines show another type of error.

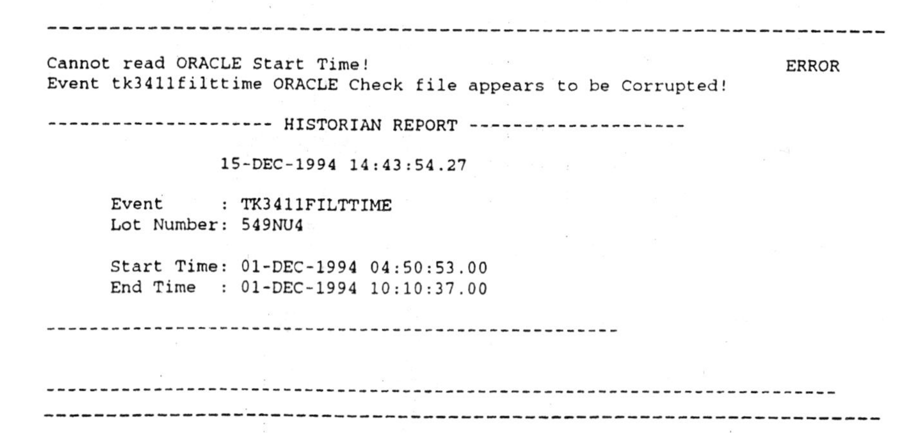

```
-----------------------------------------------------------------------------

Cannot read ORACLE Start Time!                                        ERROR
Event tk3411filttime ORACLE Check file appears to be Corrupted!

-------------------- HISTORIAN REPORT --------------------

               15-DEC-1994 14:43:54.27

      Event      : TK3411FILTTIME
      Lot Number: 549NU4

      Start Time: 01-DEC-1994 04:50:53.00
      End Time   : 01-DEC-1994 10:10:37.00

----------------------------------------------------


-----------------------------------------------------------------------
-----------------------------------------------------------------------------
```

In this case, the data were extracted from the data historian and processed by the adapter. However, the data never made it to the Oracle database. This is an example of how this tool that was designed to monitor the performance of the adapter is actually monitoring other components in the data path as well. The data shown above are very valuable to someone tracking down a problem downstream of the adapter. The event name and time stamp will show up in the error journal files.

This satisfied the original goal of simplifying the testing, but as has been pointed out earlier, real-time operations produce useful test data continuously, so the procedure described above is executed as a batch job each night and resubmits itself for the next day. This means that 100 percent of the data being processed by the adapter and all the other components in the data path are checked every day with no additional human resources required.

B. Example 2

The second example shows how data from the distributed control system (DCS) are compared with the data delivered to the data historian. In large processing plants, it is common to use configuration tools and databases to configure both DCS systems and data historians. One challenge is to keep the configurations of the DCS, the data historian, and the "gate" that connects them in synch. The situation increases in complexity as the systems become larger and more people execute changes. As changes are made either to the configuration or to the gate, a tool to verify the correct configurations is useful. Again, a single tool is used for validation and diagnostics. In this case, a server is written for the DCS and

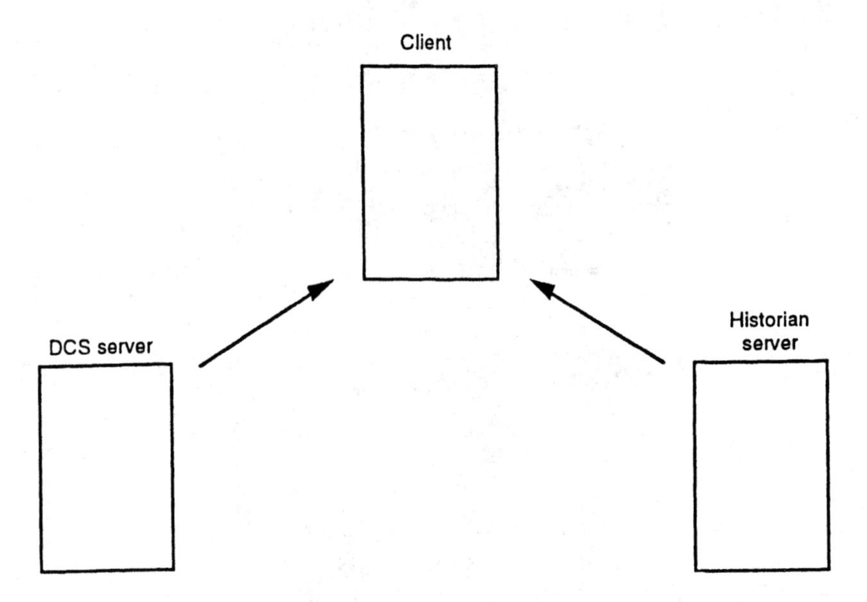

Fig. 2 Diagram of a utility to extract the same data from the DCS and the data historian.

for the data historian. A client program is written to run on the same computer that is used for the configuration utilities. Since the configuration databases are available to the client, it is simple to write a utility to extract the same data from both the DCS and the data historian. This is diagrammed below. The data can be electronically checked any time a change is made, fulfulling the data validation function, or can be checked on demand any time a question arises about the data transfer. (See Fig. 2.)

A typical report file is shown in Fig. 3. Some identification information, such as the file name and date produced, appears at the top of the report file. This is followed by specific information about all the data transferred in the ''transfer set.'' The value reported by the DCS and the value delivered to the data historian for each variable appear on the same line. The difference is calculated and displayed in the right-hand column. As was the case in the first example, reading and closely examining a few hundred of these files is tedious and better done by the computer. The report files are examined by a program that generates a summary report. In all cases, the identification information is written to the summary report so that all the transfer sets being tested are positively included. Only significant differences need to be reported. The compression tolerance is therefore taken into account when reporting differences. This greatly reduces the amount of data that must be reviewed by a person. Excerpts from the summary report are shown following Fig. 3.

DCS - Historian Comparison Report

NODE: mv142h

FILE: sys_hist:[hist_proj.bhihist.compare]mv142h_pidp_10.compare

16-DEC-1994 16:17:05.22

Tag		Value	Type	Number		Value	Difference
NODE42\INDXCIP2\FQ2144CPV	=	476.000000	PV	3509	=	476.000000	0.000000
NODE43\INDXTRAN\FT2920FPV	=	-0.000397	PV	3250	=	-0.000397	0.000000
NODE43\INDXTRAN\FT2920GPV	=	-0.005035	PV	3251	=	-0.005539	0.000504
NODE43\INDXTRAN\AT2922APV	=	4.080688	PV	3252	=	4.080688	0.000000
NODE43\INDXTRAN\LT2922APV	=	-0.370850	PV	3253	=	-0.370850	0.000000
NODE43\INDXTRAN\AT2923APV	=	4.144531	PV	3254	=	4.144531	0.000000
NODE43\INDXTRAN\LT2923APV	=	71.000000	PV	3255	=	70.980469	0.019531
NODE43\INDXTRAN\FQ2920FPV	=	18.808594	MV	3511	=	18.808594	0.000000
NODE43\INDXTRAN\FQ2920GPV	=	49.652344	MV	3512	=	49.652344	0.000000
NODE43\INDXTRAN\FQ2922FPV	=	6.298950	MV	3513	=	6.298950	0.000000
NODE43\INDXTRAN\FQ2922GPV	=	27.917480	MV	3514	=	27.917480	0.000000
NODE43\INDXTRAN\FQ2923FPV	=	6.198975	MV	3515	=	6.198975	0.000000
NODE43\INDXTRAN\FQ2923GPV	=	14.104248	MV	3516	=	14.104248	0.000000
NODE43\INDXTRAN\FT2922APV	=	0.127686	PV	3256	=	0.127686	0.000000
NODE43\INDXTRAN\SC2922APV	=	0.069336	PV	3257	=	0.055176	0.014160
NODE43\INDXTRAN\SC2922ASP	=	0.055176	TV	3257	=	0.055176	0.000000
NODE43\INDXTRAN\SC2922APO	=	30.000000	MV	3257	=	30.000000	0.000000
NODE43\INDXTRAN\TC2922BPV	=	15.211914	PV	3258	=	15.211914	0.000000
NODE43\INDXTRAN\TC2922BSP	=	15.211914	TV	3258	=	15.211914	0.000000
NODE43\INDXTRAN\TC2922BPO	=	9.999756	MV	3258	=	9.999756	0.000000
NODE43\INDXTRAN\TC2922APV	=	14.750000	PV	3259	=	14.750000	0.000000
NODE43\INDXTRAN\TC2922ASP	=	14.737305	TV	3259	=	14.737305	0.000000
NODE43\INDXTRAN\TC2922APO	=	15.216553	MV	3259	=	15.216553	0.000000
NODE43\INDXTRAN\FT2923APV	=	2.571045	PV	3260	=	2.571045	0.000000
NODE43\INDXTRAN\SC2923APV	=	59.818359	PV	3261	=	59.978516	0.160157
NODE43\INDXTRAN\SC2923ASP	=	60.000000	TV	3261	=	60.000000	0.000000
NODE43\INDXTRAN\SC2923APO	=	73.113281	MV	3261	=	73.087891	0.025390
NODE43\INDXTRAN\TC2923BPV	=	5.203125	PV	3262	=	5.203125	0.000000
NODE43\INDXTRAN\TC2923BSP	=	5.163818	TV	3262	=	5.163818	0.000000
NODE43\INDXTRAN\TC2923BPO	=	3.400208	MV	3262	=	3.400208	0.000000
NODE43\INDXTRAN\TC2923APV	=	4.989258	PV	3263	=	4.989258	0.000000
NODE43\INDXTRAN\TC2923ASP	=	4.989258	TV	3263	=	4.989258	0.000000
NODE43\INDXTRAN\TC2923APO	=	5.163818	MV	3263	=	5.163818	0.000000
NODE43\INDXTRAN\FV2922FFBPV	=	0.000000	MV	3517	=	0.000000	0.000000
NODE43\INDXTRAN\FV2922GFBPV	=	0.000000	MV	3518	=	0.000000	0.000000
NODE43\INDXTRAN\FV2923FFBPV	=	0.000000	MV	3519	=	0.000000	0.000000
NODE43\INDXTRAN\FV2923GFBPV	=	0.000000	MV	3520	=	0.000000	0.000000
NODE43\INDXTRAN\FV2922RFBPV	=	0.000000	MV	3521	=	0.000000	0.000000
NODE43\INDXTRAN\FV2923RFBPV	=	0.000000	MV	3522	=	0.000000	0.000000
NODE43\INDXFAFS\AC3073APV	=	26617.000000	PV	3368	=	26617.001953	0.001953
NODE43\INDXFAFS\AC3073ASP	=	25000.000000	TV	3368	=	25000.000000	0.000000
NODE43\INDXFAFS\AC3073APO	=	0.000000	MV	3621	=	0.000000	0.000000
NODE43\INDXFAFS\FC3073APV	=	0.003357	PV	3372	=	0.003357	0.000000
NODE43\INDXFAFS\FC3073ASP	=	3.099976	TV	3372	=	3.099976	0.000000
NODE43\INDXFAFS\FC3073APO	=	0.000000	MV	3625	=	0.000000	0.000000
NODE43\INDXFAFS\PC3073APV	=	6.778809	PV	3373	=	6.778809	0.000000
NODE43\INDXFAFS\PC3073ASP	=	16.000000	TV	3373	=	16.000000	0.000000
NODE43\INDXFAFS\PC3073APO	=	0.000000	MV	3626	=	0.000000	0.000000
NODE43\INDXFAFS\FT3073BPV	=	0.001678	PV	3374	=	0.000854	0.000824

Checked By ______________ Date ________

Fig. 3 Typical report file.

```
NODE12\INDXCLEV_7\LT0151APV     = 81.210938     PV  245 = 79.226563      1.984375
NODE12\INDXCLEV_7\FT0152APV     = 147.136719    PV  248 = 144.449219     2.687500
NODE13\INDXFARM_6\PC5201APV     = 65.128906     PV  256 = 87.718750      22.589844


==================================================================
==================================================================

            Node mv142e   18-OCT-1994 11:31:31.75

  FILE: sys_hist:[hist_proj.bhihist.compare]mv142e_pidp_11.compare


==================================================================
==================================================================

            Node mv142e   18-OCT-1994 11:32:11.28

  FILE: sys_hist:[hist_proj.bhihist.compare]mv142e_pidp_12.compare

NODE13\INDXFARM_7\FT5120CPV     = 9.360840      PV  312 = 15.200684      5.839844
NODE13\INDXFARM_7\FQ5120CPV     = 90816.000000  MV  551 = 90818.000000   2.000000


==================================================================
==================================================================
```

VII. SUMMARY—IN CASE YOU DON'T REALLY WANT TO READ THIS WHOLE THING

This section is mostly for those who skipped the geeky stuff in the last sections. Here are the main points.

Traditional validation documentation, while produced with the best of intentions, does not satisfy government, industry, or consumer mandates. An adversarial relationship between regulatory agencies and industry promotes secrecy and the inefficient use of resources.

Validation based on values—data, honesty, and integrity—serves customer interest and allows industry resources to be innovative in the design and implementation of validation tools that not only provide useful documents, but actually aid in the manufacturing process itself.

21

A Validation Plan for Process Automation

Kenneth S. Kovacs

Bailey Controls Company, Wickliffe, Ohio

Joseph F. deSpautz

INCODE Corp., Herndon, Virginia

I. THE VALIDATION PROJECT PLAN

It is highly recommended that validation be considered an integral part of all appropriate projects as early as possible in the schedule to ensure that all necessary steps have been taken during each project phase. When planning the project, utilizing a life cycle validation methodology for computer-related systems will provide the basis for a suggested validation project plan (1).

> The purpose of a Validation Project Plan is to identify the systems to be included and the procedures to be followed in a specific validation project. The procedures described in a Validation Project Plan should be consistent with established policies and should reference appropriate validation SOP's. . . . an important purpose of a Validation Project Plan is to establish specific responsibilities and expectations for each validation task (1).

In this section an example of an outline is presented with pertinent forms, worksheets, and information to assist in detailing the validation steps presented for the implementation of a validation project plan.

The documentation format should be consistent with each company's own requirements defined by its validation policies and procedures. Headers and footers should include space for the company's name, the project name, dates, section

Company: ______________

COMPUTER SYSTEM

VALIDATION PROJECT PLAN

For

Project: ______________

Approved By: ______________ ______
Quality Assurance Date

______________ ______
Operations Date

______________ ______
Engineering Date

______________ ______
General Management Date

Prepared By: ______________ ______
Title Date

Fig. 1 Validation project plan example cover sheet (3).

designations, revision numbers, page numbers, and the responsible party's name, department, and signature along with the reviewer's name, department, and signature. Pertinent headings, test names, instructions, references, text, and comments should be included in the main body of the document pages. Formats should present summary reports, documentation, detailed data, and test results in a clear manner that is logical and easy to read (2,3; Fig. 1).

II. VALIDATION MILESTONES

With all validation programs, milestones will be encountered during the validation effort of the computer-related system. In most cases these milestones involve the approval of documentation with respect to the validation effort. Pertinent milestones are represented in the validation methodology diagram in Fig. 2 and are discussed in the following sections (2,3).

A. Validation Plan Approval

After the approval of the validation plan, any revisions will follow all requirements of the appropriate change control standard operating procedure (SOP). A change control SOP specific to the validation plan will be implemented and will outline the requirements that must be followed in order to revise this document.

B. SOP Approval

An important milestone for the validation effort is the generation and approval of all validation SOPs. These SOPs shall include appropriate procedures for changing or revising all approved documents. The quality control unit will generate and clearly establish all responsibilities relating to these documents.

C. System Specifications Approval

All protocol generation, software development, prequalification testing, and final report approval shall be based upon the system specifications document. A change control SOP will be established for controlling any revisions to these specifications. Any necessary revisions to this document will be evaluated and formally approved by the appropriate personnel.

D. Protocol Approval

Qualification protocols based upon the appropriate specifications will be developed. A change control procedure for approved protocols will be established. Revisions to approved protocols will be evaluated with respect to the system specification, and all revisions will be evaluated and formally approved by the appropriate personnel.

E. System Release to Validation

Once a system is released for validation (based on the software quality assurance report [SQAR]), the system will be placed under formal change control procedures. System changes will be evaluated with respect to their impact on the system specifications, and any revision to the software after release must be approved

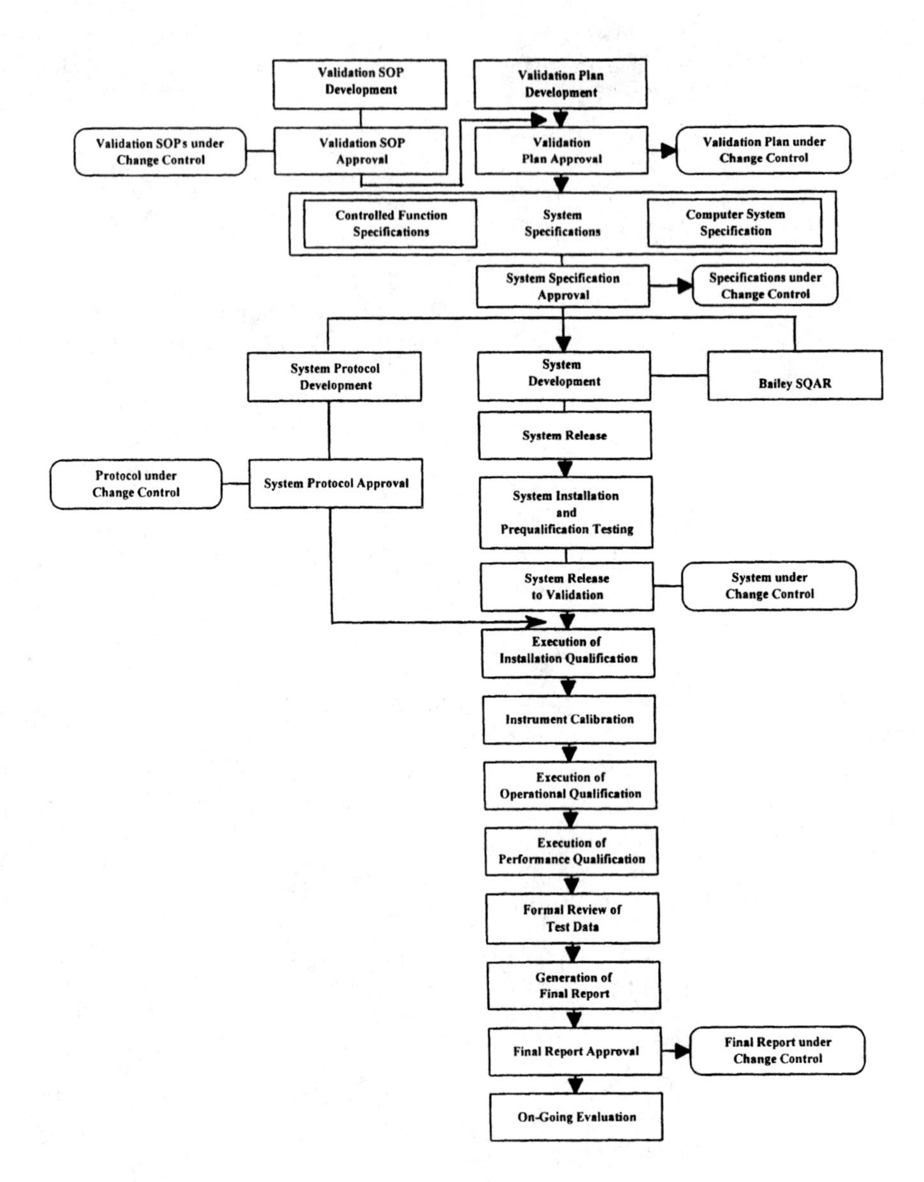

Fig. 2 A validation methodology (2).

by the appropriate personnel. All documentation of the software will be modified to reflect the changes according to a written procedure.

A milestone shall be formally noted when change management responsibilities transfer from the systems vendor to the end user.

F. Qualification Testing

All testing will follow procedures outlined in the approved validation protocols. Any deficiencies or deviations from approved test procedures found during testing will be formally reviewed and evaluations made for taking appropriate action. Change control procedures must be followed if revisions are made to approved test procedures.

G. Test Data Review and Verification

All data gathered during the testing period will be verified for accuracy. An evaluation of test data will be the basis of summary reports for final validation documents.

H. Final Report Approval

Once the test data are reviewed and their accuracy verified, final reports will be prepared that summarize the data and present conclusions and recommendations based upon the comparison of the data with the specifications. A specific change control SOP will be established for final report revisions.

III. COMPUTER SYSTEM VALIDATION PROJECT PLAN OUTLINE

The contents of a typical computer-related system validation plan should include sections with such information as the following.

A. Planning

1. Purpose: statements defining the boundaries and relationships for which the validation plan was created
2. Scope: overview, general description of systems to be validated, including location, function, equipment/processes to be controlled; and products to be run
3. Responsibilities: staffing and manpower—establishes the validation team along with the responsibilities and approvals required for each of the validation plan tasks
4. Documented policies, SOPs, protocols, instructions, guidelines, and references for executing the validation plan

5. Validation SOPs approval
6. Validation plan approval

B. Definition of Requirements

1. Methodologies: Standards, guidelines, formats, codes, or other references applicable to the validation project scope
2. Schedules: For all program tasks, with detailed responsibilities; also include schedule for validation project milestones and approvals
3. Functional requirements
4. Design requirements
5. System requirements
6. Performance test specifications

C. Selection of Vendors

1. Vendor/developer audits and evaluations
2. System hardware and software evaluations
3. Requests for proposal along with quotations
4. Vendor/system selection

D. System Design

1. Functional specifications
2. Design specifications
3. System specifications
4. System specifications approvals
5. Qualification protocol approvals
6. System design activities—hardware and software
7. Software quality assurance plan (SQAP), including detailed hardware and software test plans
8. System test plans and methodologies

E. System Construction

1. Construct and test hardware with all activities documented.
2. Develop and test software with all activities documented.
3. Integrate hardware and software for computer system.
4. Test computer system.
5. Develop factory acceptance test (FAT) and plan and document FAT results. (See the appendix of this chapter for an example of an FAT work plan.)
6. Compile system, applications, and user documentation.

F. Installation and Integration

1. Installation instructions, drawings, and documentation
2. Interconnection instructions, drawings, and documentation for the computer system and controlled function equipment
3. System start-up plan and documented implementation
4. Computerized system site acceptance and diagnostic tests along with documented results

G. Qualification

1. System release to validation
2. Qualification test plans
3. Installation qualification (IQ): overview, procedures for performing the qualification, and detailed protocols for testing the system; documentation of IQ results; summary report of IQ
4. Operational qualification (OQ): overview, procedures for performing the qualification, and detailed protocols for testing the system; documentation of OQ results; summary report of OQ
5. Documents subject to change control procedures
6. Test data reviews and verification
7. Summary report approval

H. Evaluation

1. Performance qualification (PQ): *the* step for validation providing rigorous testing for a full system challenge; overview, procedures for performing the qualification, and detailed protocols for testing the system; documentation of PQ results; summary report of PQ
2. Change control procedures
3. Security management
4. Periodic review and audit criteria
5. Provisions for revalidation
6. Disaster recovery and contingency plans
7. Maintenance programs
8. Calibration programs
9. Preventive maintenance programs
10. Training
11. Documentation of ongoing programs: system documentation, training SOPs, records for maintenance, change control, etc.; established location for storage of validation and system documentation, and computer software backup media
12. Final report review, verification, and approval

I. Summary

1. Validation project summary report
2. Reports for each of the validation steps
3. Support data
4. References
5. Relevant drawings
6. Capability studies and statistical process control (SPC) documentation
7. All other information in support of the validation effort

IV. THE VALIDATION TEAM

Team members will typically possess expertise in computer system hardware and software, process controls, quality assurance, network communications, and systems engineering. Other team members should be assigned as required to meet the objectives of the specific project. This section should list the team member by name, designate a team leader, and define their roles in the validation effort. Signature requirements and approvals for each section or task associated with the validation plan must also be documented. All personnel on this team must have the necessary experience and training to carry out their assignments. A typical validation team may include the following.

Team member	Responsibilities
Engineering	For qualification work on computer systems, networks, controls, and equipment
Management information systems	For qualification work and audits on computer systems, networks, and software
R&D	For qualification work on product manufacturing processes
Manufacturing	To operate: plant, equipment, support systems, facilities, and manufacturing processes
Quality assurance	To perform quality assurance (QA) audits for validation plan activities and computer system qualification work
Vendor(s)	To support validation team for activities associated with delivered system(s)

V. QUALIFICATION TESTING

The results of all qualification testing must be compared to predefined expectations. In the event that a test did not produce the expected results, remedial action shall be taken and retesting performed. Regressive testing is important to include following discrepancy corrections. This regressive testing is to demonstrate that earlier test results are still accurate in light of the side effects that a software modification can have on other software functions.

Software test documentation should include the following:

- A description of exactly what each test case is designed to demonstrate
- The exact data to be used for each test
- The expected results from running a test case
- Actual test results

All tests, acceptance criteria, test results, remedial actions, and retests must be documented. Qualification documentation should now be subject to ''change control'' procedures.

A. Installation Qualification

Details of the IQ should include the protocols and resultant documentation for the following:

1. Verification of installed hardware
2. Verification of installed software version
3. Verification that appropriate software backup copies exist
4. Consideration of manufacturer's installation recommendations
5. Ability to meet appropriate codes and regulations
6. Hardware checkout and testing
7. Adherence to approved design specifications
8. Verification of deliverables and other documentation, such as
   a. Equipment specifications
   b. Bills of materials
   c. Purchase orders
   d. Process and instrumentation diagrams (P&IDs)
   e. Power and fusing
   f. Connection diagrams
   g. Acceptance forms
   h. Wiring diagrams
   i. SOPs for system operation
   j. Instrument calibration records
   k. Software description
   l. Flowcharts
   m. Discrepancy resolution
   n. I/O listings
   o. Wiring and cable
   p. Location and layout diagrams
   q. Document approvals

r. Schematics
s. Vendor and user manuals
t. Source code information
u. Maintenance requirements
v. Diagnostic procedures
w. IQ test results documentation
x. IQ approvals
y. IQ summary report

B. Operational Qualification

Details of the OQ should include the protocols for the execution of specific tasks and resultant documentation for such things as the following:

- Completion of IQ
- Operating ranges
- Failure mode testing
- Operational test plans
- Interlocks and safety logic
- Acceptance criteria
- Acceptance forms
- Operating parameters
- Security requirements
- Operator training
- Functional testing
- Discrepancy resolution
- SOPs
- Document approvals
- OQ test results documentation
- OQ approvals
- OQ summary report

C. Performance Qualification

The PQ (validation phase) provides the documented evidence that the entire process, under computer control, repeatably and reliably produces an end product that meets all the predetermined quality attributes.

This phase of the program assures that

- IQ/OQ documentation and approvals are complete
- The system controlling the process is tested with actual operating conditions
- The design performance criteria has been satisfied
- End products meet specifications and quality attributes

INSTRUMENT CALIBRATION DATA

Company Name: ______________________

Location: ______________________

EQUIPMENT IDENTIFICATION			
Instrument ID:		Equipment ID:	
Manufacturer:		Serial No.	
Instr. Type:		Range:	
Calibration Cycle:		Accuracy:	
Standard(s) Used			
Manufacturer	Serial No.	Date Due	NIST Test No.

Standard	Instrument		Tolerance	
Input	As Found	As Left	Minimum	Maximum

Remarks: ______________________

____

____

Next Date Due: ______

Calibrated By: ______________________ Date: ______

Approved By: ______________________ Date: ______

Fig. 3 Instrument calibration data sheet example (3,4).

D. System Qualification (Validation) Approvals

Once the PQ is completed, a summary report for the computer-related system validation, along with the summaries of the qualification phases, should be issued. This documentation must be reviewed for completeness, discrepancy resolution, and consistency between test results and summary statements. Once reviewed by responsible personnel, the summary report can be circulated for approval within the organization in accordance with the validation plan. The objective of this step is to formally release the computer-related system for use in the manufacturing

CONTROL LOOP TEST DATA

Company Name: ______________________

Location: ______________________

LOOP IDENTIFICATION	
Loop ID:	Equipment ID:
Tagname:	Location:
Address:	Range:
Loop Type:	Accuracy:
Termination ID:	Units:
Wire Nos.:	

Standard	Sensor	Transmitter	DCS	Tolerance	
Input/Value	Output	Output	Value	Min.	Max.

Remarks: ______________________

____

Tested By: ______________________ Date: __________

Approved By: ______________________ Date: __________

Fig. 4 Control loop test data sheet example (3,4).

environment to perform its intended function as defined by the system specifications, and to ensure that the system will continue to operate consistently and reliably in a validated state.

E. Qualification Sheets-Format Examples

Figures 3–6 provide examples of the types of formats that can be used to organize data and present validation information in a clear and concise manner (3,4).

Qualification Testing Procedures Page __of ____

Project : ______________________________ Date: _______

Test Name: ______________________________ Test No.: _____

Test Description:

References:

Test Procedures:

Acceptance Criteria:

Actual Results:

Acceptance Criteria Met: Yes _____ No _____ N/A _____
Corrective Action: Yes ________ No ___

Comments:

Tested By: ______________________________

Reviewed By: ______________________________
Name Title Signature Date

Fig. 5 Qualification test sheet example format for IQ/OQ (3,4).

VI. APPENDIX: FACTORY ACCEPTANCE TESTING

A. A Sample Work Plan

Customer project management and technical personnel are expected to attend and participate in the FAT activity. This will involve a prescheduled step-by-step exercise of all elements of the test plan with appropriate documentation of all tests performed (3). Customer representatives will approve successfully completed tests and list items requiring additional work. Successful conclusion and approval of the FAT represents acceptance of the system for shipment.

Qualification Summary Report Page ___ of ___ _ ___

Project : ______________________________ Date: ___________

Summary For: IQ ____ OQ ___ PQ ___

References:

Test Category Summary Statements:

One Summary Statement for each of the relevant qualification tests is provided in this section. Results and documented information verifying that test acceptance criteria was met is affirmed in each statement.

Attesting signatures for each statement must be included in each section by the person responsible for those tests.

Comments:

Summary Report

Completed By: ______________________________

Reviewed By: ______________________________

Name Title Signature Date

Fig. 6 Qualification summary report example format (3,4).

1. Commence with the introduction of key participants along with their functions and responsibilities; review the FAT schedule, establish checkout review and approval meetings, and provide an outline of events associated with FAT procedural activities.
2. Review procedures, plans, schedules, and documentation for addressing daily punch list items.
3. Conduct a visual inspection of inventory of hardware deliverables.
4. Conduct a visual inspection and inventory of documentation.
5. Examine and verify tagging and equipment identification.
6. Examine and verify cable routing and termination connections.

7. Provide summary documentation of daily punch list items addressing installation and physical inspections.
8. Provide summary review and report of physical inspections.
9. Run system-level diagnostics.
10. Perform operational testing of system start-up initialization.
11. Load and verify system software and applications database.
12. Perform power interruption operational testing.
13. Perform transmitter voltage testing.
14. Perform system keyboards operational testing.
15. Perform loop checks.
16. Perform applications logic testing.
17. Perform checkout of display graphics and dynamic functions.
18. Provide summary documentation of daily punch list items addressing system operational testing.
19. Provide summary review and report of operational testing.
20. Provide summary review and report of FAT procedures, plans, schedules, and documentation for addressing daily punch list items.
21. Deliver pertinent documentation to customer.
22. Conduct summary meeting regarding system FAT; review accomplishments, outstanding items, plans, schedules, and documentation.
23. Execute FAT procedures for customer acceptance and approvals for shipment of the system.

REFERENCES

1. "PDA Report No. 18, Validation of Computer-Related Systems," PDA, 1995 Supplement, Volume 49, Number S1, Bethesda, Maryland.
2. "System Integration Methodology in Support of FDA Compliance," Bailey Controls Company, Wickliffe, Ohio, 1994.
3. K. S. Kovacs, *Validation Assurance and GMP Compliance*, Elsag Bailey Process Automation, Wickliffe, Ohio, 1995.
4. K. S. Kovacs, *Qualification Testing and Documentation for Computerized Systems; A Suggested Approach and Format*, Fischer & Porter, Warminster, Pennsylvania, July 1994.

22

Performance Qualification Testing of Integrated MRP/MES

Joseph F. deSpautz

INCODE Corp., Herndon, Virginia

Kenneth S. Kovacs

Bailey Controls Company, Wickliffe, Ohio

I. INTRODUCTION

This chapter addresses validation aspects of a planned manufacturing resource planning (MRPII versus MRP, which started as materials requirements planning) and manufacturing execution system (MES) integration project. We will use MRP to include both MRPII and MRP system functionalities. It should be noted that the overall project plan should include the validation activities described. Validation should not be treated as an activity separate from the project. This approach ensures that the system is designed properly, operates properly, and may be maintained properly. It also ensures that the cost of validation, both in time and money, does not negatively impact the project schedule.

Validation of the computer systems involved in the production of pharmaceutical products is a required activity. This is a requirement because the computer systems directly support the processing of product and therefore have an effect on the product quality. Regulatory agencies and industry groups maintain this position.

As computer-related systems become more complex, the validation testing requirements become more involved and complex as well. Systems are being integrated at all manufacturing domains from level 1 to level 5, being defined as control, supervisory, execution, MRP, and enterprise. To fully validate an integrated system requires considerable knowledge of the applications, the business processes being automated, and the information technology principles used in

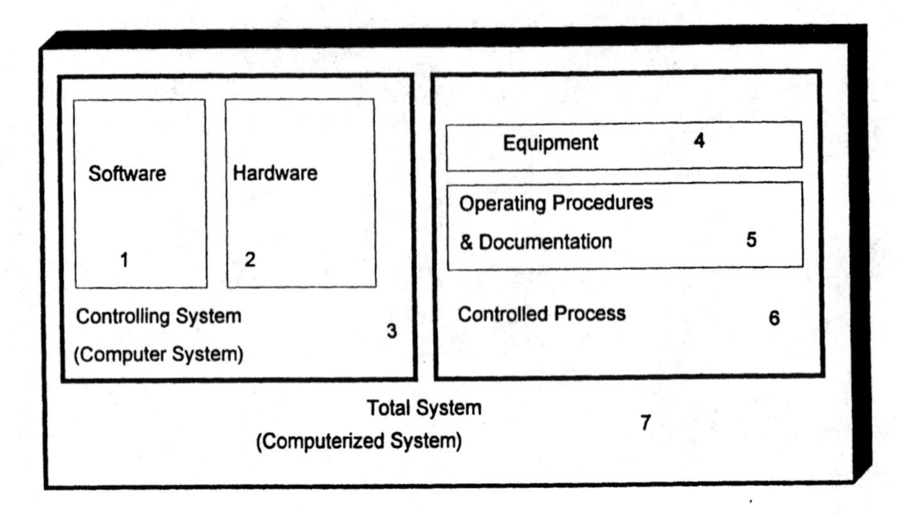

Fig. 1 Computer-related system (1).

the computer-related system. For this chapter, we are focusing on validation testing of the computer system (software and hardware), not the total system (computerized system). The distinction is exemplified in Fig. 1 which provides a block diagram of the various system components. The validation project plan for the integrated project must also be tied to the validation plan for the level 1 control system to sure total system operability.

II. MRP AND MES OPERATIONS

The scope of a typical integrated MRP-MES project includes operational activities to support, as listed below.

1. Purchasing
   a. Purchase order management
   b. Receiving reconciliation
2. Materials management
   a. Material receiving, lot and container or sublot tracking
   b. Inventory and work in process (WIP) control
   c. Grading, potency, and shelf life dating, and expiry date calculations
   d. Lot release and expiry date management
3. Recipe management
   a. Recipe creation and version control
   b. Integration with MRP specifications and inventory management
4. Batch management
   a. MRP-generated dispatch orders

   b. Production order management using recipes
   c. Recipe execution and production history data collection
5. Lot tracking
   a. Tracking of all materials, equipment, and human resources that come in contact with the product during manufacture
   b. Developing forward and backward genealogy recording
   c. Sample tracking
6. Electronic batch record creation
   a. Plant floor management/electronic work instructions
   b. Data and event collection requirements
   c. Packaging scheduling and control
   d. Quality assurance information
7. Document management and change control
   a. Repository for all required and approved documentation
   b. Issuance of documents needed for operations
   c. Repository for batch records

To test the integrated system means that the validation test protocol must provide test cases and test data sets for testing, including the following:

- Independent MRP system functionality
- Independent MES system functionality
- MRP to MES integration functionality where MES operations are dependent on the MRP system data, data dependencies, and product structures
- Corresponding MES to MRP integration functionality

Typical MRP systems will have over 120 separate transactions, of which ten to twenty are needed for integration to and from the MES environment to support the requirements defined in Table 1. The remaining internal transactions are only tested in the validation test plan if the application modules are required for current good manufacturing practices (cGMP) operations.

The MES system will generate twenty to thirty transactions to initiate, control, and record the manual and semiautomatic operations as defined in standard operating procedures (SOPs), paper batch records, and support manufacturing practices for cGMP compliance. These execution and data recording functions will generate complex real time transactions that are difficult to audit and verify by such external means as database lookups, reports, or screen captures. Examples of transaction types to support integrated MRP and MES operations are given in Table 2. These must be generated by the starting application, connect through application programming interfaces (APIs), and be decoded by the receiving application.

A. System Data Must Replicate Real Operations

The validation test plan must define protocols to test the integrated system by applying test cases in a manner that represents actual conditions, both operation-

Table 1 Typical MRP and MES Transactions to Support cGMP Operations

Integration transactions	MRP	MES
Miscellaneous receipt	✘ ✓	✓
Purchase order receipt	✘ ✓	✓
Create lot and container records	✘	✓
Move containers to proper storage locations	✓	✓
Change a lot status	✘	✓
Download a work order with material quantities	✓	✘
Create work order	✓	✘ ✓
Cancel work order	✘ ✓	✘ ✓
Close a work order	✘ ✓	✘ ✓
Cycle count warehouse location	✘ ✓	✓
Approve cycle count	✓	
Move material between locations	✘ ✓	✓
Scrap material from a location	✘ ✓	✓
Scrap material from a work order	✘	✓
Issue material to a batch	✓	✓
Miscellaneous issue to account/project	✘ ✓	✓
Report production from a stage	✘	✓
Transfer MRP work orders to MES	✓	✘
Inventory adjustment	✘ ✓	✓
Return issued material to inventory	✘ ✓	✓
MRP work order download	✓	✘
Release work order		✓
Open work order		✓

Note: ✓ indicates application will initiate transaction; ✘ indicates application will process transaction.

ally and systemically. Data dependencies are created as MRP activities, operations, and computer-related system activities create interacting transactions.

The MRP-MES database must contain data table types to support cGMP compliance and manufacturing functionality, including the following:

- Specification tables, which contain the parameter data that will not change from process to process and are usually product-independent.
- Dynamic specification tables, which are typically process- and product-specific, are entered once and used in the MRP and execution systems.
- Dynamic status tables, which are updated as a result of executing the business process rules or recording information about nonautomated portions of operations.

Table 2 Initial Specification Data and System Hardware for PQ Protocols

MRP static and dynamic specification data

1. Materials management
   a. Product codes with part masters
   b. Warehouse sites with storage conditions
   c. Area locations within each warehouse
2. Purchasing
   a. Open purchase orders with line items for receiving raw materials
   b. Receiving documents for each test case shipment
3. Accounts and projects
   a. Production account codes
   b. Production project codes
   c. Scrap and destruction account codes
   d. Scrap and destruction "reason codes"
   e. QC account codes
   f. QC project codes

MES and MRP static specification data

1. Unit of measure conversions to support the received materials
2. Internal lot numbers, examples of special numbers to be used during the receiving cycle

System hardware

1. Configured servers and workstations networked for operations
2. Online weight station integrated for automatic MES operations
3. Barcodes readers connected to workstations
4. Networked barcode printers and system printers
5. Label stock for printing labels

- History (log) tables, which are continuously updated with entries for every action taken during operational execution.

The MES production history log is the main log file, since it is a comprehensive record for compliance demonstration. Automatic creation of an activity record during a recipe execution becomes the permanent record of what has happened during the manufacture of the product. This log has sufficient detail to completely construct everything that the operator recorded and did during the activity. A batch report generator would format the production history log into reports or a batch record hard copy with different configuration and tailoring options as either a print or read only file such as an Adobe PDF format. The production history log is unalterable and all actions on it are recorded in an audit log. In the cGMP context, this record has to meet the criteria of "true copy" required by the Code of Federal Regulations (CFRs) and U.S. Food and Drug Administration (FDA)

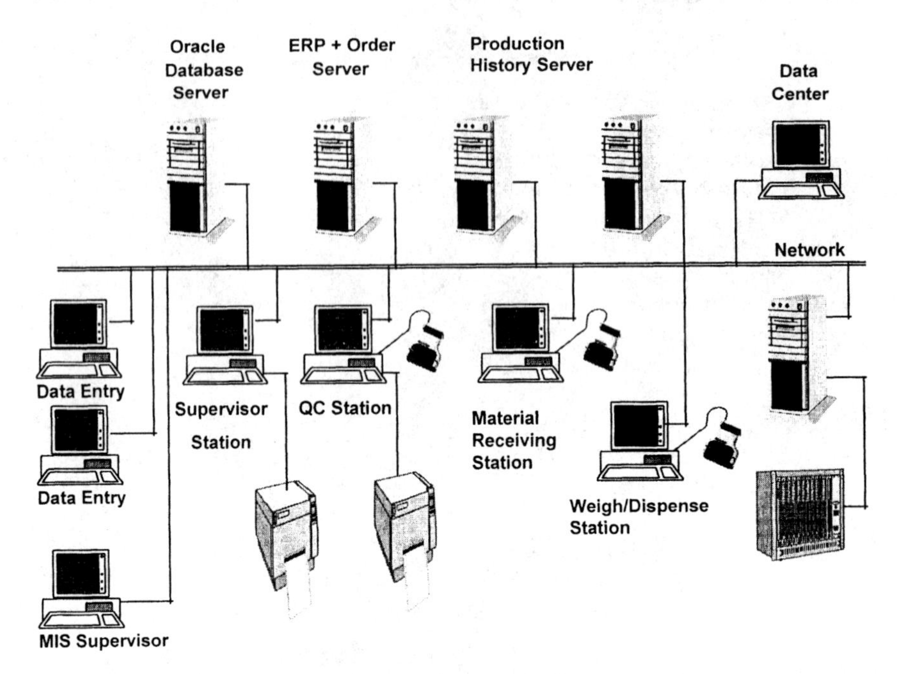

Fig. 2 Example system architecture for weigh dispense system.

guidelines for compliance demonstration. Typically these files can be archived to a WORM (write once read many) drive or CD for future access.

III. SIMPLIFIED INTEGRATION MODEL

We can use a simplified manufacturing model as an illustrative example of the complex operational and computer-related system dependencies that must be developed in the performance qualification (PQ) protocols. The example model integrates MRP and MES to perform material receiving, quality control (QC) testing, electronic material status control, MRP and MES work order creation, supervisor work order management, and warehouse dispensing of materials for production order consumption. There are a number of validated systems in use today performing the weigh/dispense operations described in the model. The system architecture showing the servers, workstations, and the manufacturing network for the example model is given in Fig. 2.

IV. VALIDATED SYSTEM COMPONENTS

For this discussion, we can assume that security requirements, plant network, operator workstations, and other equipment, such as automated scales and bar code printers and scanners, have been tested and qualified for operations during installation qualifications (IQ) and operational qualifications (OQ) testing. The static and dynamic specification database tables for integrated operations between MRP and MES have also been tested and verified to establish the initial system state. Backups of data and files have been made so that testing can be repeated.

V. TEST DATA SETS FOR THE TESTING PLAN

We need to define the test data sets for determining the initial state of the integrated system and for generating the dynamic MRP to MES transactions, inter-MES information flow, and MES to MRP transactions. The types of test data sets required to support testing the example are found in Table 2.

The MES system modules provide the execution functions, operator manual instructions, operator interactions with the automatic scales and bar code equipment, and data recording and verification practices. The MES will integrate to the MRP system for order demands inventory to be used for production, and the associated lot tracking of raw materials, as well as components and all WIP inventory. MRP will perform the material planning, master production scheduling, production planning, materials planning, and order management, if the functions are to be included in the validated system.

VI. TEST PROTOCOL SEQUENCE FOR WEIGH DISPENSE MODEL

The computer-related system has to be synchronized with operations and there are no pending MRP or MES transactions. All operational data entry from this point on is initiated from the appropriate MRP or MES workstation. Test cases of applicable MRP and MES functions can now be executed, and the results collected and verified against specifications. Figure 3 is a diagram showing the PQ testing sequence and the functional modules involved.

VII. INVENTORY MANAGEMENT (TEST SEQUENCE 1)

Except for verified static and dynamic specification data, there are no raw material balances in the computer-related system. The MRP system cannot dispatch any production orders for execution as the on-hand balances are zero. Only material received through MES workstations is allowed to be entered into inventory. Test cases are defined to allow a warehouse operator to receive the materials, verify them against existing purchase orders, select and associate the materials with the correct product masters, and create lot and container entries to start the forward genealogy tracking. Labels are printed for the warehouse operator to attach to containers and pallets as needed. Samples are taken, put in containers, labeled,

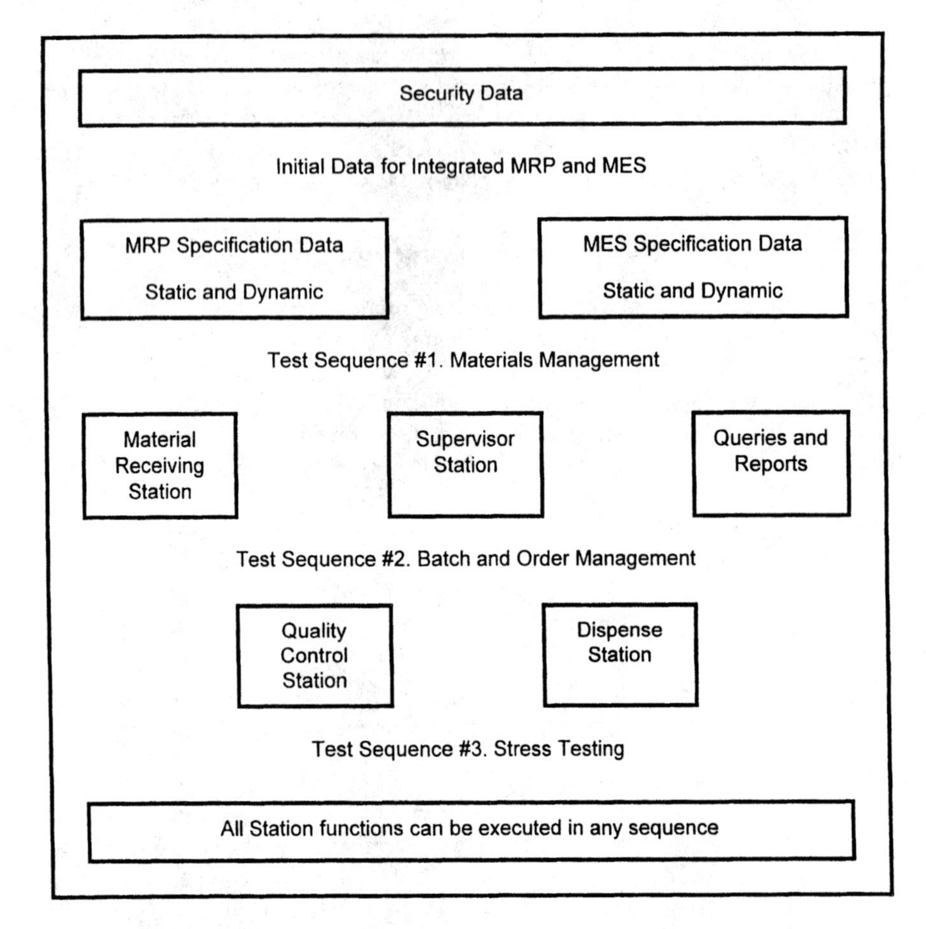

Fig. 3 Testing sequence for integrated MRP and MES dispensing operations.

and sent to QC for testing per SOPs. All material statuses are defined as "quarantine."

Electronic control of material status and expiry dating can now be managed by the system. No materials have been entered by an external source. MRP integration is performed for purchasing reconciliation, updating of inventory balances, lot and sublot genealogy, and warehouse put-away transactions in appropriate storage locations.

QA can manage all raw material release status, calculate and set expiry dates, enter potency values after sample testing has been performed, and verify the appropriate set storage conditions. By the warehouse defining the raw material status as quarantined, the quality assurance (QA) functions must interpret the status appropriately during its testing functions. Unit testing independently verifies that each module can change the status correctly. Now PQ testing will determine if the quarantine status set by the receiving module can be successfully interpreted by the QA module, which can then be acted upon as a result of the actual sample testing results (i.e., cause it to be changed to the correct "released" status).

VIII. BATCH MANAGEMENT (TEST SEQUENCE 2)

Through its planning functions, MRP can define the production orders to be managed by the supervisor on the plant floor. These dispatched orders are sent as transactions to the MES supervisor stations work flow queues. Testing will verify that the order-defined raw materials are correct and that quantity balances are adequate for the order, and will subsequently manage the status of the order to set up work queues for the warehouse to dispense materials. Integration issues such as having MRP cancel specific orders based upon the supervisor set status can be tested. The supervisor can create dispense orders based upon established bills of materials that were entered as specification data for the specific products in the dispatch orders.

The dispensing station application can now allow the warehouse operators to process production orders created by the supervisor station. They can verify materials to make the kits, dry cocktails, or shrink-wrapped, palletized supplies for each order. The warehouse operators have to rely on the electronic status and dating rules entered by QA for each product. Material verification using bar code reading equipment will ensure compliance to the status and expiry dating rules. Production history will be generated for the activities. Genealogy tables can be checked for correct lot traceability after order execution and MES-generated transactions to MRP are completed.

IX. OPERATIONAL STRESS TESTING (TEST SEQUENCE 3)

After executing the test cases for test sequence 1 and 2 test cases and verifying the results, any MRP or MES function can be executed in any order. The testing sequence has verified the data dependencies required during warehouse and manufacturing operations by the order in which test cases were executed. In performing the test sequences, the intraworkstation information flow and interstation information flow was tested and verified for the appropriate system software module. Completing the example, we have verified that material status has been successfully changed by all system modules and no module can consume or use quarantined materials or materials without a balance on hand. The system is now ready for other PQ testing scenarios. During stress testing, the data flows, data tables, and relational database tables will contain the necessary volumes and variety of transactions to determine and verify that system performance levels are above expected values.

X. COMPLETE MRP AND MES PQ TESTING REQUIREMENTS

If we now address the complete and more complex operational model of integrated MRP and MES, there are many more functions, data, and data dependencies that must be tested in the correct sequence. We can expand the test plan methodology previously presented to develop required test protocols by separating each requirement and subrequirement into the following:

- Identifying and validating the data needed prior to running the test plans (static and dynamic specification data)
- Executing the real time business process operations (using the input-process-output [IPO] charts and process flow diagrams)
- Recording and verifying the integration transactions and history log records that result from the execution operations (dynamic status data and logs)

A complete list of integrated MRP and MES operational requirements to be validated can be summarized as follows:

1. Purchasing
2. Materials management
3. Recipe management
4. Batch management
5. Lot tracking
6. Electronic batch record creation
7. Document management and change control

Each of these operational requirements will be decomposed to define the data and transaction requirements for which PQ test protocols will have to be developed to validate the system. The detail requirements are given in a number of tables that can be used as a checklist. Some of the requirements will not be in your system.

A. Purchasing

In the purchasing system, only the functions that directly interact with raw materials are validated. This includes the materials management system, production planning, and the portion of purchase order management that has the open purchase orders, line items, and other static and dynamic specification data needed by warehouse receiving for verifying incoming raw materials.

B. Materials Management

Materials management controls the activities of materials either used or produced in production. Materials are received from suppliers or produced internally. Internally produced materials (intermediates) and materials produced in processes are added to the material inventory. Product masters are typically maintained by the MRP system.

Each new lot of material received is assigned a unique internal lot number. Products and intermediates produced in production are also assigned a unique lot identifier. Transactions are created for all material moves between locations, shipments to contractors, transference from container to container, or issuance to a production order. Lot genealogy is maintained during each of the transactions.

Hazardous and nonhazardous materials are assigned a classification for handling and dispensing. Storage conditions and locations are taken from the product and analytic masters and entered on the lot and sublot records.

1. Static Materials Management Specification Data

Specification data that must be verified are all of the definitions of business rules that are implemented as algorithms, scaling factors, units of measure, and so forth. Examples of these rules are shown in the following table as a requirements checklist for inclusion or exclusion for PQ testing.

Static specification data for materials management	Req. Y/N	Test plan #	Data set #
1. Warehouse model			
a. Warehouse location definitions			
b. Storage conditions			
2. Product material characteristics			
a. Testing schedules			
b. Quality ratings			
c. Stability testing requirements			
d. Calculations for potency unit			
e. Dosage units			
f. Ratio of potency to quality			
g. Potency aging algorithms			

2. Dynamic Materials Management Specification Data

Dynamic specification data are the product masters, analytic masters, and other records that characterize the raw materials, intermediates, and finished products controlled by materials management. The master records are maintained in the MRP system and transmitted to the MES during execution functions. Examples of these data are shown in the following table as a requirements checklist for use in PQ testing.

Dynamic specification data for materials management	Req. Y/N	Test plan #	Data set #
1. Product masters			
a. Create, modify raw materials, WIP, and finished goods masters			
2. Analytical masters for product masters			
a. Create, modify new product masters			
b. Storage conditions			
c. Sample history and management			
d. Testing schedules for product			
e. Quality ratings			
f. Stability testing requirements			
3. Potency data in product masters			
a. Create, modify potency data			
b. Calculate potency unit			
c. Ratio of potency to quality			
d. Potency aging values			
4. Create, modify shelf life calculation parameters			
5. Create, modify unit of measure (UOM) conversion			
a. Volume to mass			
b. Mass to volume			
c. Bulk to number of tablets			

3. *Real Time Materials Management Status Data from Operational Testing*

A set of requirements is shown in the following checklist for inclusion or exclusion for PQ testing. Test data sets will have to be defined for each requirement using the static and dynamic specification data selected in the prior tables.

These requirements cover a broad range of inventory control activities. PQ

Status information for the operational cGMP environment	Req. Y/N	Test plan #	Data set #
1. Create, modify transaction master			
a. Warehouse moves			
b. Maintain exception history			
c. Consumption history			
d. Scrap and waste			
e. Destruction			
f. Cycle counting			
2. Received material tracking			
a. Lot, sublot, or container data			
b. Grading, purity			
c. Hold and quarantine			
d. Certification of Analysis			
e. Certification of Compliance			
f. Testing statistics			
3. Material reservations and allocations			
a. Create, modify reservations			
b. Allocate specific lots			
c. Split lots			
d. Remove allocations			
4. Shelf life dating			

5. Inventory by lot and shelf life
   a. Real time expiry dating
   b. Real time status
   c. Available to planning
6. Scheduling materials by shelf date
7. Inventory selection by lot/shelf life
8. Grading
9. Lot management
   a. Allocate lot by grade
   b. Maintain inventory balances by lot and by grade
   c. Component substitution during production
   d. Change product ID during production
10. Potency and lot activities
    a. Active ingredients
    b. Maintain inventory by lot and by potency
    c. Allocate inventory by lot and by potency
    d. Change product ID during production
    e. Scheduling recognizes potency units
    f. Formulation by potency
11. Unit of measure (UOM) conversion
    a. Stock to WIP and WIP to stock
    b. Stock to stock
    c. WIP to WIP
    d. Purchasing to stock
    e. Specific gravity calculations
    f. Recipe definitions in multiple UOMs

testing should only be performed on those applicable to operations and the scope of the integration project. The requirements are then defined in business scenarios using the existing business process practices. Test data sets can be created from existing manual records for use in validation testing. Examples of how the above requirements checklist can be formulated as operational practices are given below.

- Each new lot of material received from a supplier or made in production as an intermediate or as finished goods is assigned a unique system-generated lot number.
- If all materials are maintained in their incoming containers, the warehouse operator will track all containers into the system for the appropriate lot master after identifying the correct product master.
- All received material lot and container information will be verified by a second person before the material is allowed to be stored in its selected location.
- For intermediates, the container's asset ID will be included on the label.
- A replacement label will be a copy of the original label.
- All storage locations have specific storage conditions.
- All containers and equipment-holding material are tracked to a specific storage location.
- The system shall not let the operator enter a material in a storage location that does not have the correct storage conditions.
- Warehouse personnel will take samples using the product master sampling plan, record samples against the incoming lots, and make and apply sample labels. Sample tracking numbers will be system-generated and shown on the sample label.
- Containers of unopened materials dispensed for a specific production order can be returned to the warehouse if unopened.
- Materials cannot be transferred between production orders.
- Materials that have been weighed for a batch but are not used for that batch must be discarded.

Test scenarios can be developed to define, test, and verify the integrated system actions for each of the examples listed above. PQ testing in the proper sequence will ensure that information and actual process dependencies are properly replicated in the computer-related system.

C. Recipe Management

Recipe management allows production control personnel to create and manage product specifications, including process steps, bills of materials, bills of equipment, and operator instructions. The American National Standards Institute

(ANSI)/Instrument Society of America (ISA) (now known as the International Society for Measurement and Control) standard S88.01 on batch control models and terminology is an excellent reference for recipe management principles (2).

> This part of this international standard on batch control provides standard models and terminology for defining the control requirements for batch manufacturing plants. The models and terminology defined in this standard
>
> - emphasize good practices for the design and operation of batch manufacturing plants;
> - can be used to improve control of batch manufacturing plants; and
> - can be applied regardless of the degree of automation (2).

1. Dynamic Recipe Management Specification Data

A checklist of recipe functions is shown in the following table. The necessary requirements should be checked for PQ testing.

Dynamic status information for recipe management	Req. Y/N	Test plan #	Data set #
Recipe (formula) management			
1. Create, modify, and cost new recipes			
a. Process definitions			
b. Bills of materials (BOMs) using new product masters			
c. New bills of equipment (BOEs) using defined assets			
d. Routings and batch record instructions			
e. Formulation mixing instructions			
f. Quality specifications and tests			
g. New skills profiles			
h. Maintainance of phantom levels			
2. Create, modify, and cost new coproducts and by-products			
a. Coproduct structures (two parents)			

b. By-product structures (quantity expressed as percentage)			
c. Planning includes coproducts and by-products			
d. Waste stream structures			
3. Set and modify within recipes			
a. Bulk issue codes and release control			
b. Effective dates			
c. Lead-time offset			
d. Batch scaling based on potency and quality			
e. Alternate process flows			
f. Decimal precision (five decimals)			
g. Material cross-reference equivalence			
h. Variable product yields			
i. Single and multiple level, where-used reporting			
j. Recognized overlapping operations			
4. Simulation capability			
a. Run and confirm new recipes in simulation mode			
5. Approval of new recipes			
a. Confirm product approval lists			
b. Route recipes for approval			
c. Define and set effectivity dates			
d. Release and use new recipes			

The recipe defines a standard quantity of material that is produced in a production order. Scaling parameters allow more or less product to be made. Batches of material can also be made using one or more processes, each having one or more approved recipes. All of these conditions will have to be tested if they are going to be allowed in the running system. Recipes and their elements, bill of materials (BOMs), BOE, and so on, can be maintained in MRP, MES, or both. Typically, the actual document is controlled through a document management system. They have statuses that are assigned according to the life cycle of the recipe. Approved recipes have statuses such as editing, testing, approved, inactive, and archive, and have effectivity dates.

Recipe approval is tested through its change in status. Approval is performed through regular SOPs for routing for approval of manufacturing documents. Product approval lists are maintained for the routing of recipe changes and new specifications. Once the formal approval cycle is completed, the recipe status is available for use by production control.

Each process action has its own set of recipe parameters as required for the action, including ingredients, equipment, control system set points, and alarm limits.

Each recipe has its own set of expected products and yields and the process may produce more than one product, including waste by-products. Yields may consist of quantities, potency, volume, and so forth. As product is produced and recorded in MES, it is placed into inventory according to its storage conditions. A transaction is created that is reported to the MRP system for the maintaining of lot genealogy and inventory balances.

Revision control is maintained at the recipe level. Any change or variation in a recipe for a process represents a new revision of the recipe. No change control is maintained at the stage, step, or action levels. (Change control is implied by the recipe.)

D. Batch Management and Recipe Execution

As batch management creates and manages all aspects of production orders, it will be the focus of PQ testing of the integration between MRP and MES. Specification data, static and dynamic, may be contained in both systems or passed between MRP to MES. Using the different versions or translation of these data will create a number of data dependencies. Sequencing of execution functions will have to be recorded, as well as the actual execution results.

MES provides conversion from the transmitted MRP production orders to MES production orders. Each order is an execution instance of an approved recipe defining the materials, equipment, and other resources required for each section, stage, and action as well as the produced finished goods. Test cases will be required for each type of order with the verification contained in inventory balances, genealogy records, and MES to MRP transactions.

Processes that produce intermediates for use later in the process or in subsequent processes will create information dependencies in the materials management system. If waste is considered a process product that will be tracked by MES, reporting transactions to MRP will have to be included in the test case data sets. Finished goods and intermediates produced are reported in MRP transactions that will update inventory. Product masters must be in the MRP dynamic specification data for these products to be reported. The lists of materials with bar code entries can be made as a part of the test data sets and will aid in data input accuracy.

Events or activities relating specifically to each production order test case will be recorded in the production history log for data verification to specifications. Electronic batch record reports, genealogy tracking, and inventory reports will be used to verify the test case actions.

1. Dynamic Batch Management and Recipe Execution Status Data

Examples of recipe functions that may have to be tested are shown in the following checklist table.

Dynamic status information for batch management and recipe execution	Req. Y/N	Test plan #	Data set #
Recipe execution			
1. Create dispatch orders in MRP			
2. Transmit orders to MES			
3. Create dispatch orders in MES			
a. Standard batch sizes (parent greater than one)			
b. Verify inventory quantity extensions			
c. Nonstandard batch sizes			
d. Verify explosion calculations and inventory extensions			
4. Execute dispatch orders			
a. Lot tracking by batch			
b. Create recipe execution formula history			
c. Yields analysis by batch and by product			
5. Multiple batch number generation schema			
a. Create regeneration batches			
b. Verify explosion calculations and inventory extensions			

6. Batch record document control
   a. Nonstandard batch sizes
   b. Verify explosion calculations and inventory extensions
7. Batch record release control
   a. Nonstandard batch sizes
   b. Verify explosion calculations and inventory extensions

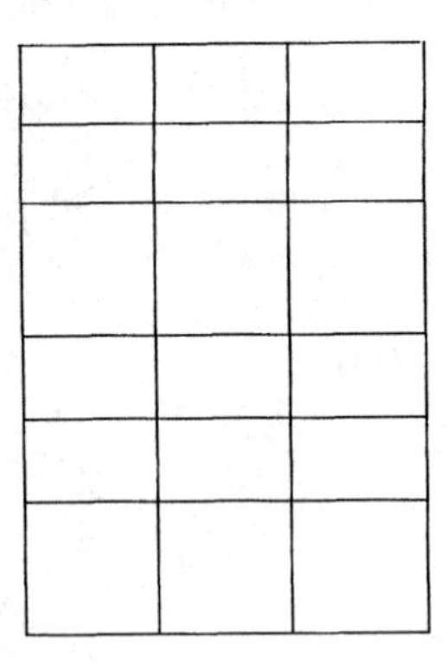

E. Lot Tracking

Forward and backward genealogy tracking is required for all materials that come in contact with manufacturing intermediates and final product. Typically, MRP systems maintain the genealogy of raw materials, intermediates, and other materials that are managed by materials management. Integrated MES and MRP operations require synchronization to capture and maintain lot genealogy. Often the dispensed materials are verified in MES as a kit, possibly checkweighed before issued, and consumed as the initial mix of the product run. MRP transactions can be created to track the genealogy of these operations.

In production, other materials are added in line to make the material balances required by the recipe that must be tested during PQ activities. Often, MRP systems cannot react quickly enough to create dispense orders for the in-line additions and product property adjustments. The MES must make material preparation work orders and matching transactions to be transmitted to the MRP as the manual operations are carried out by the operator. Scrapping and material moves to destruction of damaged or unconsumed materials need to be tested to maintain inventory balances and provide traceability of discarded materials. Often the same recipe is executed a number of times to provide the data sets for the different data and system dependencies that must be exercised.

Lot tracking is not a separate function as it results from execution and planning functions. The production history log and batch record data collection will be the repository of the information that needs to be verified and approved.

1. Split Genealogy Between MRP and MES

MRP systems are not designed for tracking the equipment that comes in contact with the product during manufacture. Clean in place (CIP) and sterilize in place (SIP) equipment cycles involve chemicals and solutions need to be lot tracked since these materials potentially come into direct contact with product through use of the equipment. Typically, MES maintains the genealogy records for these materials as well as the equipment status changes during manufacture.

2. Dynamic Lot-Tracking Status Data

Examples of requirements for forward and backward genealogy tracking are shown in the following table. These requirements are in a variety of software modules that span MES and MRP. The checklist can be used for inclusion or exclusion and trace to the test cases for PQ testing.

Dynamic status information lot tracking	Req. Y/N	Test plan #	Data set #
1. Lot tracking transactions by lot within			
a. Plant floor operations			
b. Material requirements planning			
c. Generate split, combined, graded, and adjusted lots			
d. Multiple statuses for lot in production			
2. Lot genealogy			
a. Traceability and genealogy creation			
b. Tracking by name, lot number, and batch number			
c. Complete lot traceability (forward)			
d. Complete lot genealogy (backward)			
e. For selected materials and products			
3. Track QC test for sample results			
4. Track work orders where used			
5. Track customer shipments (if required)			
6. Track vendor and incoming raw material lots through materials management			
7. Track lot, sublots, and expiry dating in batch execution			
a. Track potency and grading			
b. Record against overlapping operations			
8. Sample to batch tracking of intermediates and finished drug product			

F. Electronic Batch Record Creation

For each production order in the integrated system, MRP and MES are creating and passing transactions, while MES is producing a production history of all job activities. The electronic batch record is the official documentation containing the documented evidence that the product was made to its predetermined specifications and quality attributes. It is the recorded instance of a recipe-based production order of all of the execution and testing function. It contains the recorded data for dispensing, in-line addition, and the manual and semiautomatic instructions of the recipe in stage, operation, and action order. For PQ testing, the generated batch record should be compared with the established results to verify integrated operations. Operator inputs, recorded data, and system-generated data are recorded and prepared on the batch record for verification.

1. Dynamic Batch Record Status Data

Examples of batch record requirements are shown in the following table. These requirements are in a variety of system applications and span MES and MRP. The checklist can be used for inclusion or exclusion and trace to the test cases for PQ testing.

Dynamic status information for batch record operations	Req. Y/N	Test plan #	Data set #
Electronic batch record execution			
1. EBR recording of batch execution			
a. Materials			
b. Equipment			
c. Electronic work instructions			
d. Signatures to support the U.S. FDA guidelines			
e. Data collection requirements			
2. Integration to production history (validated)			
3. Integration to manufacturing history (not validated)			

G. Document Management and Change Control

In an electronic system, normal document management processes need to be replicated with computer-related practices and processes. These practices need to be tested during the PQ testing phase. The creation and revision process cycle is connected to an electronic information repository or vault for secure archiving and management of recipes and other objects. Revision control manages checkin/checkout object locking when recipes or elements are checked out, and access control to released versions for order creation.

Recipes need to be maintained and tested using established business rules for product approval lists, enforced action for approvals and rejections, event notification and action, substitute approvers authority (alternates), and any other manual process needed for cGMP compliance. All activities are tracked and captured in the database for in-process status, cycle time reporting, and auditing.

There will be rule sets governing the release process with automatic notification/distribution via E-mail engine, effectivity dating, archival processing rules, and maintenance.

1. Dynamic Batch Record Status Data

Examples of document management and change control requirements are shown in the checklist table below. Testing for many of these requirements is external to the integrated system. Formal test cases with a script of actions should be developed to verify the operation of these practices.

Dynamic status information for document management and change control	Req. Y/N	Test plan #	Data set #
1. Recipes, production specifications, etc.			
a. Management of recipes, versions			
b. Edit, assemble, route and approve, release, issue to plant floor			
c. Document authoring and manipulation procedures			
d. Routing and approval procedures			
e. Redlining, annotations, etc.			
f. Interface with E-mail			
g. Version control and revision process			
2. Electronic batch records			
a. Access and control of EBRs			

b. Document indexing and retrieval methods

c. Document/graphical viewer capabilities

d. Archiving processes

e. Printing

3. Security

XI. SUMMARY

Developing PQ test plans for integrated MRP and MES systems can be a daunting task. Using business process flow diagram and IPO chart techniques in the development of functional requirements and detail design specification can help simplify the task of creating test plans for the integrated system. The data analysis techniques will create the traceability matrices connecting requirements, specifications, application software, and test plan.

REFERENCES

1. Validation of Computer-Related Systems, Technical Report No. 18, PDA Journal of Pharmaceutical Science and Technology, Supplement Volume 49, No. S1, Parenteral Drug Association, Bethesda, Maryland, 1995.
2. *ISA-S88.01, Batch Control, Part 1: Models and Terminology*, ISA, Research Triangle Park, North Carolina, Oct. 1995.

23

Life Cycle Documentation for MRP–MES–PCS Integration

Joseph F. deSpautz

INCODE Corp., Herndon, Virginia

Kenneth S. Kovacs

Bailey Controls Company, Wickliffe, Ohio

I. INTRODUCTION

The purpose of computer system validation is to ensure that the system operates as desired: ''The purpose of a validation program for a computer system is to provide documented evidence that a computer has done, and/or will do, reliably, what it purports to do'' (1); ''Qualification is the procedure of collecting appropriate data that, when documented properly, provides a high level of assurance that a Computerized System will operate in accordance with the System Specification'' (1); ''Thus, computer system validation is a measure taken to ensure that both the hardware and software function as designed and that the process is controlled, or the data processed, as intended'' (2).

Validation activities and documentation are defined in the validation master plan for each life cycle project phase. Installation, operational, and performance qualification (IQ, OQ, and PQ) test plans are developed from the requirements and design specifications. Relating execution of constructed software of design specifications to functional requirements is provided by traceability matrices. The matrices contain every instance in the design that relates to a functional requirement. The test cases and data sets in the validation test plan are capable of being referenced back to the business rules and manufacturing current good manufacturing practices (cGMPs). Using a consistent numbering schema throughout narratives, diagrams, and charts will systematically create the traceability matrices. Including the numbering schema in the developed software code as comments will link the application software execution from design to requirements. The traceability matrices interrelate all levels of documentation, functional requirements, design specifications, application code, and validation testing.

II. INSTALLATION QUALIFICATION

Installation qualification focuses on the system installation. This includes, power, wiring, signal interference, delivery of all manuals, drawings, standard operating procedures (SOPs) for operation and maintenance of the system, and cataloguing of hardware and software. Simple testing to verify that the installation has been completed successfully is performed with the results recorded to show that the system meets its specifications.

III. OPERATIONAL QUALIFICATION

Operational qualification covers the aspects of loading and running the software operating systems, application programs, interface system drivers, and communication software. Operation qualifications could include reexecuting the factory acceptance tests on the systems installed on-site with the newly installed software. Unit tests of each software module, including the configuration (procedure), are performed, and the test results are recorded and verified to meet the specifications. Test cases are executed to verify that each server configuration meets specifications.

IV. PERFORMANCE QUALIFICATION

Performance qualifications verify that the integrated system is performing its intended functions while installed in its cGMP operating environment. Tests are performed on the entire system as opposed to the unit testing of subsystem or commercial applications. As in production, subsequent or downstream activities are dependent on prior or upstream activities. These dependencies have to be factored into the test plan replicating actual conditions as much as possible. The business rules must be tested in the integrated system as they occur in the operating environment. Each application has embedded procedures, configuration parameters, calculations, and algorithms to model the business process rules. The behavior of these procedures has to be tested as an integrated system.

With the integrated system in the actual operating environment, PQ testing can begin after the IQ and OQ testing has been completed and approved. Operating personnel should perform the testing. System performance has been documented that the computer-related system functions as specified.

V. MANAGING THE INTEGRATION PROJECT FOR VALIDATION TESTING

The integrated system must be documented in specific terms to achieve business benefits. Projects that are defined in broad terms have little chance of reaching closure on any single phase of the system development life cycle. We all know anecdotal stories or have personal experiences of systems that never exited from the requirements, design specification, or construction phases. Reference 3 describes some of software's chronic crises: ''Studies have shown that for every six new large-scale software systems that are put into operation, two others are canceled. . . . And some three quarters of all large systems are 'operational failures' that either do not function as intended or are not used at all.''

Definition of an achievable scope and the detailing of exact system specifications is critical. Similarly, the process that is being automated must be defined to a level necessary to achieve business benefits. A clear understanding of the process and what is essential to the running of the process is required. Only value added functions are incorporated in the design, while removing work practices that provide little value will result in the maximum benefit.

Attempting to integrate across organizations (i.e., to automate the entire site at one time) can become unmanageable. The scope should be segmented to manageable and achievable phases. The availability and skills of personnel assigned to the core and extended teams, the degree of reengineering incorporated in the planned system, the cost of the project, and the timelines for commissioning the system often limit the project scope to realizable expectations.

VI. CONVERTING BUSINESS PROCESSES TO SYSTEM TERMS

System specifications should be as detailed as possible and modeled after the existing procedures. In pharmaceuticals, producing the drug product is only a piece of what is needed. Process equipment parameters, process settings, SOPs, drawings, safety information, and other master batch record documentation defining the recipe for producing the drug product must be identified in the system model. The test data sets must come from this repository of documents and cGMP operating procedures. A cGMP-based data model, business process flow diagrams, and IPO (input-process-output) charting are some of the complementary techniques used to convert business processes to requirements and detail design specifications.

VII. cGMP DATA MODEL

With a cGMP process data model and resulting physical database, the functional requirements can be more easily met. The data model shows the entity relationships between information entities and how they relate in a cGMP environment. Lot tracking with both forward and backward genealogy is an example of missing functionality in many commercial systems that is essential for pharmaceutical manufacturing information management. The physical database must be included in the design since it must be validated as a part of the integrated system. Using the design principle that no business process rule is defined in the construction phase, the validation test plan can be developed during the functional requirements and detail design phases of the software development life cycle (SDLC). Using the validation test plans as a basis for testing, OQ or unit testing can be formalized and used for construction testing. Performance qualification testing can become the expanded testing of the different applications integrated together module by module.

The manufacturing resource planning (MRP)-manufacturing execution system (MES) database should be a comprehensive, process-driven database supporting pharmaceutical manufacturing operations. It must have tables for materials, processes, human resources, equipment, specifications, and traceability requirements. The database should contain the following data table types to support cGMP compliance and manufacturing functionality:

- Specification tables, which contain the permanent data that must be read before specific process rules can execute. Warehouse and production product storage conditions, material saftey data sheets (MSDS), SOPs, and manual instructions to perform a line clearance or start a production lot are examples of specifications. These table parameters will not change from process to process and are usually product-independent.
- Dynamic specification tables, which define materials, processes, process equipment, and such assets as scales, instruments, and storage containers. Master records that define the physical, analytical, and process characteristics of raw, work-in-progress (WIP), and finished materials, definitions of asset masters, and recipes for making products are examples of dynamic specification tables. These data are typically process- and product-specific, and are entered once and used in the MRP and manufacturing execution systems.
- Dynamic status tables, which are updated as appropriate when system actions occur. Lot masters and sublot or container records for a new lot of material, raw material status changes as a result of QC testing, and the MRP generation of production orders are examples. These data have to be entered or created by execution functions. Operators at workstations or MRP will initiate these data transactions. The resulting information is the result of executing the business process rules or recording information about nonautomated portions of operations.
- History (log) tables are the production history of the integrated system. Log files are continuously updated with entries for every action taken

during operational execution. These tables are updated whenever a material status is changed or a transaction is made verifying material consumption in a production order or the execution of a recipe recording data, signatures, and operator-acknowledged exception conditions.

VIII. DOCUMENTING PERFORMANCE QUALIFICATIONS FOR COMPLEX SYSTEMS

In typical integration projects, there will be commercial applications that are self-contained or stand-alone modules, custom software to address specific business processes, and kernel product applications that are used to model business processes when executed. MRP systems are an example of self-contained applications. They can be operated separately with data being entered through keyboards and screens. Well-established application programming interfaces (API) exist for interfacing to and from the MRP system. Process automation and manufacturing execution are examples of custom and kernel applications. The trend is toward the latter.

How, then, is one to define validation plan test environments (test protocols, test plans, and test data sets) in which there are different lexicons for the variable entities, business rules, system algorithms, data manipulations, and transactions? One approach is to use a requirements definition methodology that can link to design specifications and validation testing. Key parameters that are needed for all three levels of documentation (functional requirements, design specifications, and PQ testing) are the following:

- Identifying material data and information elements as well as the source of the data
- Defining the process that is going to convert materials or create information
- Identifying outputs from the conversion process, material lots, production quantities, or created information
- Determining the destination of the converted materials or information

Business process flow diagrams and IPO charts are examples of analytical tools that can link requirements through testing for complex integrated systems. Linking the three sets of documentation with a consistent numbering system will create traceability from requirements to design documentation to validation test plans. The links can be formalized into traceability matrices for testing and verification purposes.

The business process flow diagrams show the people and process activities integrated with the computer-related system functions. Figure 1 is an example of a business process flow diagram for solid dosage operations.

Each process operation is a production order driven by a transaction order from MRP. The production order recipe is the one or more paper batch records

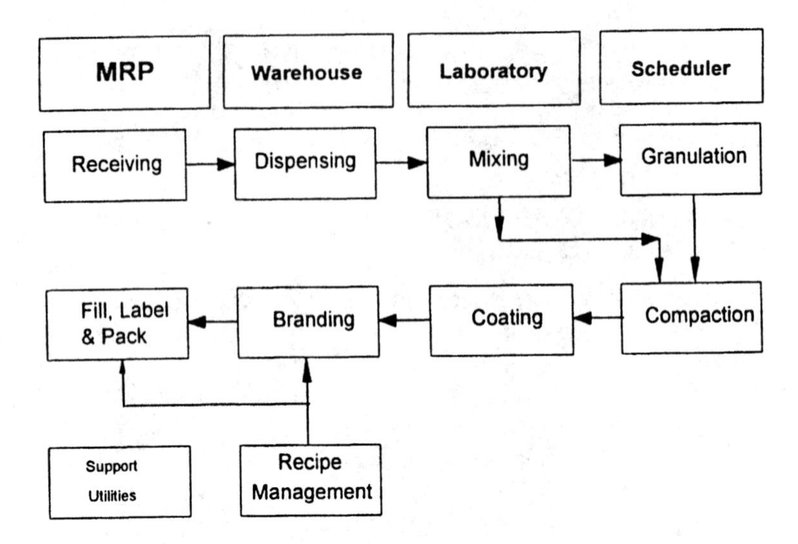

Fig. 1 Business process flow for solid dosage operations.

that are followed by the operator performing manual and semiautomatic activities. Each work flow activity in the flow diagram is decomposed in an IPO chart that defines the what and how for each business process work flow activity. Automatic, manual, and computer system functions are defined and identified on the IPO chart. The IPO chart form is defined in Fig. 2.

The sources/input data and destinations/output information are identified during the process decomposition steps and are related to the physical database tables. The IPO charts describe in detail the business process rules of each activity. Typical requirements for integrated MRP to MES and process control system (PCS) projects include the following:

- Inventory control activities
- Purchasing transactions
- Recipe information flow
- MRP and MES production order management
- How lot tracking will be created
- Transactions from MES to MRP for completed orders
- Interfacing to scales
- MRP transaction to process control system
- Where testing instrumentation is used
- Process control inputs and outputs
- Equipment line setup and checkout
- QA transactions for sample tracking and results recording

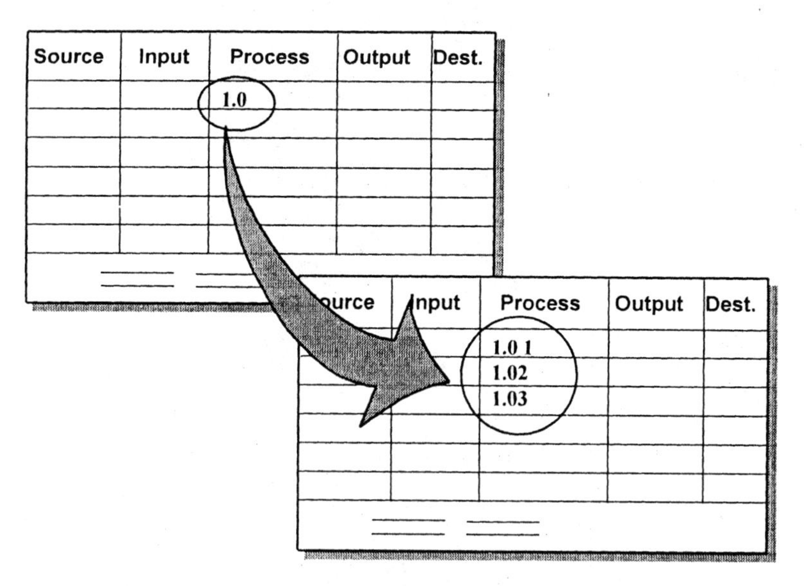

Fig. 2 Input–process–output charts linked for traceability.

IX. DOCUMENTING INTEGRATED PROCESS AND SYSTEM OPERATIONS

During system integration, the MES information bus is linked to plant floor devices through a plant floor network, usually separate and secure from external communications. There may be direct network ties through proprietary data highways for specific types of automation and instrumentation. The MRP or other plant-level systems are integrated to the MES system through wide area networks or other local area networks connected by routers and bridges. As the MES system is the connecting link between plant-level business systems and automation equipment, the test protocols will involve all of the enterprise domains–controls and supervisory, execution, MRP, and enterprise. Test plans will have data transactions that originate in MRP and need to be communicated to the control or supervisory level. These can be transmitted through the MES layer to maintain a consistent transaction history or directly if suitable audit trails can be maintained in MRP. The top-down information flow from MRP is represented in Fig. 3 as connected IPO diagrams.

The MRP system is the source of the inventory, production planning, and specification data used by the MES. MES will use this information to verify execution parameters, materials, recipes, and any specifications required for the manufacture of the product. The transactions between MRP and MES will have to support activities for the following:

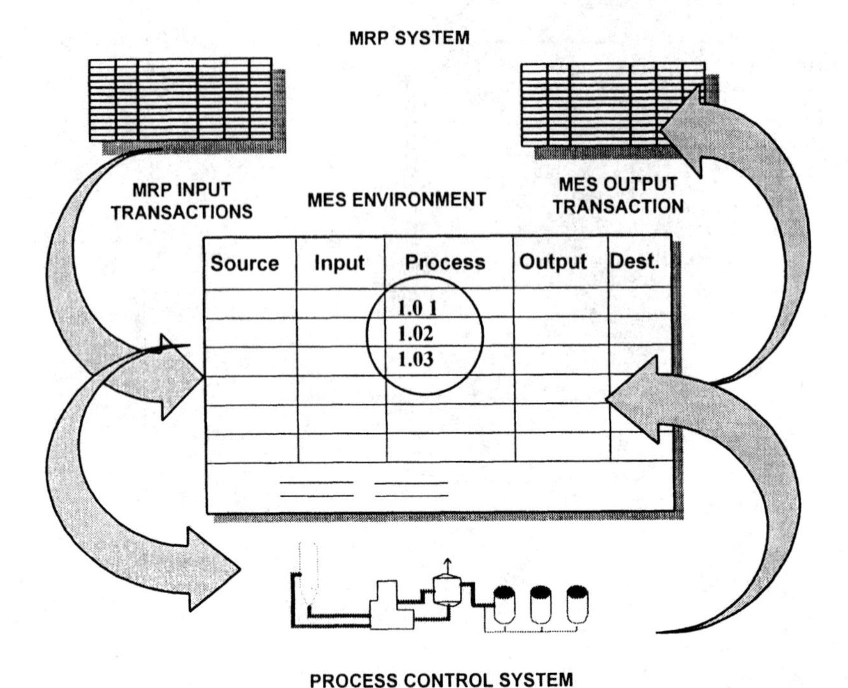

Fig. 3 Information and data flow from MRP to MES and process control domains.

1. Purchasing
2. Inventory control
3. Recipe management
4. Batch management
5. Lot tracking
6. Electronic batch record creation

Linking requirements and specifications will define these transactions for the test protocols/test plans. The IPO charts with the linking hierarchical numbering schema will aid in PQ test plan development and execution. All conditions have to be tested as the traceability matrices define the information and process flow paths. If a new MRP system is installed or an existing divisional or corporate system used in the plant, revalidation of the system environments can be readily accomplished. We assume that the new application will have been unit or subsystem tested successfully at this point. We would develop new test plans for the test protocols to support the new business process rules. We would use existing

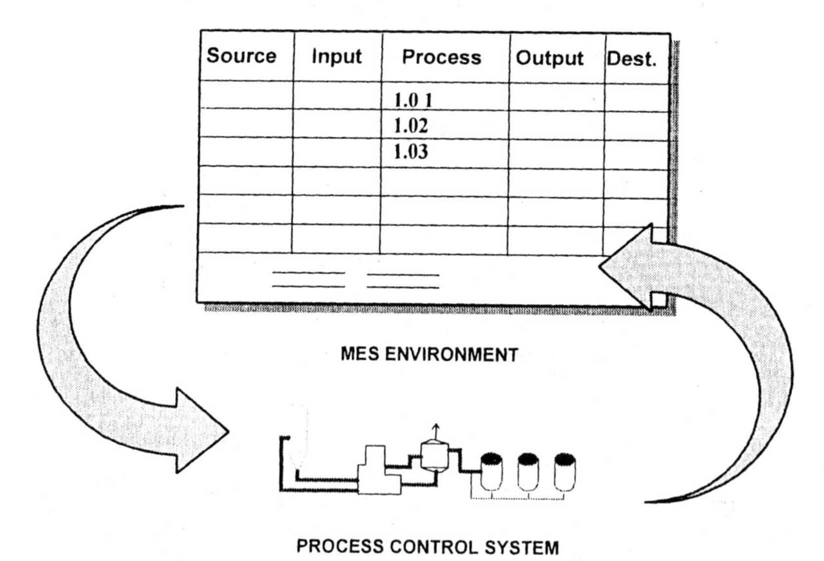

Fig. 4 Traceability between MES and process control.

IPO charts to show the transactions from the new MRP system to the MES. The developed test cases and test data sets are reusable for the new MRP system after the translations for the new lexicon are made to the test plan.

X. MES TO PROCESS CONTROL

MES and the process control system (distributed control system, programmable logic controller [PLC]) will be used for simulated and live OQ and PQ testing. OQ testing will ensure the instrumentation is properly connected and defined in the real time database and the proper connectivity to MES is present for recording exceptions and required batch record data. Testing includes verifying the following:

1. Tagging and aliasing
2. Point naming, relative addressing
3. Hierarchy of configurable points
4. Logical parameters
5. Report templates
6. Add, move, copy, and delete database online
7. Data historian operations
8. Alarm classes
9. Alarm class state processing

Table 1 Documentation Outline for Validation Life Cycle

Phase I: Concept and Definition
1. Project scope: business and manufacturing requirements
2. Project plan
3. Program team matrix
4. Documented policies, SOPs, protocols, instructions, guidelines, and references for executing the validation plan.
5. Validation master plan
   a. Glossary of terms
   b. Factory and site acceptance test plan outlines
   c. Validation checklist
6. Schedules: for all program tasks, with detailed responsibilities and project milestones.

Phase II: Functional Requirements Specification
1. Functional requirements specification
   a. Narratives, high-level business process flow diagrams, and IPO charts
   b. Traceability linking process flows to IPO charts
2. Business process improvements plan

Phase III: Selection of Vendors
1. Vendor/developer audits and evaluations
2. System hardware and software evaluations

Phase IV: Detailed Design Specification
1. Refined project plan
2. Design specification
   a. Narrative, detailed business process flow diagrams, and IPO charts
   b. All business rules defined
   c. Database tables and fields defined
   d. Expanded traceability linking functional requirements to design documentation
   e. Written factor and site acceptance test plans are completed, along with procedures, methods, and acceptance criteria.
   f. Software quality assurance plan (SQAP), including detailed hardware and software

Phase V: System Construction
1. Approved unit test plans.
2. Approved factory acceptance test plan; documented FAT results.
3. Unit tests completed, data recorded and verified against specifications.
   a. Review of functional specifications
   b. Engineering design to specifications
   c. Defined release criteria
   d. Factory acceptance testing and review
   e. Review of test results
4. The software quality assurance report (SQAR) ensures that the applied system released for delivery meets established specifications.

Table 1 Continued

Phase VI: Qualification Testing
1. Perform installation qualification (IQ) testing
   a. Perform IQ test plan: record test data, verify against specifications, approve
   b. Validation master plan checklist items approved
   c. IQ approval
2. Perform operational qualification (OQ) testing
   a. Execute site acceptance testing (SAT), record, and approve
   b. Perform OQ test plan: record test data, verify against specifications, approve
   c. Validation master plan checklist items approved
   d. OQ approval
3. Perform performance qualification (PQ) testing
   a. Perform PQ test plan: record test data, verify against specifications, approve
   b. Validation master plan checklist items approved
   c. PQ approval
4. Completion of phase VI
   a. Change control procedures in place detailing configuration management and document version control
   b. Rollout plan approved

Phase VII: Operations and Plant Rollout
1. Update system documentation under change control
2. Training of personnel impacting system operation
3. Contingency plans and disaster recovery plans approved
4. System audits and reevaluations approved
5. Provisions for remedial action and revalidation plans approved
6. Maintenance program in place

   a. Meaning, acknowledgment, instruction formatting
   b. Severity actions and data storage
10. Alarm filtering
11. Templates for alarm classes
   a. Ranges, value thresholds, delays, deadbands, acknowledgments
12. Trending
13. XY charts, multiple pens, color coding, limits

Using the same IPO charts, the test plans to execute each integration test protocols can be formulated as they would occur in operations. These test plans will be additional IPO charts for integration testing of data acquisition, data transmission, data processing, data storage, and data retrieval between the MES and the process control system. Traceability is supported by the numbering convention. This integration testing is illustrated in Fig. 4, in which information is flowing to and from the MES and process control system.

This bottoms-up analysis will provide the schema for developing the test plans for the hardware–software interactions between the MES and the process control automation. The same approach would apply to any plant floor automation that will be integrated to the MES. Automated scales, bar code wands and printers, and automated instrumentation can be tested in a like manner.

XI. DOCUMENTATION CHECKLIST

Table 1 is an outline of the documentation developed, reviewed, and approved to complete each validation life cycle phase. In an executable plan a checklist document is prepared to ensure all the project documentation is prepared, assembled, reviewed, approved, and filed properly. Examples of the detail forms, test parameters, and testing philosophy is given in various chapters for process control, MES, and MRP systems.

REFERENCES

1. Validation of Computer-Related Sysytems, Technical Report No. 18, PDA Journal of Pharmaceutical Sciences and Technology, Parenteral Drug Association, Bethesda, Maryland, Supplement Volume 49, No. S1, 1995.
2. C. A. Kemper, Vendor support required in control system validation, presented at the PDA International Congress in Basel, Switzerland, 1993.
3. W. W. Gibbs, Software's chronic crisis, *Sci. Am.*: 86–95 (Sept. 1994).

24

Research and Development Automation

Jeffrey S. Gramm

Glaxo Wellcome Inc., Research Triangle Park, North Carolina

I. INTRODUCTION

Pharmaceutical R&D spending has been doubling every five years, which is equivalent to a 15 percent yearly increase. This trend can not sustain itself indefinitely. R&D will have to become more efficient, just as manufacturing has. This will mean that management will expect more productivity with equal or less spending. R&D is still vital for innovative pharmaceutical companies in that future competitiveness and profits depend on a continuous pipeline of new products. Pharmaceutical firms have large investments in their internal R&D facilities and personnel. In order to get more value of each R&D dollar spent, management will institute a number of cost savings policies and implement concurrent R&D. Concurrent R&D will incur more risk but shorten the time to market for new products by paralleling as many activities as possible. This change in the way R&D is done will necessitate implementing new ideas. These will essentially be ways of empowering the researchers already employed so that they can become more productive. The automation professional is well versed in these methods due to the fact that they have been implementing them in the manufacturing environment since the 1980s. The techniques have been refined based on actual experience. Automating the R&D environment will be an integral piece in making research more competitive. In fact, competitiveness in R&D will determine which technology companies will survive, just as manufacturing competitiveness determined the survivors of the 1970s and 1980s.

II. RESEARCH AND DEVELOPMENT AUTOMATION ENVIRONMENT

In order to determine the trends for the future it is instructive to look historically at R&D automation. Early automation consisted of manual agitators, heating mantles, cooling baths, thermometers, and glass reactors so scientists could visually see how the chemistry was progressing. Chemical analysis was done by manually taking samples. Most researchers had one or more technicians who continually tended to the experiments. The technicians would set up the equipment, run the reactions, make observations, isolate materials, run chemical analyses, clean up, and set up for the next day's experiments. Chemistry tended to be less complex and typically was easily accomplished in an eight-hour day. Since labor was inexpensive and automation equipment was expensive and bulky, most research was accomplished manually. With the advent of electronic controls equipment became smaller and easier to use in the lab environment. The first variable to be controlled was temperature. Instead of a technician manually jacking up cooling baths or heating mantles under reactors to maintain a specified temperature, the temperature controller, using high and low switches on the thermometer, would raise and lower the heating or cooling medium. Technicians were freed from the mundane task of temperature control for the experiments. This enabled them to tend more experiments. It also provided for more reliable temperature control, which led to better correlation of experimental results. Lab automation continued to mature with the advent of microprocessor instrumentation and controls. The control systems were smaller, cheaper, more reliable, and had a lot more capabilities. During this period temperature control became more sophisticated by using thermocouples, Resistance Temperature Devices (RTDs), and jacketed glass reactors. Many other parameters were controlled using volumetric flow sensors, agitator speed control, electric scales and pumps for mass flow control, pressure sensors, and even online analyses for heats of reaction and chemical analysis using gas chromatographs (GC). The technician required higher-level skills to run the equipment. Results were more reliable and variables were controlled to the extent to which strategies for experimentation were implemented by the development scientist. This enabled the scientist to determine which variables affected the reaction and to what extent. The strategies also help plan experimental parameters to minimize the number of experiments required to determine variable interaction. Scientists tended to use terminals on the company's mainframe for storage of information and experimental analysis. All information had to be manually transferred from the lab notebook to the computer. Sometimes analyses were automatically stored via the first lab information management systems (LIMS). As computer technology developed, personal computers (PCs) were integrated into the lab environment. This enabled researchers to automatically collect, archive, and analyze data in their lab. This created researchers who controlled the destiny of their automation environment. It also created islands of automation, just like the manufacturing environment. This isolation was also promoted by company management information system (MIS) departments because they didn't want their networks loaded down with continuous streams of process information. Most software that was used early on was custom and written either by the scientists or dedicated resources working for them. This caused a support problem in that if a critical team member left, the software he or she was using might be unusable and nonsupportable. The applications tended to be local and not integratable into the sitewide networking/computing environment. During this whole development scientists were becoming more knowledgeable in using automation and the benefits derived therein.

During this period numerous companies started manufacturing equipment for the lab environment. On the whole this equipment was not as robust as that made for manufacturing. This was due to the fact that lab equipment typically needed to be more compact and was used only during forty hours a week for short duration (one to eight hours). As the simpler chemical entities were discovered and patented, researchers started synthesizing more complex entities. The complexity of the chemistry required more complex processes and thus automation requirements. With the advent of biotechnology these requirements were magnified by the fact that living entities required tightly controlled conditions for longer duration. Chemical and biological reactions now require time frames greater then a typical eight-hour day to complete. Unmanned operations have become more commonplace, thus requiring increased equipment reliability and off-site alarm and monitoring.

From an economic standpoint automation systems can be easily justified from the cost of material and personnel, not to mentioned increased drug development time due to mishaps. Material cost can be substantial, depending on raw material costs and the extent of preprocessing that has been invested into the ingredients being used. Typically during drug development a reaction content can range in cost from several hundred dollars for the first steps in a reaction sequence to several thousand and even tens and hundreds of thousands of dollars. In biological processing, media and cell cultures costing several thousand dollars are normal. But loss of biological cells can be very detrimental if they need to be replicated. From the standpoint of personnel costs, a typical researcher's overhead is worth $10,000 to $20,000 per week. Finally, time to market is critical to a product's success and profitability. Normally this is not accounted for early in the R&D cycle. When this analysis is done, losses can easily be from $1 to $100 million per month. This large figure is due to the fact that with novel therapies, the first company to market a drug captures substantial market share. Also the patent life of any compound is limited; after which, genuine competition greatly erodes profitability. With the renewed emphasis on concurrent R&D, every delay early on will affect subsequent efforts and ultimately product launch date. The mere cost of rescheduling parallel and serial activities will be very disruptive and costly. Due to these factors automation can be easily justified in the R&D environment.

III. FUTURE AUTOMATION TRENDS

Based on the current state of the art of control technology and the progressively stringent and critical requirements of the R&D environment I see future trends to be the following:

1. The continuing computer integration of R&D activities to provide better control of activities and interaction between functional areas in R&D and with interfaces to safety, manufacturing, drug approval, and marketing.
2. Implementation of control systems that are maintainable and tightly integrated into existing site networks.
3. Use of more reliable/robust industrial instrumentation and systems instead of current laboratory-grade components.
4. Control, monitoring, and alarming in the numerous areas in which researchers work. Lab, office, and home capabilities for around-the-clock unmanned operations.
5. Use of real-time experimental analysis software using numerical methods, along with expert systems.
6. Use of expert systems to help plan operating conditions and experimental strategies.
7. Increase in government regulation (EPA, OSHA, FDA). Direct access by safety and health departments to employee exposure and waste treatment records.
8. Integrated scheduling management to help drive drug R&D in a more efficient manner.
9. Use of industrial methodology in development that can be directly moved to the manufacturing environment.
10. Increase use of online in situ analytical technology such as fiber optic and automatic sampling.

The key to all the activities, from controlling experiments on the lab bench to archiving information to analyzing information and sharing it with other functional areas in the corporation, is what I call computer-integrated R&D (CIRD). Efficient and effective integration of R&D in the total pharmaceutical enterprise will depend on a properly implemented CIRD system. This effort needs to be carefully and logically thought out in order to get the desired results. All the other aspects stated above depend on this phase of the process. Any inefficiencies incorporated here will hinder the ultimate effectiveness of the system. It is vital that the solution is fully documented and uses standard components to maximize the value to the enterprise.

Implementation of standardized solutions that are maintainable and tightly integrated into an existing installed base has become more critical due to limited resources, the number of groups with which one is interacting, and globalization of R&D efforts. Information needs to be disseminated worldwide and sometimes to R&D efforts in other companies that have joint development agreements. This integration requires that the information be imported and stored and retrieved in standard formats. Current technology has evolved to client–server networking, which is ideally suited to the control environment. Server computers tend to be maintained by the site information technology (IT) department. Client computers are both on the researcher's desktop and in the lab processing reaction and analytical information. These client computers tend to have common software such as Windows@-based word processors, spreadsheets, and databases. If this is the case, then the control systems should be Windows@-based for ease of communication, maintainability, and compatability maximization. There are numerous network systems as well as programming software, operating systems, and server hardware. Since IT and engineering groups are under the same fiscal restraints as the rest of the organization it behooves us to standardize as much as possible to minimize hidden life cycle system costs.

Reliable components in all areas of the CIRD system are necessary because of the increasing demands of the chemical and biological processes. Biological reactions tend to have durations in days and weeks. The biological entities being processed tend to have very tight operating ranges for a number of variables, such as temperature, dissolved oxygen, nutrients, pressure, agitator speed, and pH. The instrumentation monitoring these parameters must be reliable and accurate. If any of the instruments fail during a run the whole batch can be lost, therefore industrial instrumentation that is designed for running seven days a week, twenty-four hours a day (7 by 24) should be used. Additional critical instruments that have a high probability of failure or drift during a reaction, such as pH or dissolved oxygen, should have redundant sensors. The control system should also be industrial- not lab-grade. Programmable logic controllers (PLC), single loop digital controllers (SLDC), supervisory control and data acquisition (SCADA), and distributed control systems (DCS) can be used in the labs and pilot plants. Recent advances in all these control systems have provided for highly capable compact equipment that meets R&D requirements. The level zero and level one control components are critical because as long as the processes are being controlled in a predictable manner the results and products from the process can be used. But any failure at this point can ruin the entire process, resulting in lost time, money, and material.

Currently most analyses are made by manually taking samples. The trend is to automatically run analyses in situ; this can provide for more data points and faster reaction to upset conditions. These analyses will occur with automated sampling mechanisms in current analytical devices.

Researchers are busier than ever and have numerous work environments other than the lab. They tend to have detached offices and home offices. Thus it is critical that they have access to their information in all of these work areas. When processes are occurring they also need to be alerted to problems so they can be resolved without loss of the reaction components. Alerting key people can be accomplished via automatic pagers or phone calls. Currently the pager works better because it is mobile, but the future will see mobile phones becoming commonplace, thus ending extensive pager use. It is also important to view all this technology as a tool; that is, the people using it should not need to read manuals to use it. In order to accomplish this all components should be standardized and intuitive. Windows@ systems are good examples.

The researcher's time is very valuable; thus to optimize these highly qualified people we need to relieve them of mundane tasks so they can concentrate on the higher-level task. We can also assist them with making these decisions as well by presenting and analyzing information. This can occur in real time as the reaction/process is occurring, prior to starting the process, or after completion of the process. For instance, during the reaction the control system could plot critical variables versus time and compare them to a desired result or previous run. If deviations start to occur the researcher can be alerted and the control system could even suggest solutions if expert systems were developed. Prior to starting the process the system could suggest operating parameters based on previous runs or experimentation strategies. Postprocess analysis correlation using statistical methods will give better insights into variable influences. The key to implementing each of these capabilities is the ease of data transfer to the appropriate program through standard data formats and warehousing.

Due to the ever-increasing number of regulations, safety and health personnel must be apprised of operations on the R&D site. EPA currently regulates chemical usage. Biological regulations are in their infancy and can be expected to grow as we better understand the risks and parameters to monitor. Currently it behooves companies that want to be good corporate citizens to monitor themselves and maintain records of decontaminated or burned waste. If a problem arises in a municipal waste treatment system the corporation with the highest profile will be suspected first. Thus companies should be prepared to present evidence proving their waste discharges did not cause the problem. Therefore I believe industry needs to be proactive on monitoring, recording, and controlling biological waste treatment. This is a lesson that we should have learned from the chemical industry before us. Employee health profiles during the course of their employment at a company would be greatly enhanced, given access to process records. FDA of course has Good Laboratory Practice (GLP) and Good Manufacturing Practice (GMP) guidelines, depending on the phase of product development. Automatic batch record archival provides for increased comfort by FDA regulators that you are in control of your process. Of course this also means that your systems were developed properly and are well-documented, but this requirement is necessary for long-term maintainability and thus should be in place as a good engineering practice (GEP). Ultimately, much of the information obtained in R&D is collected and submitted in a new drug approval (NDA) application. Currently computerized NDAs (CANDA) are become the trend for future applications. CANDA development would be shortened in a CIRD environment. Any data that need to be submitted and all numerical correlations would already be in a computerized format ready to be appended into the CANDA.

Due to the effort to speed up R&D drug development time scheduling, project management of R&D activities will become of the utmost importance. Each of the individual functions in R&D as well as the groups that interface with R&D will need to be better coordinated. This will likely be accomplished by drug project management personnel who will guide drugs through development and schedule the limited resources so that the company obtains the best value for its investment. This scheduling will need to track activities as they happen and update downstream activities that are affected by perturbations. Access to the computer records of planned and completed activities will be important for the R&D project manager to accomplish their task.

When a drug is in final development, engineers will need to design a manufacturing facility for large-scale production. Many of the techniques and methods used during development will have to be implemented in the manufacturing facility due to the fact that they were incorporated in the NDA, therefore it essential for quick start-ups that the development environment use the same procedures and equipment as manufacturing. From the automation standpoint, if industrial instruments, control systems, and software are used in development then the same systems can be ported directly into the manufacturing environment with most of their documentation required for validation. Currently this does not often happen, but efficient operations will force this new reality into organization thinking. Barriers between the development and engineering departments need to be broken down so the two groups work harmoniously as a team. This will shorten start-up times and increase the quality of manufacturing operations. It should also help in obtaining FDA approval of the manufacturing site.

The key to implementing these future trends will be employees who think globally and work as a team with other departments versus thinking locally and working against other groups. The only way corporations will succeed will be via coordinated efforts and commitment from all the departments, employees, and management. CIRD will be one of the essential tools to enable this coordination to occur efficiently and effectively.

25

Plant Design and Engineering

Jack Conaway

Winners Consulting Group, Amherst, New Hampshire

The cost of developing new drugs and getting them approved for production and marketing is astronomical. In order to recover these costs and run a profitable business, pharmaceutical manufacturers expect design/construction firms to use the latest in plant design systems to help reduce their plant development costs and modification investments (1).

In order to reach expense goals for plant operations, owner/operators of pharmaceutical plants are relying on an evolving set of facilities management applications (2). The leading companies know that plant design, engineering, and facilities management are parts of a single plant engineering life cycle (3). They have realized that further reductions in operation costs depend upon linking plant design, engineering, and facilities management systems and sharing plant data across the entire plant engineering life cycle.

I. DEFINITIONS

Plant design may be defined as the development and documentation of requirements and specifications for a new plant or modifications to an existing plant. Plant design typically includes the site as well as the structure of the plant; its utilities; heating, ventilation, and cooling systems (HVAC); environmental, health, and safety systems (EHS); and the material handling, process, and packaging equipment in the plant. The output of plant design is used in the construction or modernization of a plant. It is also useful in the remainder of the plant life cycle.

Facilities management refers to engineering activities performed in the plant to support its operation. The Association of Facilities Engineering (formerly the American Institute of Plant Engineers—AIPE) offers a somewhat expanded definition of facilities engineering.

- Selection of plant sites and real estate
- Modernization of building and grounds
- Development and operation of facilities, including
  - Machinery and equipment
  - Plant facility
  - Environmental protection and resource recovery
  - Safe and healthy work environments
- Maintenance of facility, machinery, and equipment

Plant design and engineering is defined here as the combination of the above definitions.

II. THE PLANT ENGINEERING LIFE CYCLE AND ENTERPRISE

A pharmaceutical business life cycle includes many tasks from the discovery of a new drug through its manufacture. (See Fig. 1.)

The plant engineering life cycle comprises the later phases of the business cycle with emphasis on design, construction, operation, and decommissioning of the plant. Distribution and support of the new drug is accomplished via shipments to local warehouses that supply doctors' offices, hospitals, and retail outlets and is not normally considered to be part of the plant engineering life cycle.

The plant engineering life cycle is supported by a number of companies working together in a plant engineering enterprise, as shown in Fig. 2.

Discovery
Research
Testing
Process Development
New Drug Application
Plant Design
Construction
Operation — **Plant Lifecycle**
Distribution and Support
Decommissioning

Fig. 1 The pharmaceutical business cycle.

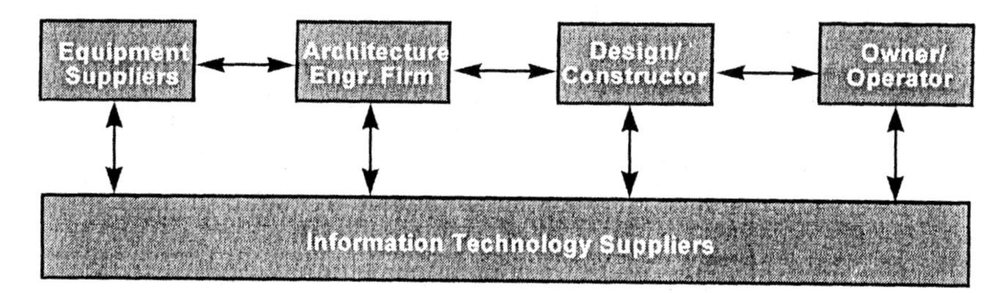

Fig. 2 Plant engineering enterprise.

If the process for producing the new drug requires new equipment to be developed, this work is undertaken by equipment suppliers who pass their designs and products on to the other members of the enterprise. Architectural and engineering firms use this information in the design of the plant, which is passed on to the construction firm that builds the plant. In many instances, the plant design and construction phases are accomplished by one large Architecture, Engineering, and Construction (A-E-C) firm that is responsible for program management of the design/construction project, including the recruitment and management of other suppliers. The as-built designs then pass on to the owner/operator (pharmaceutical manufacturer) who operates the plant until it is sold or decommissioned. During this cycle, information technology (IT) suppliers provide a variety of hardware and application software (design, analysis, maintenance management, document management, safety and environmental compliance, etc.). IT suppliers may also provide services for integrating the plant design and engineering systems, both together and with manufacturing planning and execution systems.

III. PLANT DESIGN AND ENGINEERING REQUIREMENTS

The high cost of new drug development and competitive challenges in the pharmaceutical industry require that plant design activities be accomplished in the minimum amount of time without sacrificing accuracy. Once the plant is in operation, safety and environmental compliance, product liability, and public relations issues require that plant engineering be carried out in an efficient and quality manner.

To support rapid plant design, a robust set of textual and graphic specifications are needed, including the following:

- The overall plant structure
- Plant layouts representing subsystems such as structural steel, brick and mortar, HVAC equipment, and utilities

- Piping and instrumentation diagrams (P&IDs)
- Equipment designs
- Process models, simulations, and work instructions

To support efficient and safe plant operations, application systems need to be in place for

- Preventive maintenance
- Maintenance management
- Space planning, costing, and chargeback accounting
- Safety and environment compliance

For the design, construction, and plant engineering phases of the life cycle, training is required that may combine video with textual and graphic data. Documentation creation and management is also required to provide context and preserve information for all phases of the life cycle.

IV. CURRENT APPLICATION SOLUTIONS

Most A-E-C firms and pharmaceutical manufacturers have given up trying to satisfy plant design and engineering requirements with their own in-house application software. This approach has become slow and expensive and in the long run cannot keep up with the functionality of commercially available software. Internal Information Systems (IS) groups in these companies are focused on developing applications that are not available commercially, proprietary project databases, and computer infrastructure and integration between the third-party applications. The emphasis is on customizing third-party applications to fit into internal processes and life cycles.

The commercial software industry provides applications and services for plant design and engineering in the following segments:

- Plant design
- Specialized design and Computer Aided Engineering (CAE)
- Project management
- Maintenance management
- Space management
- Engineering Environmental Health and Safety (EHS) document management systems (EDMS) and product data management (PDM)
- Business office

The heart of this application domain is the plant design application with its large project/plant database. These are expensive, complex applications that have been developed over many years and have many auxiliary modules.

Most of these application segments have high-end and low-end applications. The high-end applications have been around longer and were typically developed for mainframe and minicomputers. Today they often operate in UNIX or IBM environments. The aggressively developed high-end systems have migrated to client–server implementations over time with client software on PCs and workstations. High-end applications have full functionality, scalability, higher price tags, and in many cases, older programming technology.

Low-end applications were originally developed in PC environments. Some remain on standalone PCs. Others have gained scalability and functionality, migrating to client-server computing, mostly in Windows and NT network environments. In some market segments, low-end applications have moved up-market, leaving the low price points to PC-based applications with reduced functionality. These third-tier applications do not generally satisfy the rigorous requirements of the pharmaceutical industry and are not widely used.

V. PLANT DESIGN SYSTEMS

Most design/constructor firms use a single high-end plant design system that shares data with other applications through a centralized database. The database contains 3D geometry data describing the plant structure and other project and component data. The plant structure data are often interfaced with low-end drafting systems used for schematic work or design work among other enterprise partners. Owner–operators and equipment suppliers tend to use low-end drafting systems.

Plant design systems include a wide range of capabilities and modules, including

- 2D CAD and schematics
- 3D modeling, walkthroughs, and simulations
- Interference checking
- Bulk material and weight takeoffs
- Equipment and instrumentation lists and bills of material
- Piping design
- P&IDs
- Process flow diagrams
- Steel/structural design
- Concrete design
- HVAC layout and design
- Electrical design and cable raceways
- Standard component catalogs

Plant design systems are also supplied with interfaces to popular low-end drafting systems (e.g., AUTOCAD and Microstation) and the specialized design and CAE systems described below. Maintenance of interfaces between these applications as new versions come online is one of the most difficult challenges in integrating applications throughout the plant life cycle.

Plant design applications generally support some integration standards such as Initial Graphics Exchange Standard (IGES) data transfer and access to relational databases via standard query language (SQL). Data sharing continues to be difficult, however, because each plant design system has its own proprietary database. Published application programming interfaces (APIs) help link plant design systems to other applications. APIs are not much help, however, in large enterprises with multiple applications of each type. Unfortunately, this is a common situation in the pharmaceutical and A-E-C industries, in which there have been consolidations through merger and acquisition. These companies should reduce the number of applications with overlapping functionality. Many appear to be waiting for common data formats and business objects to solve this problem, but these will be a long time in coming.

Exciting new capabilities for plant design systems include virtual reality interfaces to walkthrough and simulation software, parametric design capabilities, and integrated workflow. Care will have to be taken in implementing workflow, however, because it is too early to determine how this will be accomplished in the future. Workflow is also starting to be integrated with project management systems, EDMS and PDM systems, and as business office software running across Internet protocols.

Perhaps the most dramatic capability of future plant design systems for end users will be Internet/Intranet front ends and access to remote databases and electronic commerce.

VI. SPECIALIZED DESIGN AND CAE SYSTEMS

Some detailed design and analysis of piping, structural frames, concrete, and specialized structures is done with individual applications from separate third-party vendors or developed in-house. Mechanical CAE systems of the finite element variety are used for stress, thermal, and deflection analysis of a wide variety of plant components. The most popular of these specialized design and CAE packages are supplied with interfaces to the major plant design systems.

VII. PROJECT MANAGEMENT SYSTEMS

Project management systems are of extreme importance to A-E-C firms charged with managing the thousands of activities that comprise the design and construction of pharmaceutical plants. Large A-E-C firms use high-end project management systems backed up by proprietary project databases and custom project consolidation software. The central project database is often linked to programs that track resource skills, availability, and charge rates, and the financial systems of the firm that keep track of the consolidated project business. A-E-C firms also use low-end project management systems for small projects and interface the results to the central database.

Plant owner–operators have smaller projects to manage, and tend to use the popular, low-end project management systems for this purpose.

Project management systems have capabilities for

- Project modeling and analysis
- Scheduling
- Resource management
- Cost management
- Presentations and reports

Modeling and analysis allows the development of work breakdown structures and process flows, and what-if and risk analysis. Scheduling utilizes precedence diagramming or critical path methods (CPM) to determine timing and relationships between activities in the work breakdown structure. Resources are assigned to activities, and capacity analyses are performed to compare the availability of existing resources with project requirements. Budgeting of activities, tracking of actual costs versus budget for activities and the entire project are performed on an ongoing basis. Also, cost variations to plan and cash flows are determined as part of cost management.

Project management client software has its own predefined presentation and report formats, including activity bar (Gantt) charts, work breakdown lists, histograms, and time histories for trend analysis. This output may also be integrated with desktop business office software for reporting purposes.

Cross-functional program management software for PCs is also available that combines the budget, schedule, and responsibility data from project management systems, process models from business process reengineering (BPR) applications, and teaming relationships on projects to get a complete picture of the cross-functional program.

VIII. MAINTENANCE MANAGEMENT SYSTEMS

Maintenance management systems, also known as CMMS, are used for reactive and preventive maintenance of facilities and their production machinery. CMMS contain capabilities for

- Work orders
- Labor management, including skills, availability, and labor rates
- Scheduling of work orders and consolidation of maintenance schedules
- Inventory management for tools, supplies, and repair parts

- Resource tracking
- Report management, including inventory control, maintenance histories, and documentation for all maintenance transactions

Integration is often provided to popular CAD drawing systems, Enterprise Resource Planning (ERP) and financial systems, EHS systems, and EDMS.

CMMS is available on a variety of platforms, including legacy mainframe and minicomputer systems, client–server systems with PC clients, and modules of large ERP systems or mainframes.

IX. SPACE PLANNING SYSTEMS

Space planning systems use CAD capabilities and standard icons for office equipment to further detail plant layouts, calculate floor areas, and determine space costs based on costs per square foot. With the large amount of downsizing, facility consolidation, and churn, there is an increasing demand for these systems. Space planning is supplied as an add-on to CAD applications by some CAD vendors and by smaller specialized PC software vendors who are also often distributors for popular CAD applications (mostly AutoCAD). Most space planning applications run in a PC environment.

X. ENVIRONMENT, HEALTH, AND SAFETY SYSTEMS

Pharmaceutical bulk manufacturing generates several hazardous materials as by-products: spent organic solvents, still bottoms, and other ignitable toxic wastes containing acetone, methanol, benzene, chloroform, carbon tetrachloride, and phenol. In addition, fugitive emissions such as ammonia may be released into the air.

In order to operate a pharmaceutical plant, operators must get permits to generate, treat, and recycle hazardous wastes and emissions. Permits are dependent on being able to demonstrate that procedures and supporting EHS systems are in place to satisfy federal, state, and local regulations. Typically this requires maintaining records of waste generated, stored, and treated; work instructions and processes and their change control; equipment validation; out-of-spec process deviations; and management notifications. Trend analysis is also performed on manufacturing records for both quality and preventive maintenance purposes. Records on the training of all employees on work instructions, procedures, and EHS systems must be maintained.

Under the U.S. Superfunds and Reauthorization Act (SARA), corporations must report annually to the Environmental Protection Agency (EPA) on the quantity of toxic chemicals released into the environment. Reports include air emissions, off-site waste transfers to waste treatment and recycling facilities, wastes generated, and types of waste treatments conducted. The data from each corporation is then added to the EPA's publicly available database. SARA Title III (Emergency Planning and Community Right to Know Act) also requires that information related to potential chemical hazards be provided to local governments and the public and encourages emergency planning through local emergency planning committees (LEPCs).

Obviously, EHS performance is a public and community relations issue of the first magnitude to pharmaceutical manufacturers as well as being an important government regulatory issue.

There are approximately 1200 sources of information on regulations, standards, and software for EHS (4). Most of the EHS software systems only support one or two of the following areas of EHS:

- Air quality
- Water quality
- Toxic wastes
- Hazardous materials
- Pests
- Noise
- Natural and cultural resources
- Workplace health and safety and so on

Fewer than ten EHS systems address nearly all of these areas. Most EHS systems run on PCs.

XI. ELECTRONIC DOCUMENT MANAGEMENT SYSTEMS

In order to support the various phases of plant design and engineering, many documents and records are required, including the following:

- Facilities manuals
- Maintenance manuals
- Equipment manuals
- Process descriptions
- Work instructions
- Batch records
- Manufacturing safety data sheets (MSDS)
- Safety and environmental reports

Most of these documents can be created with PC software, either office suites or desktop publishing, or else more specialized applications. However, desktop software does not normally have the capability to manage the documents. In the highly regulated pharmaceutical industry, documents must often be managed across the entire plant engineering life cycle.

EDMS systems perform a number of document management services, including the following:

- Storage, retrieval, and access security
- Review and approval
- Revision control
- Configuration management
- Redlining and markup
- Archiving
- Process modelling and workflow

EDMS systems manage metadata or ''data about data'' to store and retrieve documents. Metadata contain information about document files (e.g., author, document date, revision number) that allows users to select and retrieve documents. Documents that the EDMS manages may be loaded into its electronic vault or may be electronically or manually resident in some other location. Remote electronic documents can be accessed using distributed database technology or middleware. Pointers are returned to manually stored documents such as paper reports and drawings, microfiche, and aperture cards.

In addition to metadata-based attribute searches, some new systems support ''fuzzy searches'' of document text content to rapidly return documents containing key words or phrases. This type of document search is well represented on the Internet by search engine and Web browser software, and can be expected to gain prominence with Internet front ends to EDMS systems.

EDMS systems typically allow document access security to be controlled by information regarding the check out, editing, and approval authority assigned to particular individuals. Lock mechanisms are also included to prevent simultaneous edits of a single document.

Review and approval is typically accomplished by assigning these responsibilities to particular individuals and automatically notifying these people when action needs to be taken regarding a document. Some systems include electronic signatures to signify approval. Revision control allows new revisions to be considered and managed simultaneously with older revisions of the same document without getting the versions confused. Configuration management assures that as key information changes in a document, all dependent data are changed automatically to maintain consistency.

Redline and markup capabilities allow users to append notes to documents and to mark them up as part of an editing process. These capabilities may be resident in separate viewer modules available from a different set of specialty software vendors. Some markup software emulates the yellow Post-its that are used with paper documents.

With the large number of documents and revisions, an archiving strategy is important to manage storage capacity and costs. EDMS systems have automatic archiving that is customizable to each organization's requirements.

Workflow capabilities automatically take documents through a work process. There are three types of workflows: administrative, production, and ad hoc. Administrative workflow automatically routes documents through administrative procedures such as review and approval. Production workflow routes documents through business processes such as plant design, construction, or equipment maintenance. EDMS systems may have internal workflow capabilities that allow administrative workflow and can often be set up to handle production workflow. Some kind of process modeling capability may be required for the latter.

PDM systems, developed originally to manage complex product data in the discrete manufacturing industries, may be an alternative to EDMS systems. High-end PDM systems have all the capabilities of an EDMS system, plus they manage information about a ''product'' structure and its bill of materials. PDM systems may be used in place of an EDMS if the plant engineering enterprise believes that it is important to manage plant data at the component (rather than the drawing or schematic) level. This concept, referred to as ''plant as product,'' is examined in Ref. 1.

XII. BUSINESS OFFICE SYSTEMS

Business office systems run in a PC desktop environment. They supply word processing, spreadsheet, business charting, and presentation graphics software. These software packages may be obtained separately, but are increasingly purchased as integrated office suites selected as office standards for a whole company or division (5). If document creation is also done in a PC environment, other capabilities may be added, such as image scanning, optical character reading, photo editing, and desktop publishing.

In a PC Windows environment, output from all of these software packages can be combined with output from plant design and engineering applications, such as CAD drawings, MSDS, and instrumentation lists, to create a wide variety of required documents.

Modern business office software also contains collaborative applications: electronic mail, electronic notes, conferencing, ad hoc work flow, and groupware authoring tools to tie together distributed team members across a network.

XIII. STANDARDS FOR PLANT DESIGN AND INTEGRATION

To create a set of integrated applications that can support the plant engineering life cycle, two types of integration are required, as shown in Figs. 3 and Fig. 4.

Vertical integration is made possible by having the elements of technology

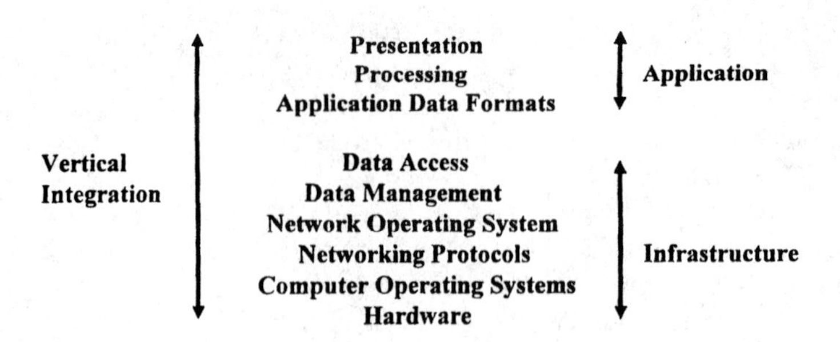

Fig. 3 Vertical IT integration.

standardized as much as possible and selected so that they are easily layered on top of each other (See Fig. 3). Vertical integration is particularly important in creating a unified infrastructure that can form the basis for application integration.

Horizontal integration involves the linking of applications along the plant engineering life cycle by sharing or exchanging application data (See Fig. 4). Application protocols that are necessary to complete horizontal integration have generally lagged behind the development of standards for the underlying Information Technology (IT) infrastructure.

Each layer of the IT stack in Fig. 3 has associated standards that enable vertical and horizontal integration. The standards may be de jure(i.e., created by an official standards body), industry (i.e., created by industry consortia), or de facto (i.e., created by the dominant success of particular products in the marketplace). Because of the long cycle of development for de jure and industry standards (eight to fifteen years), de facto standards for the IT layers are beginning to emerge concurrently with the emergence of industry titans such as INTEL and Microsoft.

Infrastructure standards have generally developed faster than application standards. Typical infrastructure standards are

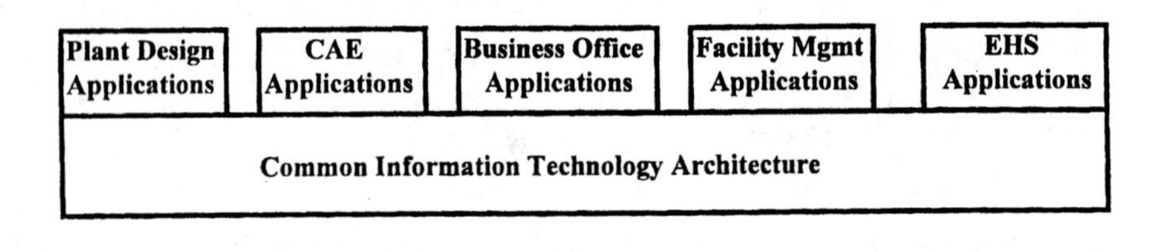

Fig. 4 Horizontal IT integration.

- Data access—open database connectivity (ODBC) and SQL
- Data management—Oracle
- Network operating system—Microsoft NT
- Network protocol—transmission control protocol/Internet protocol (TCP)/IP
- Operating system—Microsoft Windows
- Hardware—INTEL chips

Infrastructure standards are independent of plant design and engineering applications. Their selection should be based on strategic considerations at the business division or enterprise level, which should support the selection and development of plant design and engineering applications.

Application-level standards present a particular challenge for plant design and engineering. The presentation layer standards are coming along nicely, but the processing layer standards and standards for application data formats continue to lag the implementation of new technology. Application data format standards are particularly critical since they aid the transport of data between applications and are necessary to realize the dream of data sharing between multiple application clients.

Presentation standards allow common user interfaces and interface styles to be available to multiple applications. They also allow output from multiple applications to be combined in a single display or document page. The Windows operating system and the popular graphics user interface (GUI) development environments such as Visual Basic and Powerbuilder can provide the common look and feel to multiple applications in a plant engineering life cycle.

The unified display of output from multiple applications is already available for business office applications via object linking and embedding (OLE) from Microsoft in Windows and NT environments. Standard extensions to OLE for CAD drawings have been developed by the Design and Modeling OLE Consortium, a group of vendors led by Intergraph and Microsoft. These extensions provide the capability to graphically combine CAD representations from multiple vendors and to embed CAD drawings in documents with spreadsheets, business charts, presentation graphics, and word processing from business office suites.

The *processing* layer of an application performs calculations according to the programming of particular algorithms. Unfortunately, the geometric algorithms in plant design and CAD systems have not been standardized. This can lead to differences in the calculation of geometry and the location of points in space. Problems in calculating interference between parts may result. This should not generally be a concern in pharmaceutical plant design. If it is a problem for a particular design, a work-around solution may be found in the use of smoothing routines, which have the ability to bound geometric variations.

Standardization of *application data formats* for plant design is being addressed by the PlantSTEP consortia in the United States, the PISTEP and ECLIPSE efforts in Europe, and the ProcessBase project of the European ESPRIT Program. PlantSTEP and these other efforts are supporting the development and use of the Standard for the Exchange of Product Model Data (STEP) standards of the International Standards Organization (ISO).

Also known as ISO standard 103039, STEP specifies the application protocols that may be used to share or transfer plant and process data between multiple applications. Pharmaceutical plants will be able to make use of several of the general STEP protocols as well as those developed specifically for use in the A-E-C and process industries. The latter are listed below along with their availability dates.

Step protocol	ISO draft standard availability
AP 221: Process Plant Functional Data and Schematic Representation	October 1997
AP 225: Structural Building Elements Using Explicit Shape Information	April 1998
AP 227: Plant Spatial Arrangement	November 1996

AP 221 deals with the standard representation of P&IDs, HVAC, and electrical systems. AP225 covers the detailed design of structural elements of the plant. AP 227 deals with the shape, material, and functional aspects of piping systems. It also specifies the location of piping and related plant systems that impact piping design.

A separate standard deals with the representation of standard components for process plants (ISO standard 13584: Standard Parts Library). Several draft elements of this standard are under review.

From the information above, it is evident that many of the draft application data standards for process plant design and engineering will not be ready until 1997 or 1998. Potential users can expect a further delay as new standards are refined and incorporated into popular plant design and engineering applications. Eventually, horizontal integration at the processing and application data layers will be addressed by standard, networked objects, but this dream is further in the future. Companies that want to implement application integration for plant engineering today may be forced into using alternative strategies based on middleware until these standards become implemented.

The predominant middleware standard for combining presentation data for PC computing is OLE from Microsoft, as discussed above. OLE does not address integration of applications at the enterprise level, however. Microsoft has developed enterprise integration middleware called ActiveX based on its component object model (COM). ActiveX only supports Microsoft operating systems. In the rare instance in which all systems are running Windows and NT, ActiveX would be a good choice for future planning. In a multivendor IT environment, the preferred standard is the Common Object Request Broker Architecture (CORBA) from the Object Management Group (OMG). Bridge software is also becoming available to connect OLE and COBRA environments.

XIV. ISO-9000 AND PLANT DOCUMENTATION

Other standards that may aid in the development of plant engineering systems, particularly in the area of documentation and document management, were developed in the quality movement.

One of the most popular quality initiatives that applies to all industries is ISO-9000. The ISO developed this pragmatic set of standards and guidelines. ISO-9000 is based on earlier quality standards developed by the British and the U.S. military. Today, certification to ISO-9000 is a must for suppliers to the European Economic Community (EEC). In the past few years, many U.S. companies have put out the banner indicating that they too have been certified in one of the ISO-9000 standards.

The requirements of the ISO-9000 series of standards can best be summarized by three guiding principles;

1. Explain what you do.
2. Do what you say.
3. Be prepared to prove it.

To satisfy the first principal, *Explain what you do*, each company must document its policies, work processes, and procedures, including all process steps used to assure quality with their associated measurements.

Normally, the pursuit of ISO-9000 leads to the creation and management of a large number of documents that must be kept up to date over time at each facility. Each plant creates its own master quality manual which explains the quality policy and program and gives an overview of the quality system that has been put in place across all functions of the plant (e.g., marketing, R&D, plant engineering, purchasing, manufacturing, and distribution). Interactions with trading partners are also described. The quality manual refers to separate, more detailed documents describing processes and procedures that in turn refer to detailed work instructions. Quality records are also kept for each quality assurance step in the quality system.

To satisfy the second principle, *Do what you say*, the company must institute communication and training programs for all employees so that they fully understand the facility's quality policies and program and are able to carry out the their specific duties according to plan. This is done at a number of levels, including the following:

- Top management demonstrating its commitment to the program
- Training in quality systems and procedures
- Training in work instructions
- Communication of the results of quality records
- Continuous improvement activities and the communication of improved business results

Key communications and training information must be stored and kept up to date as well.

Documentation is also very important in satisfying the third principle, *Be able to prove it.* At this stage of ISO-9000 implementation, auditors who have been certified by registrars check on all aspects of the quality system and its documentation. This is normally done the first time by internal company auditors and consultants as they ready the plant for an outside audit. The outside auditors provide initial audits and follow-up audits until the plant reaches certification. Periodic postcertification audits are held on a continuing basis. No certification is granted if one major nonconformance to the standards has failed to be corrected. Auditors not only check on the documentation (quality manual, processes, procedures, and work instructions), but they examine quality records and question workers on corrective actions and documentation that were made after quality problems arose. Auditors interview workers in the plant to determine if they are following work instructions and have the proper equipment, knowledge, and training. Surveys of ISO-9000 audits have consistently revealed that lack of proper documentation is the number 1 reason for loss of certification.

Failure to reach ISO-9000 certification can have very important negative business consequences for a plant and its parent company. Many audits are requested by customers of the plants to decide on preferred vendors and award of major contracts. They invoke the fourth principle of ISO-9000, *No certification no sale.*

In the past, ISO-9000 has been used to ensure that environmental and safety policies and procedures are satisfied as well as quality procedures. Until now, however, no explicit rules regarding these subjects have been included in the standards. A draft standard called ISO-14000 is now available that specifically addresses these issues. The EEC is moving rapidly to adopt ISO-14000 standards as an overlay on the existing ISO-9000 standards.

In 1996, document creation software with built-in templates for ISO-9000 compliant documentation became available.

XV. DISTRIBUTED CLIENT–SERVER COMPUTING

Client-server computing relies on the segmentation of application software to make more efficient use of computing technology. User interfaces can be operated on inexpensive PCs and official databases and management applications can reside on a smaller number of more powerful server computers. The body of the application can run on PCs or servers or be split between them, depending on how much computing resources are consumed, what parts of the application need to be close to the user, and the need for data sharing. Servers can also be used to share specialized or expensive resources such as high-speed printers or compute engines.

With the proper selection of IT, client–server applications can be integrated into a unified, application system over an enterprise network consisting of local area networks (LANs) linked into wide area networks (WANs). Some large companies maintain their own WANs, but it is more typical for pharmaceutical companies to access an external WAN. Increasingly, companies are using the Internet as a WAN to connect multiple sites as well as to tap into information and conduct commerce with external sources. (See Fig. 5.)

Most plant design and facility management applications today are developed to client–server models. By combining this new style of computing with data standards (e.g., STEP) and/or object-oriented encapsulation standards (e.g., OLE and CORBA), a distributed client–server application system that supports the entire plant engineering life cycle can be implemented.

The casual user no longer needs to understand where applications or servers reside or where the processing is done, and data originate in response to commands entered via his or her desktop. The primary system design parameter becomes the user's desktop performance. With faster chips and higher network bandwidths, performance is no longer an issue.

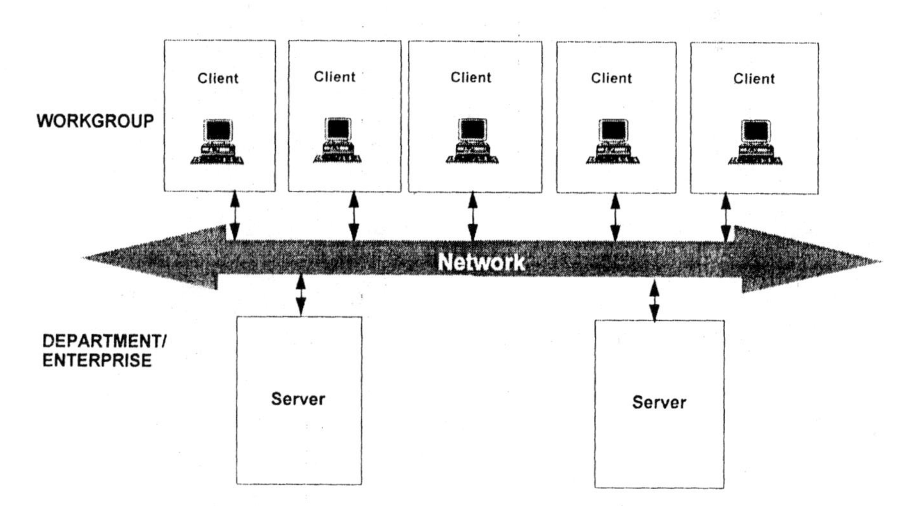

Fig. 5 Distributed client-server computing.

XVI. PUTTING IT ALL TOGETHER

Integration of the plant design applications and databases in a distributed client–server environment is illustrated in Fig. 6.

Reference 1 found that large A-E-C and some process manufacturing firms are moving in this direction. Most are running client applications such as 2- and 3D-CAD, analysis, project management, and desktop publishing software in a PC-Windows environment. These systems are increasingly integrated at a presentation level through Microsoft's OLE technology. With design and modeling extensions to OLE, CAD drawings may be combined with output from business office suites and electronically inserted in compound documents.

While some UNIX workstations are being retained as clients, mostly for high-end simulation and walkthrough applications, many companies are moving UNIX boxes to server functions or replacing expensive workstations with the new Intel-based PCs. They are backing up these systems with legacy servers operating in UNIX or proprietary mini/mainframe environments. Most of these companies have plans to replace legacy servers with NT machines. Large servers that store high volumes of design files and documents are accessed through EDMS or PDM systems. At this time there are very few PDM systems in this environment, but more are expected in the future (1).

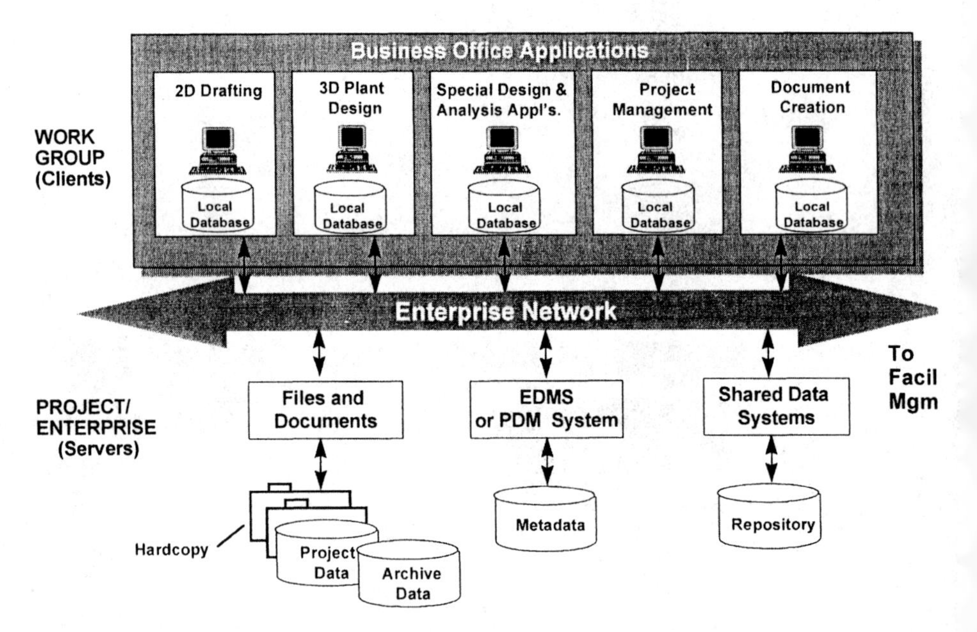

Fig. 6 Integrated plant design system.

In the enterprise networking arena, the trend is toward TCP/IP networks moving to NT as a network operating system. This means that many companies will be replacing proprietary networking protocols and network operating systems with this technology. The TCP/IP protocol is also used by the Internet. This allows the extension of Internet technology within the enterprise (i.e., Intranets) to be an important part of the enterprise network in the future. With the rapid development of plant design applications with Web browser front ends, traditional client-server architectures may be largely superseded by Internet technologies in the future.

At present, facilities management is much less integrated than plant design. Proprietary systems with dumb terminals have given way to workstation-based systems, which have been almost totally replaced by the PC (2). Most of the applications are built on top of popular low-end CAD systems such as AUTOCAD and run standalone. If they are networked, they are probably on a different LAN in large corporations from the LAN for plant design applications, but they should be on the same enterprise network. This allows the facility management applications such as space planning to access the latest plant CAD files electronically.

In the future, we will probably have integrated facility management systems similar in architecture to integrated plant design systems. Figure 7 illustrates what

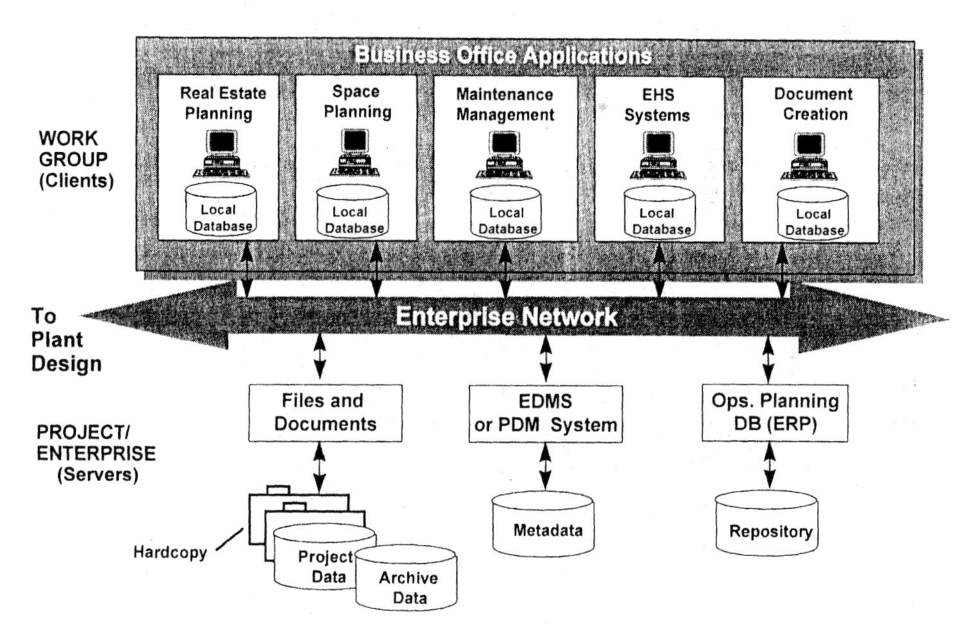

Fig. 7 Integrated facility management system.

a future facility management system might look like. As in the plant design system, client applications, corporate real estate, space planning, maintenance management, EHS, and desktop publishing are integrated through the object-oriented capabilities of the office suite software. Reference 2 also suggests that the environment outside the plants will be connected to facilities management through links with Geographic Information Systems (GIS). There is also the exciting possibility that intelligent building control technology will be linked to facilities management applications, much as ERP systems are linked with Manufacturing Execution Systems (MES).

Some aspects of integration will depend heavily on the organizational structure of the company using the system. For plant owner-operators, for example, it is not clear whether EHS systems will be part of the facilities or manufacturing departments or be shared between these two groups. Figure 7 shows a link to ERP servers. This recognizes the fact that many ERP systems have maintenance management modules for production systems that may need to be coordinated with facilities maintenance. The maintenance costs calculated by the CMMS should also electronically feed the financial modules of the ERP system.

It will be important for facility management applications of the future to access the same server data as the plant design applications if integration across the plant engineering life cycle is to be achieved.

REFERENCES

1. J. Conaway and G. Wilson, *Plant Engineering: 1995 and Beyond*, International Data Corporation, 1995.
2. E. Teicholz and T. Ikede, *Facility Management Technology*, Wiley, 1995.
3. *The Data Asset Approach: A Model for Plant Lifecycle Management*, EA Systems, 1995.
4. *Environmental Software Catalog*, International Environmental Information Network, 1996.
5. D. Card and M. C. Lofredo, *PC Office Suite, Word Processor and Spreadsheet Market Review and Forecast*, International Data Corporation, 1996.

26

Logistics

Joseph J. Kowalski

Capitol Management Consulting, Inc., Hopewell, New Jersey

I. INTRODUCTION

In the past ten years we've seen more changes in warehousing and distribution than in the previous fifty years. The momentum is just beginning.

Pharmaceutical firms are focusing on business process improvements to ensure success in the twenty-first century. Their vision is to leverage "core business process" into a successful enterprise.

Some major initiatives include forward planning, benchmarking, vertical integration, outsourcing, cost containment, continuous improvement, reengineering functions, financial restructuring, and employing just-in-time inventory management.

The goal of the "transformed" enterprise is customer delight! Improving customer satisfaction and service is paramount. Critical success factors are providing value-added services and rapid response time. These are the "deliverables" of efficient distribution and warehousing activities.

Direct communication with the customer employs computers using networks (local and wide area) to achieve seamless information integration. A paperless environment is desirable, with instant access to vital data. Firms are moving rapidly into wireless communication and electronic data interchange (EDI) to achieve additional cost savings and customer benefits.

Emerging technologies are expected to be fully integrated into the distribution and warehousing environments. Automatic identification (bar-coding) is well underway in outbound shipping and it is expected to be the operating standard internally and throughout the supply chain. Automatic vehicle and retrieval systems, high-speed sorting, and interactive training are enabling firms to achieve rapid response and increase storage density.

Further along the technological ladder are artificial intelligence, virtual reality, and voice-activated applications. Each one will transform how we distribute and warehouse goods.

Suppliers are playing a broader role as firms become more selective. Companies are reducing the number of suppliers and adopting longer-term arrangements. Key dependencies are emerging through strategic alliances, partnerships, joint ventures, and outsourcing of critical activities or supplies. Risks are outweighed by ensuring mutual benefits to both parties.

Moreover, regulatory influences are deepening, so that firms must consider the multitude of government issues globally. Firms are looking to Current Good Manufacturing Practices (CGMPs) in Food and Drug Administration (FDA) and United States Department of Agriculture (USDA) environments as elements of key business process and expanding their systems to include Environmental Protection Agency (EPA), Environmental Control Regulatory Act (ECRA), Code of Federal Regulations (CFR) 48, Occupational Health and Safety Administration (OSHA), American Disabilities Act (ADA), and International Standards Organization (ISO) 9000. By incorporating these statutes into their business practices, companies can achieve both compliance and business harmony.

Product tracking and traceability is essential in regulated environments. The regulatory agencies and firms are moving quickly to electronic submission, document control, and approvals. This movement is catalyzed by electronic interchange and computer networks.

II. DISTRIBUTION PLANNING

A. Site Selection

In pharmaceutical distribution supply sources and customer locations must be considered for optimum efficiency. Generally they can be distilled into the following ten key considerations:

1. Markets—proximity and trends
2. Materials and services—raw materials, supplies, and professional expertise
3. Labor—density, legislation, demographics, skills, and unionized or union-free
4. Transportation—air, overland, water, small package, rail, rapid transport, and courier
5. Government—tax base, solvency, special incentives

6. Environmental—regulations, conservation initiatives, and master plan
7. Utilities—power, fuel, telecommunications, water, waste disposal
8. Community—housing, public transportation, traffic patterns, education facilities, recreational, and cultural
9. Emergency services—medical, fire, police, and hospital
10. Overseas access—enterprise zones, freight forwarders, brokers, agents, preparation, storage, and packaging

To determine where distribution should be located a simple comparison table is essential. By comparing several alternative sites to the existing source a service and cost matrix can be developed.

Advantages and disadvantages of each alternative can be revealed and form the basis for the "best" business decision for each supply chain element.

Companies can avoid serious mistakes by incorporating site selection using this method. A simple evaluation table for distribution, supplier, or warehouse sites follows.

Criteria	Current	Alternate
1. Location		
2. Facility size		
3. Operating cost per SF		
4. Outbound volume		
5. Inbound volume		
6. Geography served		
7. Freight cost		
8. Days transport		
9. Fixed cost		
10. Variable cost		
Summary		

Cost and time to the customer can be determined to solidify where supply points should be located. Using this method encompassed the entire supply chain from the supplier to the manufacturer, distributor, and customer.

Alternatives beyond site selection can be considered for maximum response at minimum cost. External distribution and public warehousing or services advantages can be evaluated to achieve optimum market penetration and efficiency.

III. WAREHOUSING

A. Management System

The warehouse is the "jewel" of the decade. It presents the single largest opportunity for firms to improve their bottom lines and services. The primary objective of a warehouse is to provide customer service. This objective is further defined by these necessary functions.

- Has utility for material, goods, and products
- Makes goods available when and where demanded
- Provides a protective shell for inventory
- Determines quantity and variety of inventory to carry

Various types of warehouses are strategically located to provide desirable service. Whether the facilities are internal, a distribution center, public warehouses, contract warehouses, or rolling warehouses, they all must meet the service and budget tests.

B. Management

Warehouse management consists of two layers—management and staff. Reporting relationships are moving closer to a financially driven structure that supports markets economically.

Essential activities in warehousing are

- Receiving
- Sorting
- Inspecting
- Storing
- Picking
- Checking
- Packing
- Loading
- Shipping

In total, each activity is supported by maintenance, security, safety, and housekeeping services. These are in turn managed by the essential business systems in information, finance, inventory management, and materials location.

The twenty-first century warehouse role is incorporating many customer and materials management activities. Order processing, special packaging, pick-and-pack kitting, price marking, repackaging, import/export services, customer and/or supplier EDI, customer billing, and logistics consulting are all offered by today's forward-thinking companies.

C. Cost Containment

Opportunities to reduce operating costs are under careful scrutiny. Major waste factors are receiving special attention. Areas that can yield measurable improvements are

- Reduced slow-moving or obsolete stock
- Elimination of unplanned line stoppage due to missing or no inventory
- Labor consolidation
- Enhanced database accuracy through automatic identification
- Consolidated freight in and out
- Reduced physical inventory requirements requiring less storage space.

Careful review of warehouse functions can reveal additional opportunities for cost reduction. A simple table is used to illustrate the financial and percentage of total burden of each function. Subsequently, an activity-based cost approach can be applied to determine which function consumes the largest amount of the cost and would be a target for the greatest savings.

Function	Cost	Percentage
Receiving		
Sorting		
Inspecting		
Storing		
Picking		
Checking		
Packing		
Loading		
Shipping		
Support		
Total		

D. Productivity

Pharmaceutical firms are focusing on improving warehousing by building flexibility into the system to ensure rapid response capability.

Internally, material placement to maximize storage density and picking efficiency should receive careful attention. Material access is essential to productivity in that work is minimized and product flow maximized.

Firms are going beyond inventory placement by reviewing item-stocking quantities and movement. Early warning programs are in place to detect unfavorable trends and inventory inaccuracy immediately.

The dynamics of warehousing incorporate inventory management as a key performance factor. Counting is frequent and cycled to include stock activity and balance.

The objective is to eliminate storage whenever possible!

E. Technology Utilization

Programs are available to reduce cost and improve efficiency. Let's look at several that are underway in pharmaceutical firms.

1. Automatic storage and retrieval. Although this requires substantial capital investment, the payback can often be justified by reduced storage space, improved inventory accuracy, and productivity.
2. New picking methods. Incorporating pick-to-light technology productivity can be improved in a paperless environment. Bar-coding in picking, location management, and work measurement all yield favorable results.
3. Supplier certification. Materials testing and checking are absorbed by the supplier, thus eliminating customer checking. Quantities and contents are ''certified.'' Compliance can be audited randomly for reinforcement.
4. Automatic identification (bar-coding). No single technological advancement has had more favorable impact upon pharmaceutical firms. The applications are numerous and all can yield measurable improvements. Some examples are
   a. Material marking
   b. Invoicing
   c. Incoming inspection
   d. Material location
   e. Order processing
   f. Material traceability
   g. Employee productivity
   h. Capital goods management
5. Automatic packaging. Packaging and transportation can be consolidated to deliver optimum quantities in the most efficient manner. Logistics software exists to maximize transportation loading and material access to ensure effective customer service.
6. Materials storage and movement. The variety of choices for equipment are numerous. To make the ''best'' selection several factors must be considered. These factors are the basis of developing equipment requirements. Essential considerations are:
   a. Types of items to be stored
   b. Load sizes
   c. Physical obstacles
   d. Aisle access
   e. Travel distances
   f. Movement frequency
   g. Product variety
   h. Space height, width, and length
   i. Operation duration
   j. Environmental restrictions

Keep in mind that equipment considerations go beyond the traditional forklifts. Powered and nonpowered equipment should all be evaluated in selecting the "best" application.

Specialized equipment is emerging that encompasses "dock-to-stock" activities. New designs are available in transportation vehicles, storage configurations, materials movement equipment (conveyors, chutes, cranes, etc.), and support structures (bins, drawers, nests, racks, tubes, docks, doors, etc.).

F. Impact of the Computer in Warehousing

Computers are revolutionizing how warehouses function. Firms quickly realized that mainframe-driven systems with "dumb" terminals are ineffective. Client–server applications have emerged as the power tool of warehousing. Using PCs with standalone and connectivity to servers or a mainframe achieves the best of both worlds. Data are linked for overall management, information is instantly available online, and activities are calculated in real time.

The changes in the operating environment of warehousing includes customers, warehousing, and suppliers. All must function with accurate and timely information. Changes can be implemented immediately, expectations communicated, requirements documented, operations controlled, problems identified and solved, time utilization improved, and performance measured.

Warehousing is driven by forecasts, orders, distribution, and inventory plans. They respond by moving goods from dock to stock in the most efficient manner possible.

Current trends indicate that the twenty-first century warehouse will rely even more on direct information. Moreover, warehouse support activities—equipment utilization, storage space management, productivity, efficiency, training, and rapid response to customer requirements—will continue to be high priorities.

Efficiency is the prime focus of the "new-age" warehouse. Each activity is carefully examined as to its value added. All functions and tasks are queried as to whether they can be sped up, consolidated with others, or eliminated. Consequently, warehousing operations are streamlining functions and eliminating time-wasting steps.

The computer provides the device to eliminate tedious or repetitious operations. Bookkeeping and data entry can be automated, vehicles programmed and directed, and stock location, placement, and inventory quantities managed.

Linkage to the business systems becomes transparent in a computerized warehouse.

When using EDI, information synergy is obvious. Suppliers monitor material levels and ship when quantities reach agreed-to minimums. Invoices are transmitted electronically, material data sheets and certificates of accuracy are online, and material locations can be preassigned prior to receipt. Customer orders can be "pulled" and shipped and invoiced electronically—instantly. Less material handling is the measure of warehouse efficiency.

G. Systems Applications

Financial, warehousing, customer, and supplier performance measurement is essential in the modern center. Employing EDI, bar-coding, and integrated application within ''connected–integrated'' systems ensures maximum effectiveness.

Firms are planning expanded systems to handle the changes and volume of transactions. Some key considerations in planning system changes are response time, speed, and memory of the existing systems. The need to plan for future needs with accurate forecasts and business systems is critical.

As the role of the warehouse expands, the system's capability must meet the business needs. In addition, disaster control becomes more apparent to protect the business. A word of caution—automatic backups, disaster control testing, and alternative plans should be validated regularly. Customization, if necessary, should be minimized and documented. These special requirements place special risks on effective disaster control if undocumented or unmanaged.

H. Material Location

The pivotal element in warehouse inventory accuracy is the location system. Whether the criteria are random, designated, or a hybrid of both, it is the essential control element.

The location system in a regulated industry should contain the following information:

- Quantity
- Item description
- Value
- Square or cube dimensions
- Weight
- Unit of measure
- Date received
- Expiration date
- Batch, lot, or serial number
- Special circumstances or notations
- Restrictions
- Who put it away
- Quality status (e.g., quarantine)

I. Inventory Management

The single largest cost of warehousing is the cost of goods—inventories. Firms have adopted just-in-time philosophies to reduce inventory quantities. How much should be on hand? The lowest possible amount to provide the highest level of service!

Reducing inventories can be achieved through requiring supplier receipts certification instituting consignment stocking, reducing and avoiding slow-moving or obsolete stock, standardizing operations and components, and managing inventory turnover.

Inventory turnover is measured in two ways—financial and physical. The traditional inventory turnover calculation that incorporates sales-to-inventory investment is important; however, physical movement must also be captured to evaluated storage space utilization.

Slow-moving and obsolete stock must be avoided. Firms are developing early warning systems to control inventories. The causes of unwanted stock are: lack of demand (lost business), overpurchase or production, and product changes (revisions or modifications without an existing stock disposition plan). Firms have discovered that these causes are controllable and consequently have made dramatic reductions in inventory, but eliminate unwanted stock without risking customer service.

J. Performance Measures

Warehouses are undergoing dramatic changes to meet market demands. Firms are realizing that warehousing is a strategic advantage to customer satisfaction. A set of "world-class" indicators to measure performance are the following:

1. Customer satisfaction or service percentage
2. Number or percentage of orders canceled
3. Number or percentage of orders incomplete
4. Order cycle time
5. Order size, range, and volume
6. Cost of goods/sales to warehouse cost
7. Inventory turnover (financial and physical)
8. Inventory damage ratio
9. Inventory accuracy ratio
10. Equipment utilization
11. OSHA accident rate
12. Employee productivity
13. Employee attendance

K. Summary

The changes in warehousing are dramatic and measurable. Firms realize that this portion of the business process can be a valuable competitive ally.

27

Bringing Distributed Control Systems into the World of Client–Server Batch Control

Anthony R. Gonzalez*

Pfizer Pharmaceutical Group, Brooklyn, New York

Mark Castro*

Pfizer Pharmaceutical Group, Groton, Connecticut

I. INTRODUCTION

In industrial environments that are continuous-process and batch-dependent, there are more pressures for increased data collection and refinement of information provided from traditional automation systems. At BW Manufacturing, Inc., there were definite trends developing not only for increased data requirements, but for a higher level of data refinement and information development to support the biotechnology processes executed daily. In biotechnology manufacturing and other regulated industries, these pressures have been fueling the intense interest in the Instrument Society of America (ISA) S88.01 standard for recipe management and process control.

S88.01 is the most recent and comprehensive effort to address standardization of batch and recipe management fundamental approach and methodology.

II. S88.01 OVERVIEW

The foundation of the S88.01 specification† is the presentation of batch models, primarily the following:

---

*Formerly with BW Manufacturing, Inc., West Greenwich, Rhode Island.
†*Batch Control Part 1: Models and Terminology*, Instrument Society of America, Oct. 23, 1995.

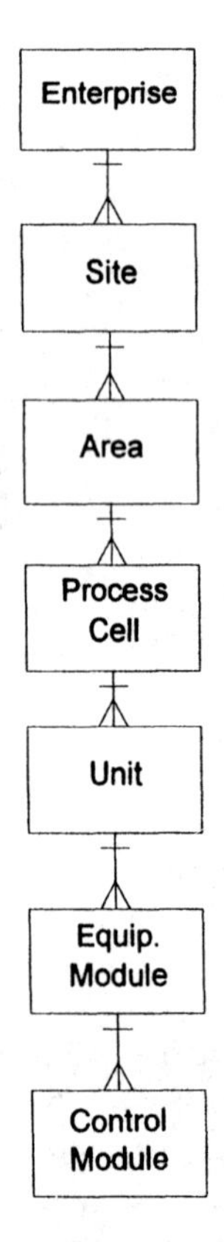

Fig. 1 Physical model of the process plant.

- Batch processes
- Batch procedure
- Physical models

As with any complex, multifaceted problem, analysis and eventual understanding is aided by structured models that organize the problem domain. This structured organization facilitates communication of the problem between people by revealing inherent order within the problem, hiding unnecessary detail, and emphasizing relevant factors for a given problem area. (See Fig. 1.)

The physical model of the process plant is hierarchical. It defines specific physical levels: enterprises, sites, areas, process cells and units, equipment modules, and control modules. Each level groups all of its elements to form an individ-

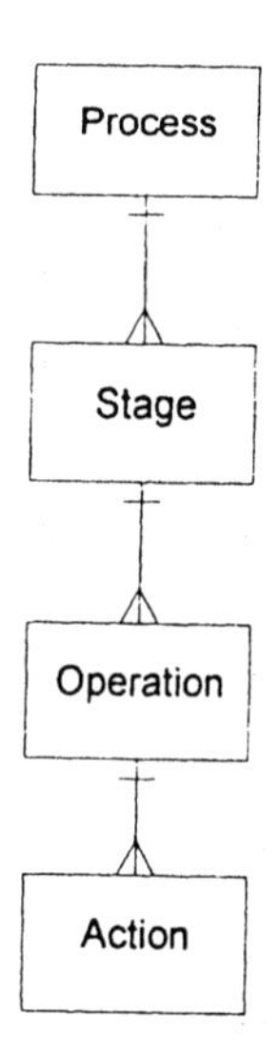

Fig. 2 Procedural control model.

ual element of the next level up in the hierarchy. These levels are determined by different factors, depending on the level. The higher levels most likely are determined by higher-level business needs and are possibly mapped to physical business organizational structure. The lower levels are determined on the basis of physical equipment functionality, the equipment's independence on other equipment, and to a certain degree, the control abstraction desired by formation of a control group.

The batch process model presents a hierarchical association between the elements of a batch process. These elements combine to create a model of actions required to create a product. This *nesting* of processes orders levels of processes into stages, operations, and individual actions. As we shall see, these levels will be mapped to corresponding levels within the physical model. (See Fig. 2.)

The *procedural control model* defines the actions required to manufacture a product defined by the process model using the manufacturing resources defined in the physical model. There is a close association between the control and process models. Each level of the process model maps to a level of procedural control that is then mapped to a physical model level to form a given *control capability*. (See Fig. 3.)

Coordination control handles the execution of the individual procedural control entities. It includes the direction, scheduling, and synchronization of control entities as well as resource arbitration between entities. This type of control or-

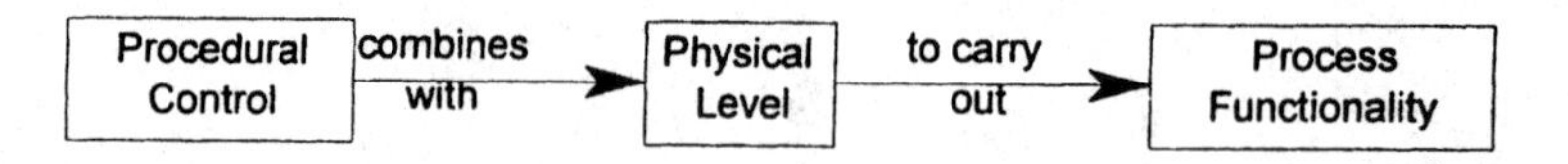

Fig. 3 Coordination control model.

chestrates the groupings of separate procedural control much like a manager coordinates his or her subordinate's activity, resources, needs, and communication flow.

Recipes define the processing activity required to manufacture a product. The recipe is also a process specification document. S88.01 emphasizes the following concepts: recipe independence on equipment and transformation of a general recipe to an equipment-specific control recipe. The first concept stresses the need to start with recipes that are process-centered and separated from the manufacturing implementation of those processes. The second concept focuses on a methodology that transforms those process-centric general recipes to a control recipe that contains all the information required to manufacture a product on a given set of equipment. This transformation is a sequence of information-gathering activities as the recipe is instantiated down the physical model and specific manufacturing data are added to the recipe. (See Fig. 4.)

The general recipe does not contain any information that connects it to a specific physical model. A general recipe can be applied to any subgroupings within the enterprise model. The coordination control of the recipe (whether manual or automated) will direct and schedule the recipe to a specific site, process cell, area, and so forth. As the recipe is directed, physical model-level information is gathered and becomes part of the initiated recipe. This information includes specific equipment resource assignments, level-dependent control detail and capabilities, specific raw materials, and their quantities.

In biotechnology, processes such as media and solution preparation, fermentation, and purification are batch-specific and are classic applications for distributed control system (DCS) implementations for process control. The graphics, trending, and data collection capabilities are ideal for producing batch data and reports for regulatory documentation of specific batch processes. Process control repeatability and the ability to apply consistent control strategy throughout the scale-up process in product development are key features that a DCS can provide to batch-driven processes. Most DCS have similar hardware components, configuration and control loop capabilities, and functionality. At BW Manufacturing, a Fisher–Rosemount Systems DCS is in use, and terminology used in regard to DCS applies to this system.

This area of recipe management is very complex and the following sections are intended to show the basics of a DCS and compare this environment to that

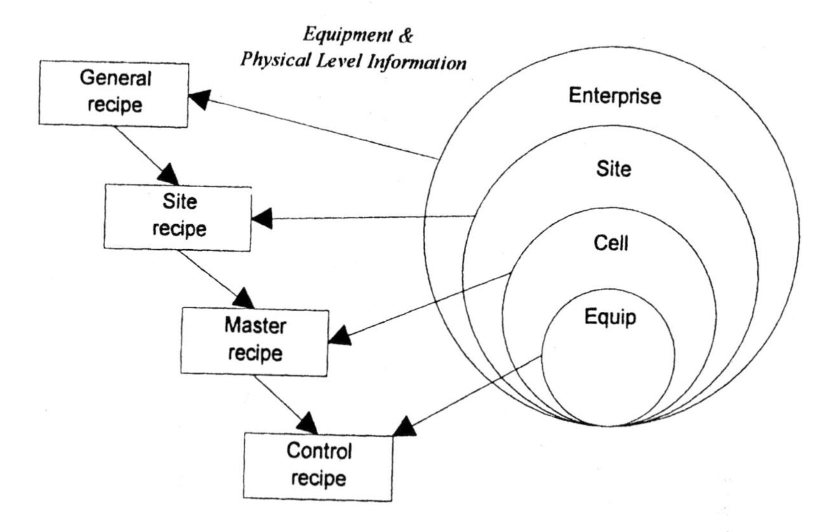

Fig. 4 Sequence of information-gathering activities.

of a DCS architecture employing client–server principles. We will discuss information management benefits of client-server architectures. We will also discuss the validation methodologies that are required for both traditional DCS architectures and how client–server technology can streamline the validation process and yield a more modular and flexible framework to design and implement batch process control.

III. TRADITIONAL DCS APPROACH TO BATCH CONTROL

Let us now discuss the development and design of a traditional DCS control strategy for a production operation performing batch processes. The process development cycle for a batch process will not be the focus in this section. What we will focus on is the use of the process design or specification to develop the control strategy or automation specification for operations controlled by the DCS. Specification and design of a DCS application can vary from industry to industry and from company to company within the same industry.

The process of development starts with the process developer writing a process specification that is process-, time-, and condition-specific and material-based. The automation or system engineer then begins to transform this process specification into the automation specification. As the automation specification is developed, the process developer and operations staff are brought into the loop to review and give feedback on the automated process. But now we must ask

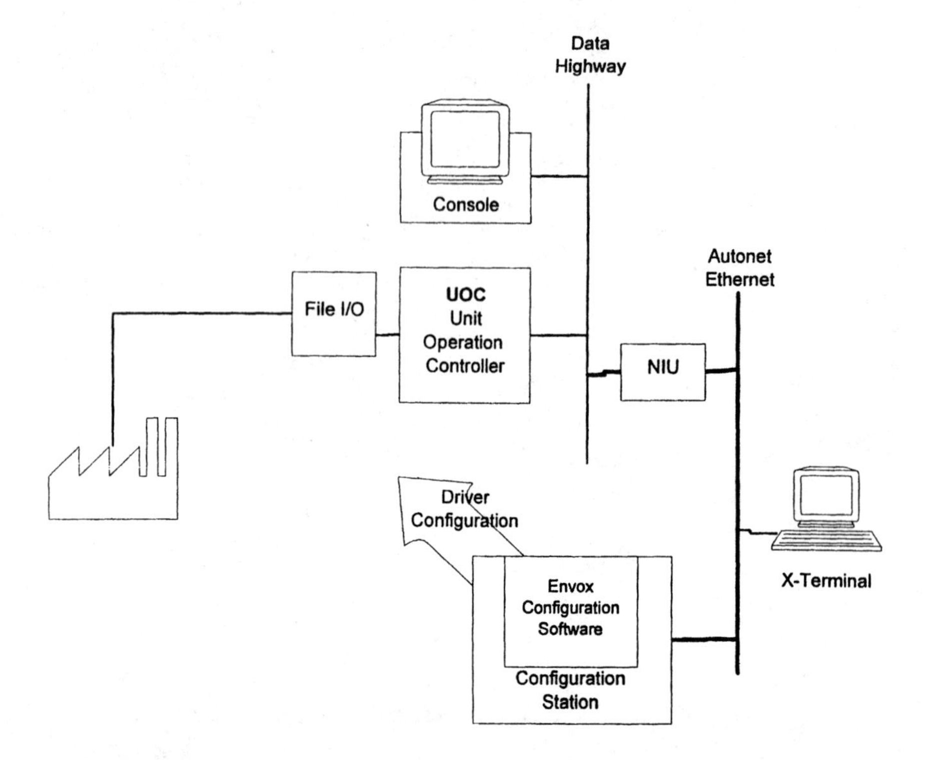

Fig. 5 Traditional DCS architecture.

the question, "What is the DCS composed of, and how are batches controlled and executed?"

The answer to this question is contained in the three major components of the DCS.

- Configuration tools
- Batch operations
- Control loops

A traditional DCS is depicted in Fig. 5.

The configuration tools are the tools that allow the automation or systems engineer to program the DCS source code. Details of the system such as process instrumentation, DCS equipment, data collection requirements, resource allocations, and batch operation executables are programmed into the source code to create the process configuration. Since process equipment and specifications are tightly coupled in the process configuration, any change in either will cause the necessity of revising the configuration. The batch operations are the executable process steps that are carried out by the DCS controller. Batch operations are sequences of states that process equipment transitions through to attain the specified process results. If we address the network architecture of a traditional DCS host computer (as illustrated in Fig. 1.2), we can see how the DCS host is integrated to the other system hardware components via the DCS data highway and the enterprise ethernet. The configuration host computer is used to program and download the process configuration to the DCS unit operation's controllers and consoles. Consoles are connected to both the data highway and the enterprise ethernet.

The unit operations controller (UOC) is connected to the data highway and communicates to termination cards on specific process equipment for configuration downloading and data collection from instrumentation.

The control loops describe the instruments and equipment specified in the configured source code programming. The automation or systems engineer programs these loops to be either process- or product-specific, or in modular generic code that can be applied to multiple product or process configurations. Control loops are independent entities and are invoked to control a process when needed by the batch operations. Control loops have been developed in groups to increase programming efficiencies. Although programming can be positively impacted, there are validation issues that outweigh the small programming gains.

In this DCS model, data exist in many areas and in many states. Field instruments monitoring physical equipment conditions transmit a current to termination cards that convert the current to a digital format. These digital values are polled by the UOC, and are stored in data registers. The information in these registers are reviewed by the control loops and batch operations for control strategy decisions such as invoking of control loops or process sequencing. Data from these registers can be output to a console or a database. The database would be residing on the configuration host computer and facilitated by a network interface unit (NIU). Batch reports can be generated from the controller, database, or console for review and operator action.

Since a traditional DCS has all process-determining parameters imbedded in the configuration source code, validation must include review and challenge down to the source code level. If grouping of control loops has been a programming practice, even small changes in DCS operations can impact many areas within the configuration. The extent of the validation is that each control point and control loop is checked and tested and each batch operation is verified. Also, alarms, system failure, and recovery procedures are examined and tested to prove that the DCS responds as specified in the automation specification. Depending on the nature and extent of the changes to the process, process qualification (PQ) may be required.

The earlier in process development that the automation strategies are introduced, the more benefit will be attained from a traditional DCS. Just as important as the review of process development for its impact on scale-up is the impact of process development on the automation strategy. The ideal situation would be to have automation configurations that were scaleable and only required volumetric parameter changes as a process moved through the scale-up stages into commercial batch production. With physical plant differences causing configuration point differences being the norm, a common DCS configuration will not work from research to manufacturing without some configuration modifications. This is still a big step in the right direction, as opposed to starting the specification process from scratch. Upgrades to process, process equipment, efficiency improvements, and DCS technology keep these systems in a virtually continuous mode of change.

In order to cope with a dynamic process environment, automation and systems engineers need to find new ways to be able to accommodate change and reduce its impact on workload and regulatory compliance. The quest for systems that will adapt more readily to dynamic environments led us to seek out a new DCS architecture.

IV. CLIENT–SERVER TECHNOLOGY

The principle in adapting a DCS into a true client–server architecture is to restructure the traditional system into two distinct layers, that of process and equipment functions. This establishes the key tasks in designing the restructured system into development of process recipes and specification and development of equipment drivers. The separation of process recipe and equipment control is the key element in developing a true client–server relationship. An equipment driver is a discrete software module that provides access to and control of a specific control loop or control functionality. The equipment driver concept will be discussed in detail later in this chapter. It is important to understand that a driver provides a specific functionality of control that is used in conjunction with the physical equipment but does not require knowledge of the actual process being performed.

Process recipes are broken down into procedures, operations, and phases. These steps perform the batch processes necessary to produce final product. Also, the recipe specifies the data collection, process parameters, sample requirements, and operator instructions necessary to successfully make product. One way to distinguish whether control information should be driver- or recipe-based is the following:

- If information is specifically related to type or design of equipment and independent of any recipe running on the equipment, the information should be included in the driver.
- If information is specifically related to the recipe and independent of any equipment involved in the process, the information should be included in the recipe.

For example, a parameter for temperature control is specific to a process and its process recipe, but the use of a defined control loop with specific valve numbers to provide temperature control is dependent on the physical equipment design of the production site to be used. For any control statement the recipe calls for, the driver is responsible for knowing how to provide that control for that physical equipment design. In summary

- Recipes are independent of the equipment that they will interact with and control.
- Equipment drivers take instructions and parameter information from recipes and use this information to control within a specified range for their stated function.
- Now you come to having client–server environments that are *functionally equivalent* versus DCS that must be *identical* in order for recipes to be transportable.

In a full client–server environment, the recipe server provides requested recipes unit server functionality and accepts completed batch journals into data storage. In addition to this primary role, the server also maintains revision and validation status for every recipe in the database.

Figure 6 shows the hardware architecture for a single-suite client-server environment. A systems person is assigned the responsibility of inserting recipes into the recipe server. This safeguards the database to ensure that the revision of the recipe is correct and that the recipe has been certified by quality, production, and engineering as suitable for implementation.

The unit server sends recipe phases to the control system or user interface. The server also logs security, data points, and recipe phase completion. The unit server is responsible for execution and management of all units within a suite. Resource allocation is designed to minimize risk and the opportunity for failure. The modules that make up the unit server will be discussed in the section on application interfaces.

The data storage concept employed is to create a relational database that is composed of all information related to product and its process. In application, a data warehousing concept is a collection of databases and access methods that are utilized in all phases of the manufacturing processes. Recipes are managed and served to requesting unit servers. Completed batch journals are logged into the database. A critical component in the use of the data storage with batch information is *read-only access*. Information may be added to the batch database, but never modified.

Validation of a client–server environment has advantages over a traditional DCS in its inherent modularity and its segregation of process from equipment. The equipment drivers are equipment–specific and oriented so that they model the behavioral characteristics of the equipment and instrumentation they control.

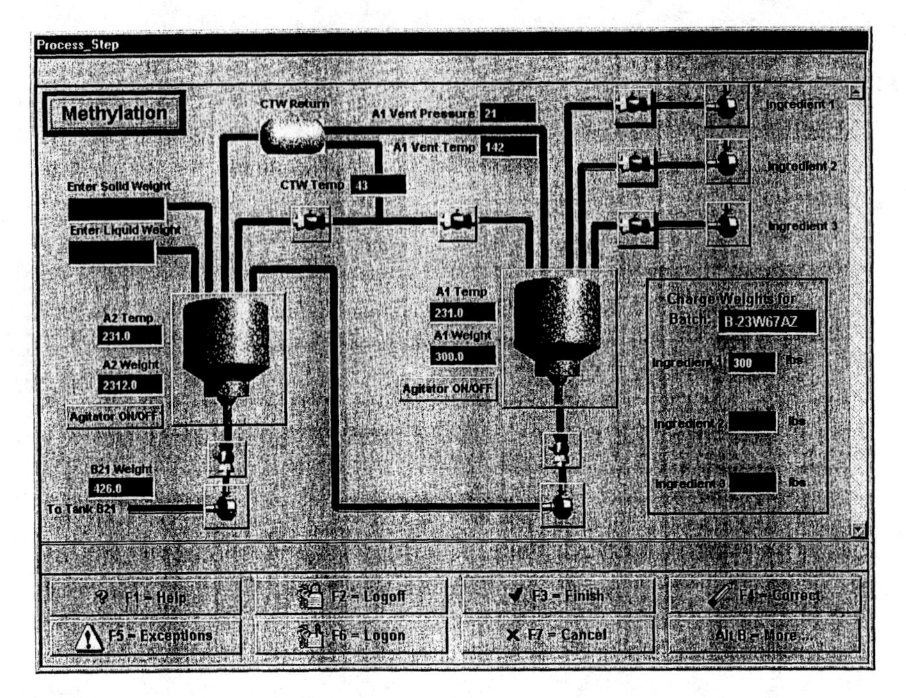

Fig. 6 Operator windows.

In this environment recipes can be written to include "validation tasks" that perform different challenges and record the results of those challenges in order to validate driver functionality. The process recipe becomes simpler to validate because there are fewer process-related variables to transition. The equipment drivers have already been validated and the recipes work within those driver limits. The recipes can also be modified to include additional data collection to support process validation. Following the validation approval, the data collection can be commented out of the recipe or removed. An additional benefit of the client–server environment is that validation test requirements are stored and documented in a reusable format so that recipe validation is significantly streamlined for future recipe revisions. Portability is an inherent part of the client–server environment. The use of design standards for equipment and drivers throughout a company can ensure maximum portability and utilization of configuration software with minimum additional configuration cost. When recipes call for a specific task to be performed, the driver takes care of any local customization.

V. USER INTERFACES

X Windows technology plays a key role in delivering the client–server information and automation user interface windows. The information and automation windows provide user access to the functions of the client–server environment. X Windows technology has enabled tremendous advances in access and delivery of automation throughout a facility. X Windows terminals can be used to access multiple information screens within a system and/or multiple system screens. In the client–server environment the operator relies on two primary windows, shown in Fig. 6. Operators can move from window to window as their monitoring and information needs change. The unit server has a session monitoring each recipe that is in progress. The control system allows access by the operator to view any unit that is in operation.

The control system provides several essential functions.

- Graphics
- Data access
- Driver communications
- Alarms

The graphics are typical DCS graphics with set points, color-enhanced equipment diagrams, and trends. In this configuration they are provided by Fisher-Rosemount's Operator Work Place (OWP) software, which provides operator console access from a remote terminal. This is direct control system communications by which the operator can view the status of equipment and answer alarms. The communication software, the client–server, and the control system are provided by Fisher-Rosemount's Computer Highway Interface Program (CHIP). CHIP is configured to have points that are evaluated by the process controllers and stored in CHIP for access by data-logging programs. Process alarms are always handled directly by the control system. Equipment limits, failures, and process limits are detected by the drivers and the process alarms are posted.

The operator acknowledges the process alarm, reviews the condition that caused it, and initiates a corrective response. For example, if a temperature alarm is set to post when the vessel rises 5 degrees above the set point, a process alarm will be generated. Product alarms are generated when processes deviate from product specification limits. Those would be added control limits that monitor additional control process data. The operator would determine what action would resolve this (perhaps a heater circulation outlet has been restricted) and implement the correction. Recipes do not implement equipment alarms, but product alarms can be generated. Recipes, however, can change alarm levels. Control systems are best suited to deal with process alarm issues.

The unit server provides functions that deal with

- Recipe processing
- Unit status
- Data evaluation

When a recipe is requested for execution a master recipe is invoked and coupled with quantity and equipment assignments data to form a control recipe. The operator assigns the selected equipment unit where a recipe is to be performed. The operator initiates the recipe and begins to monitor the recipe phase execution, interacting with the user interface screens whenever operator input is required. The unit server role in information gathering is distinctive to the client–server environment. Prior to this, system engineers were relegated to using awkward methods of soliciting information from operators within a framework that was designed to do low-level process control.

The problem was that the DCS had very limited ways to deal with operator-generated information, which accounts for most of the information contained in batch reports in a regulated environment.

The unit server also *maintains* a unit status to provide supervisors and operators with current information of the unit's status at any point when necessary. This can be used to place equipment in and out of service. In order for any unit to accept a recipe for processing it must be ''available'' for service. This is very helpful in a multiproduct facility in which such common resources as waste and buffer solutions can be viewed as shared resources by multiple process current status of units is beneficial for service-related tasks such as repair and maintenance. The data-logging functionality of the data-logging unit server has two destinations.

- Trend graphics
- Batch record journal

The unit server can dynamically trend data as they are logged from the control system. A recipe can also use control system data for calculations and recipe branching decisions. For example, a material charge might be based upon the present level of material in a reactor. In the case of a branching decision, the recipe may determine from instrument data analysis an additional processing phase to be executed.

The information window is a unit server function (noted in Fig. 8 below), that allows an operator to control species. The recipes may be run in automated or manual mode. The recipes may be suspended, restarted, or terminated through this interface. Every function point in the information window is security checked to determine that the person attempting the function is authorized to do so. Recipe tracking allows the executed recipe phases to scroll backward and forward so that the operator can see the history and future tasks assessed with that recipe. The phases are time stamped as completed.

Parameter tracking shows the parameter values that the unit server is sending to the critical system for a recipe phase.

Recipe links to external systems can be provided through a recipe in the client–server environment. Since the recipe has access to information of events that have and will occur, a LINK recipe statement can be used to initiate transactions to external systems. For example, the LINK will create a transaction that can be sent to a lab entry information system to record and log the event of a sample being taken. The important point of this interface is that it is parametric, not programmatic. Changes in the recipe or equipment drivers will not change the LINK function. The data you select may change, but the basic interface remains constant.

VI. APPLICATION INTERFACES

The recipe server receives complete recipe databases from the recipe notebook. The notebook is an application that allows the process developer to select both recipe verbs and parameters. The Recipe Definition Language is detailed in Section. The server manages all recipes in a relational database. Access to this database is managed by a security module to verify and track recipe usage.

Batch execution processes are the core of the BBC. The BBC architecture interconnects any DCS, PLC, control PC, or controller as a low-level control system and integrates a common recipe execution process that receives as an input control system independent recipes. The recipe is independent of the control system with which the batch execution process is currently in communication. The recipe commands do not directly control the process equipment, but instead send calls and parameters to the equipment drivers, which in turn are ultimately responsible for the control of the equipment. Figure 7 illustrates the relationship between the batch executor, unit driver, and process equipment.

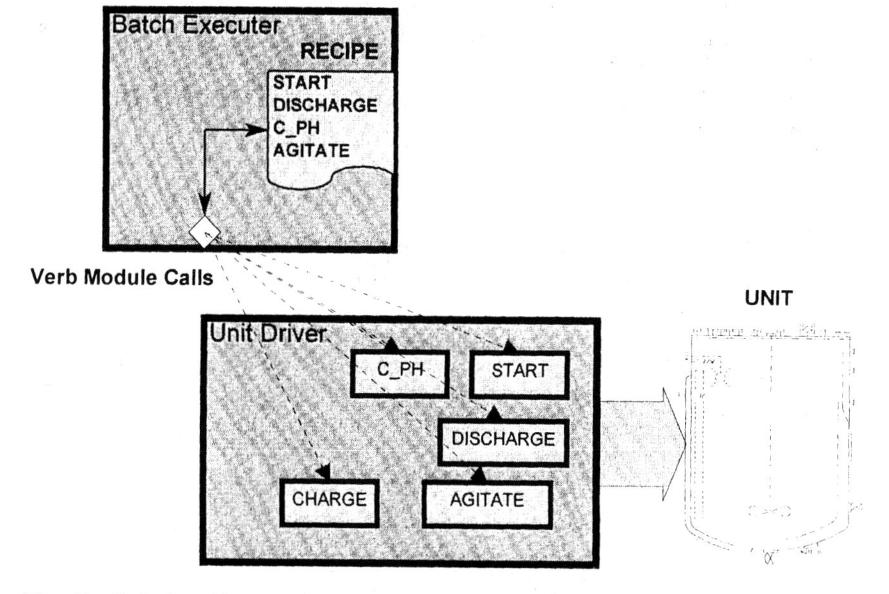

Fig. 7 Relationship between the batch executor, unit driver, and process equipment.

CHIP provides the unit server with access to the control system data points. This is how the BBC communicates with the controllers.

The CHIP and the distributed control system hide controller access method details and addressing overhead to instrument data and provide higher-level object information by grouping information into related object groups. Instead of dealing with raw instrument data, the unit server accesses information that relates to equipment and units.

VII. CONTROL SYSTEM DRIVERS

Control system drivers are the recipe application programming interface (API) to the control system. They are calls that recipes can make to initiate and manage control of process equipment. The drivers are the result of applying software engineering practices of modularity and decoupling into the BBC architecture.

For every unit under control in a process domain there is a control system driver that is configured for it. Each driver provides a set of calls or automation verbs that a recipe can call. Each one of these automation verbs can have a set of parameters for which a recipe can define or request a specific control activity. For example, a bioreactor may have one unit system driver that provides separate automation verbs for temperature control, pressure control, pH control, sterilization, and material transfer management.

The temperature control verb has parameters for the set point, an engage/disengage switch option, and process alarm limits. In the example just described, if a recipe makes a call to the temperature control verb with the engage switch parameter enabled, the driver initiates loop control with the set point and alarm limits, and control is returned *immediately* to the recipe. It is then the driver's responsibility to maintain the requested temperature control. This is an example of an asynchronous driver verb that processes concurrently with the control recipe. In the case of the sterilize verb, it may be desirable for the recipe to wait for the completion of the entire sterilization phase before the recipe initiates the next verb call. The sterilize verb would be developed as a synchronous verb that causes the recipe to block until the driver completes the verb activity.

Interunit communication is needed to operate a process train made up of separate units. This can be seen in the case of material transfer from one unit to another. This scenario requires the upstream unit processing a discharge verb, to be synchronized with the downstream unit processing a charge verb. Each verb call can be from separate recipes being executed by independent batch execution processes on the recipe server. When either the discharge or the charge verb starts, it waits for a synchronization signal from the corresponding verb driver to start. When received, the transfer initiates and continues until either verb specifies the completion of the activity (depending upon the specification of the drivers and the current parameters' values). If during the transfer either unit senses problems, it can abandon the transfer, signal the other unit of an abnormal termination, and inform the batch executive of an aborted step.

Alarms are used to indicate abnormal conditions. The BBC system has a two-layer alarm architecture. Equipment alarms are responsible for notifying when equipment limits are being approached (e.g., the working pressure limit of a bioreactor).

The control drivers are responsible for the management of equipment alarms. Process alarms are responsible for notifying when product quality parameter limits are being approached. It is the responsibility of the batch executor to manage the process alarm conditions established by process alarm recipe statements. An example of this two-layer alarm architecture would be the pressure status of a bioreactor under operation. The bioreactor has a working pressure limit of 50 psi. The reactor has an overpressure rupture seal set to activate at 45 psi. The control driver for the reactor would logically have an equipment alarm built-in set at 40 psi to alarm when the rupture seal is close to rupturing. The product that is currently under production has a pressure range of 8 to 10 psi during the SEPARATION phase. The recipe for the product would contain a product alarm verb that would alarm when the pressure is not within the 8 to 10 psi range. The two-layer alarm schema modularizes alarming responsibilities into equipment and product, making them independent. This simplifies the configuration development for a new product to just what is required for the product leaves out details of the equipment. The equipment alarm details are engineered into the unit control driver.

VIII. RECIPE DEFINITION LANGUAGE

The Recipe Definition Language (RDL) is used to construct process recipes. By using this standard way of expressing the process knowledge, process engineers, process developers, operators, and automation engineers can all examine the recipe and understand the process actions and information transactions required to make a product.

RDL is composed of server verbs, client verbs, and rules for constructing parameters (parameter syntax). Server verbs are processed by the batch executive recipe server. They handle recipe navigation and built-in language functions. Client verbs are executed by separate client processes. The operator and automation system are clients to the recipe server. Operator verbs support operator interface activities. Automation verbs are verbs that call driver verbs. Figure 8 shows how the server and client verbs interact.

Operator client verbs interact with the operator and manage information flow between the operator and the batch executive recipes server. The verb operator information request (OIR) is used to prompt the operator for batch information. This information may be used later in the recipe for batch record formulation or

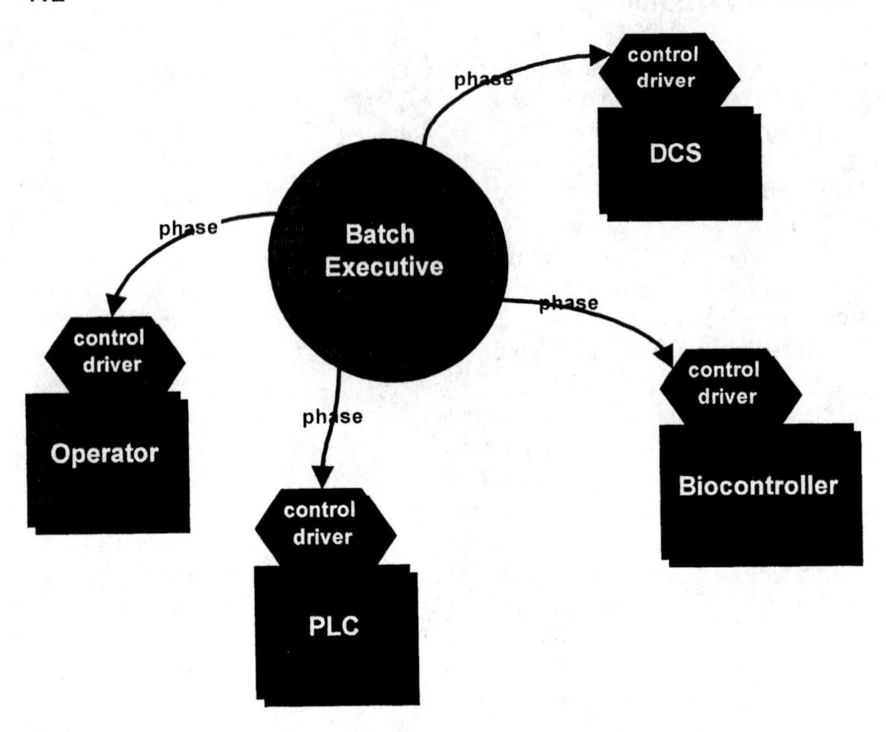

Fig. 8 How the server and client verbs interact.

for storage in the batch journal. The MANUAL verb informs the operator of a manual procedure to follow.

The automation verbs make calls to the control system driver verb. The automation verb is called and the appropriate parameters are sent as described in the control system driver section.

Server verbs can be classified into navigation, language, and information verbs. Such navigation verbs as WHEN, GOTO, WAIT, and LABEL are controlling the sequence of verb execution. Such language verbs as OPERATION and PHASE provide recipe segmentation, which promotes effective organization of recipe verbs. Such information verbs as PRINT, LINK, and LOG handle information management for a running RDL recipe. PRINT can be used to generate reports or bar code labels for product identification. LINK is used to integrate the external information system with the BBC system. Examples of external systems are laboratory and maintenance information systems. The LINK call creates transactions that are sent to the external system.

The LOG verb manages data logging of selected control system data points. The data are stored in the batch journal in a relational database structure. With a separate call of the LOG verb, the server can start logging a data point, change the sampling rate, and stop the logging. These activities are controlled by different parameter values to the LOG verb call.

The behavior of a verb can be managed with each call-through by setting the appropriate parameter values for the verb. The template of a verb can have any number of parameter values that must be specified when the verb is called. For example, the LOG verb may have an ENGAGE parameter that can be set to either ON or OFF. Calling the LOG verb with the ENGAGE verb set to ON will start the logging of the data point specified by another parameter.

Verb	Parameter name	Parameter value
LOG	Point Name	PR4-PIC01
	ENGAGE	ON

Later on in the recipe, in the recipe cleanup section, another call to the LOG verb with the same data point will stop the logging of the data point.

Verb	Parameter name	Parameter value
LOG	Point Name	PR4-PIC01
	ENGAGE	OFF

The real power of verb parameters is revealed with the understanding that parameter values are evaluated at execution time and values can be constants, variables, or expressions. In the previous LOG example, the OFF and ON parameter values are fixed constants that are determined when the recipe is created. Examine the following recipe excerpt:

Verb	Parameter name	Parameter value
OIR	PROMPT	"Enter Data Point to Log"
	TAG	$ANSWER
LOG	POINT_NAME	$ANSWER
	ENGAGE	ON

In this example, the OIR prompts the user for the data point to log. The user would enter the name of the data point into an input field on the operator interface. The point name is stored in a recipe variable called $ANSWER. The LOG verb then uses this variable as the value of the POINT_NAME parameter. Therefore, the point name for the log verb was determined at recipe execution time. This capability enables flexible control of process activities as information gathered during the batch from operators, equipment, and external system is used to determine and process the details of verb calls.

The RDL parameter syntax defines the rules for constructing parameter values. Mathematical calculations, variable assignments, and string operations are examples of some of the powerful capabilities that can be realized through the RDL parameter syntax. Calculations can be used to determine the amount of material to charge a bioreactor to reach a cell density of 3.4 × 10**6 given the current volume in the reactor. An OIR would allow operator intervention in an automated calculation procedure, if required.

An RDL recipe development platform called the *Recipe Notebook* has been developed to allow rapid creation of recipes. This tool guides the user during the development process with ease-of-use features similar to a spreadsheet. The Recipe Notebook permits modeling recipes so that once a basic framework has been worked out, variations on the initial recipe are easily constructed. Once the recipe has been developed it can be printed out for detailed verification. When ready, the recipe is moved to the recipe server with a single press of a button.

The Recipe Notebook is bound to an industry (biotechnology, pharmaceutical, chemical batch process) by the dialect of RDL that is selected. Multiple RDLs may be used at a given facility without collisions as long as the verbs are registered and uniquely defined. For transfer from site to site identical RDLs must be used.

IX. CONCLUSIONS

The BBC, Recipe Notebook, and RDL configuration methodology hopefully embodies all the principles for batch control that S88.01 intended for its batch control standard. In developing this application architecture in a biopharmaceutical environment, BW Manufacturing has created an environment that promotes reduction of system development for new processes and increased system quality assurance through streamlined but not compromised validation as an integral part of the system.

Control vendors will hopefully develop varied modular products that customers can integrate to their own client–server architectures to provide standard functionality and further economies of scale. A few possibilities, such as libraries of validated drivers, database functions, and analytical add-ons, would enhance the client–server DCS environment dramatically and bring process automation to new levels. This philosophy could be adapted by equipment vendors by providing control drivers specific to customer design specifications, which would allow customers to concentrate on recipe development and process development strategies.

The adaptation of control systems into a client-server environment may be seen by all regulated industries as well as regulatory agencies as a much improved methodology in which to implement control for biopharmaceutical, pharmaceutical, and chemical processes. Also beneficial will be the increased assurance that system validation will be current and not compromised.

28

Batch Process Automation

Teddy H. Tom

Moore Products Co., Spring House, Pennsylvania

Kenneth S. Kovacs

Bailey Controls Company, Wickliffe, Ohio

I. BATCH PROCESSES

Batch is "A process that leads to the production of finite quantities of material by subjecting quantities of input materials to an ordered set of processing activities over a finite period of time using one or more pieces of equipment" (1). This definition of a batch process recognizes that the amount of material produced in a single batch is finite. Batch also "means a specific quantity of a drug or other material that is intended to have uniform character and quality, within specified limits, and is produced according to a single manufacturing order during the same cycle of manufacture" (2). Unlike a continuous process, extending the run time of a batch process does not result in the production of additional product. Products manufactured in batches are dependent on three factors: the sequence of process actions used to produce the product, the quantity and quality of the material used in each process action, and the operating parameters used in executing each process action. Changes to any of these factors can alter the product produced. This has the implication that multiple products can be produced using a single recipe procedure in the same set of process equipment.

Batch processing is discontinuous. Equipment is started up, raw materials are fed to the equipment semicontinuously or on a batch basis, the material is acted upon by the equipment to produce the product, the unit is shut down, and the product is removed from the equipment. The cycle is then repeated for each batch.

The definition also provides for the production of a batch product in multiple pieces of equipment. Because the product can be made in one piece of equipment, multiple steady states are possible in a unit. Whether a product is produced in a single unit or in multiple units is dependent on the equipment capabilities and the provided batch plant production paths.

II. SIMPLE BATCH CONTROL SYSTEMS

Simple control systems can be integrated with manual operations to provide a solution for smaller, single stream batch processes with a limited number of simple recipes. The implementation, validation, and maintenance of these types of controls is usually straightforward. With simple batch control systems, batch records must be assembled from batch sheets, data logger and recorder information, and manual entries on standard forms.

A. Single Loop Controls

The least complex control system consists of single loop controllers with sensors installed in the process to monitor the specified parameters. Combined with a controller output connected to a process controlled element, a feedback loop is created to regulate the process to a specified setpoint. The three-mode algorithm capabilities of proportion, integral, and derivative (PID) on these controllers provides a very precise control loop that can be tuned for specific processes and operating environments. PID algorithms remain as a basis for all modern batch control systems. Advances in loop controller technology now provides units that are readily available with multiloop, logic, and autotuning capabilities.

These controllers as stand-alone units do not provide the automatic recording of data and information required for good manufacturing practices (GMP)-compliant batch records. Setup, calibration, tuning, and testing of these controllers is straightforward. Standard manufacturer's manuals and operating information, along with functional requirements, system specifications, process operating instructions, and the controller configuration information, should be sufficient to generate the protocols for the validation qualification testing required for these controllers.

B. Programmable Logic Controller Systems

Programmable logic controllers (PLCs) are microprocessor-based systems that provide a means of controlling processes via Boolean-type statements referred to as ladder logic. More advanced PLCs may provide for programming with sequential function charts as well as with ladder logic. Typically, input devices wired to the programmable logic controller are processed and acted upon per the program logic. Resultant output signals are produced to control the process through field devices also wired to the PLC system. PLC input/output modules are available for virtually every type and level of analog, discrete, or pulsed control signals. Sophisticated PLCs provide functionalities such as PID controls, networking, file transfers, and sequencing.

Programmable logic controllers as stand-alone systems do not generally provide sufficient memory to efficiently capture process data and information required for GMP-compliant batch records. Setup, calibration, tuning, and testing of these controllers is straightforward. Standard manufacturer's manuals and operating information, along with functional requirements, system specifications, process operating instructions, and the program logic, should be sufficient to generate protocols for the validation qualification testing required for PLC systems.

C. Data Loggers and Recorders

Where the capture of process parameter data is required for batch records, data loggers and recorders provide an inexpensive solution for simple batch processes. These components can be specified for compatibility with virtually all standard control signals, such as 4-20 ma, 0-10 VDC, 1-5 VDC, and RS-232 interfaces. This signal compatibility allows ease of installation with loop controllers and PLCs. Process recording systems can be as simple as a strip chart recorder or as sophisticated as computerized multiloop data loggers with hard disk drives for data storage. Software packages can also be integrated with the computerized systems to provide data retrieval and analysis.

Qualification testing of these units is also straightforward, and the methodologies utilized for loop controllers and PLCs will suffice for these components as well.

III. COMPUTERIZED BATCH CONTROL SYSTEMS

As the complexity of controlled equipment, connected input/output signals, recipe requirements, and batch record histories increases, more complex batch control systems are needed. With industrial computer technologies providing greater capabilities at reduced costs, computer hardware is rapidly becoming a commodity item. Software functionalities should be viewed as the differentiating factor when evaluating computerized batch control systems. Open computer architecture provides the greatest flexibility in the implementation of this type of batch control system. Computerized process control systems allow the application of pertinent hardware and software for executing multiple recipes, controlling complex batch processes, and storing and archiving data and information for GMP compliance.

A. SCADA Systems

Supervisory control and data acquisition (SCADA) systems are generally available as separate software packages running on stand-alone computer systems. A variety of SCADA features and functions provide for acquiring data, displaying and controlling processes, and generating reports. Software modules or third-party batch software packages are available for many SCADA systems to provide recipe execution and batch management in conjunction with the control and data acquisition capabilities of the basic SCADA software.

SCADA software running on personal computers requires software drivers to interface to third-party applications, systems, or networks. The availability of these application driver interfaces allows the SCADA systems to exchange data with a wide variety of PLCs, input/output hardware, third-party software packages, and loop controllers. SCADA systems provide scalability from one node to multiple nodes communicating on a network.

A computer system validation plan is required for SCADA systems. Due to the multiple hardware platforms, software packages, interfaces, and databases associated with an integrated SCADA system, a well-planned and implemented validation program is a necessity.

B. Distributed Control Systems

A distributed control system, or DCS, is a computer-based industrial process control system consisting of one or more CRT display operator stations and multifunction controllers that communicate via a data highway network. Open architecture DCSs in general utilize computer workstations to provide the technology required for running graphics, global databases, and integrated software packages. They also enable operator interfaces running in different environments (e.g., NT or UNIX) to coexist on the same network.

Distributed Control System features and functions provide for acquiring data, displaying and controlling processes, and generating reports. Integrated batch software modules are available for many DCSs to provide recipe execution and batch management in conjunction with the control and data acquisition capabilities of the process control software.

Using software drivers to interface to third-party applications, systems, or networks allows the DCS to exchange data with a wide variety of PLCs, input/output hardware, third-party software packages, and loop controllers. Scalability is available, since one computer workstation generally can drive multiple X-Window CRTs operating in a client–server mode. Multiple computers are easily connected through a network for communications.

A computer system validation plan is required for DCSs. With a global database, integration of a DCS with multiple hardware platforms, software packages, interfaces, and information systems should be straightforward. A well-planned and implemented computer system validation program is a necessity.

C. Software Functions

Batch process automation software for pharmaceutical applications requires functionality enhancements to meet GMP compliance issues as well as batch control requirements. Basic software functions should include the following:

- System security access and identification for all users
- Version control for batch recipes
- Flexible report generation for batch records
- Online standard operating procedures (SOPs)
- Alarms with message and reporting capabilities
- Ability to capture operator comments in batch record
- Comprehensive batch record historical database
- Ability to provide complete batch audit trails
- Event summary logs
- Availability of real-time statistical process control (SPC) with alarms
- System status displays
- Utilities for backup and restore

With basic functionalities the system should be properly secured from unauthorized entry, provide process alarms and messages, generate reports as needed, and allow real-time production analysis. A comprehensive historical database, batch records, recipe version control, and online SOPs, are all beneficial for both generating GMP-compliant documentation and providing audit trails for the batch process.

IV. TRADITIONAL BATCH AUTOMATION

Traditional batch automation begins with the desire to optimize the production of an identified product. This product is manufactured using a recipe that in its most basic form consists of a formula and a procedure. The procedure is a set of sequenced process actions that are necessary to make the product. The formula consists of the set of raw materials called for by the recipe and the parameters that are to be used in the procedure. In traditional batch automation, the equipment used for producing a product is first identified and qualified for use. The next step consists of determining how each of the desired process actions required to manufacture the product is executed in the identified set of process equipment.

Once the strategy for making the product in the selected set of equipment is determined, the control instructions for producing the product are written. When completed, these coded instructions are functionally tested to prove that when applied to the equipment, the code causes the desired product to be produced. In this scenario, each time a new product is introduced into the plant, a new unique set of instruction codes is written and tested.

A major disadvantage of this method of implementation is evident when physical changes are made to the physical process layout (e.g., the addition of a valve in the feed line for adding a component). The user has to revisit each of the recipes affected by this physical change and make appropriate instruction code revisions to reflect those changes. Each of these recipes will have to be retested to confirm that it still produces the intended product.

V. MODULAR BATCH AUTOMATION

A. Modular Batch Concepts

Modular batch automation results in the creation of sets of control instructions that are reusable in creating multiple recipes. This is possible because these sets of control instructions are recipe-independent and equipment-specific. Each of these sets of control instructions represents an equipment capability. Examples of equipment capabilities include mixing, adding a material, heating, and cooling. Each capability can be defined by the user once the physical equipment layout has been determined.

A recipe is simply a sequenced set of equipment capabilities. For example, a mixer recipe may involve the addition of two materials, mixing of the material, and transfer of the resulting solution to another part of the process.

In modular batch automation, the user first identifies the capabilities of each equipment unit in the batch facility; for instance, a reactor in the plant that has an agitator, a heating and cooling coil, piping to add raw materials a and b, and drain piping. Because of its physical properties, this reactor will then have the capability of mixing, heating and cooling, feeding components a and b, and draining. This information is then used to develop independent modular groupings of control instruction code that carry out each of the identified equipment functions. Each coded module can be functionally tested to confirm that it performs properly. These modules are stored in a library of equipment functions and become the building blocks for the creation of recipes.

When a product is introduced into the plant, the recipe is constructed by selecting the appropriate modules (or function blocks) from the library and linking them in the proper sequence. Recipe testing now involves confirming that the modular sets of control instructions are linked in the proper sequence to produce the product.

Previously we noted the difficulty that can be encountered in traditional batch automation if the physical layout of the plant changes. In modular batch automation, if a physical change in the plant occurs, such as the integration of an additional valve in the feed a line, the user can simply go to the control instruction set for ''add a'' and make the appropriate code change there. This control instruction set is then tested and will be automatically implemented in all the higher-level recipes that use the add a process action. This can greatly simplify the ongoing validation requirements in a GMP-regulated batch operation.

B. Modular Batch Automation Benefits

There are a number of benefits associated with automation using the modular batch concept. They include the creation of reusable recipe building blocks, the development of recipes independent of control logic, and the simplification of recipe functional testing for ongoing validation. It is important to remember that the recipe building blocks are reusable because they are equipment-related functions and are totally independent of the recipe that is to be automated.

Following the concepts of modular batch automation allows personnel to create recipes without having to code in the language of the system. All that is necessary from the recipe creator is the knowledge of the sequence of process actions necessary to produce the product. Recipe creation then becomes simply a matter of selecting the preconfigured recipe building blocks and coupling them in the appropriate order.

Recipe testing is simplified because it is not necessary to check the control instruction performance, since this was done when the recipe building blocks were first created. The testing now revolves around proving that the order in which the modular recipe blocks are executed meets the performance criteria for making the product.

VI. IMPLEMENTATION METHODOLOGY FOR MODULAR BATCH AUTOMATION

One methodology for implementing a modular batch automation project consists of the following steps:

- *Generation of an equipment functional definition.* This document identifies the process equipment components that constitute the batch operation and describes process actions that can take place within each identified major piece of equipment.
- *Development of a process and instrumentation diagram (P&ID) using this functional definition.* This diagram shows the layout of the major equipment and instrumentation pieces, the physical connections between the pieces of equipment, and the support equipment required to carry out the identified process actions. This step and the previous step are usually iterated to satisfy the category of product to be produced and the existing site constraints, such as the utilities available.

- *Segmentation of the P&ID into equipment entities.* This step determines the flexibility of the batch equipment by identifying equipment modules such as units, piping headers, and shared equipment modules.
- *Implementation of the equipment database.* In this step, the segmented batch plant equipment is defined and mapped to the control system using the equipment database. Equipment attributes are defined to allow the control system to allocate the appropriate equipment module for use during the execution of a batch recipe procedure.
- *Implementation of the software control loops and logic.* This includes definition and development of the strategies to be used in controlling the batch equipment. This step includes the definition of equipment interlocks, safety logic, process graphics and displays, trend screens, and required reports.
- *Creation of the basic recipe building blocks.* Most control systems refer to these blocks as phases. Each building block represents an equipment process capability and is written in the control language of the target control system. These building blocks are stored in a library of basic building blocks or in a phase library.

These steps can be carried out without any knowledge of any of the products that will be manufactured in the batch equipment. Again, all of the steps described thus far are equipment-dependent and recipe-independent.

- When a specific product is identified, a library of operations can be created from the recipe building blocks. An operation is a user-defined grouping of recipe building blocks or phases.
- If strict ISA S88.01 (1) conventions are followed, unit recipe procedures are created by grouping operations that execute in a unit.
- Sequencing the appropriate unit recipe procedures produces the batch recipe procedures. These batch recipe procedures in combination with the batch recipe header, formula, equipment database, and safety and compliance sections, complete the development of an S88.01-based batch recipe.

VII. STRATEGIC ENTERPRISE MANAGEMENT AND INTEGRATION

A. Integrating the Enterprise

In order to meet the needs of their customers in a timely manner, individual departments, groups, or organizations within an enterprise must communicate real-time information. Activities within the enterprise that are linked and dependent upon each other can be managed intelligently with the availability of this real-time information. In order to link batch systems to enterprise information systems, a strategic enterprise management plan is a prerequisite. Turning a vision into reality requires planning. With an agreed-upon strategic plan meeting the needs of all enterprise users, implementation of the plan is user-driven. Once everyone involved in the planning stage understands the justification and the benefits derived from "strategic enterprise management," implementation will never be quick enough for those awaiting their part of the overall system.

Computer system open architecture technology allows multiple vendors to communicate via industry standard network protocols. Software application protocol interfaces (API), required for integrating different vendor software packages, are commonly imbedded in the standard package or offered as off-the-shelf options. With the available power and reliability of today's computer systems, imagination is the only limitation to the possibilities of what could be included in an enterprise integration strategic plan. In reality, company resources are normally the factor that limits what will be included in the strategic plan. Because of resource limitations and the desire to allow new technologies to be assimilated by the enterprise, a phased project approach is highly recommended for the implementation of any enterprise computer integration project.

Benefits from strategic enterprise management will be different for each user. Envision a manufacturing facility in which real-time information is available on a need-to-know basis. Incoming raw materials can be entered into inventory by product, lot number, manufacturer, quality certification, specifications, and an internal identification number through bar code scans. Quality assurance (QA) product release information can then be posted as soon as the raw materials meet QA requirements. A real-time raw materials inventory with storage locations could be available online. Of course, all data are automatically entered for record keeping and reporting. Security would be an integral part of this system, with all operating personnel having their own bar-coded or magnetic access card, along with a password or personal identification number (PIN). If procedural questions arise, online SOPs would be available as a reference. Procedure checklists could also be online, with appropriate personnel "filling in the blanks."

A scenario such as this can be formulated for every activity within the enterprise. Production information regarding yields, quality, and equipment can be obtained within seconds. Operating personnel can be easily prompted through preparatory work in production. Detailed batch process records can provide full traceability of batches through the production process from raw materials used to label information on the packaged product. Strategic enterprise management can provide the means for rapid release of batch materials to decrease product time to market, identify potential problems before production interruptions occur, assure that product quality specifications are satisfied, and simplify GMP compliance issues.

In a truly integrated open environment, the process automation system passes appropriate information to the enterprise systems as required. These enterprise systems may include integrated manufacturing execution systems (MES), enterprise resource planning (ERP), manufacturing resource planning (MRPII), or point solutions, such as laboratory information management systems (LIMS), maintenance management, document management, and production scheduling, just to name a few.

It is imperative to remain focused on the enterprise "vision" requirements to ensure that as each part of the system is implemented, full compatibility will still be achieved after all phases of the strategic enterprise management (SEM) system are integrated. Since the individual systems must ultimately operate as a single SEM system, proper planning, integration, and testing are required to assure that other parts of the system are not negatively affected as new parts of the system are brought online. This should be an integral part of the validation qualification testing for all systems.

B. Batch Data Analysis: Trending, SPC, and Spreadsheets

Trend analysis of batch data is useful while running the batch and for historical comparisons. Knowledge of a typical or theoretical data parameter trend line for a particular batch can provide insight as to how the batch is progressing as compared to an "ideal." Should questions arise in the future about the quality of a particular batch, accessing the historical batch database to analyze the data by batch identification number is invaluable.

Real-time SPC provides a means to analyze product attributes and process parameters during production. Much has been written regarding the use of SPC techniques for QA. Information derived from taking production samples to a lab for analysis can be hours old by the time it is returned to the production floor. By integrating SPC algorithms with process controls and alarms, a real-time online system can be implemented to perform corrective changes or provide process alarms based upon statistical parameters. For example, rules can be readily established to monitor sensor inputs and take corrective action or alarm if a specific number of identical inputs is obtained. A condition like this could occur with a faulty sensor or a resistive fault in wiring and still indicate that the process is "normal." In this case SPC could provide an alarm condition before the process itself is out of control.

Batch data analysis can be invaluable for

- Providing up-to-the-minute reporting of actual manufacturing operations results along with the comparison to past history and expected business results for performance measurement and ongoing improvement on an enterprise basis. Performance results can include such measurements as resource utilization, resource availability, product unit cycle time, conformance to schedule, and performance to standards.
- Providing real-time analysis of process and batch measurements collected from manufacturing to assure proper product quality control and to iden-

tify problems requiring attention. Through analysis, actions may be recommended during the batch run to correct problems by correlating the symptoms, actions taken, and results to determine the cause.

The performance analysis function compares actual manufacturing data to process specifications and the historical database for process improvement, optimization, and troubleshooting. Performance analysis shall be specifically configured to generate information for batch records, such as actual variances versus allowable variances, actual yields versus theoretical yields, and ongoing process capability indices showing process consistency and reliability to operate within specifications. Performance data can also include real-time and historical process data, batch cycle times, in-process sample test results, and finished product test results.

Statistical tools provided in enterprise management systems will allow performance analysis of data to generate control charts and process capabilities for production control and continuous process validation (CPV) of repetitive processes. In addition, QA analysis of data and batch record data for LIMS can be performed as stipulated in SOPs and communicated within the enterprise as required to meet operations and regulatory requirements.

C. Batch Tracking

A materials management function in an enterprise provides access to information regarding the status, quantity, location, and disposition of materials at all times. Tracking and controlling inventories of raw materials, intermediates, QA samples, spare parts, and other materials used is provided for the manufacturing facility. Information can include component raw material suppliers, lot numbers, quantities available, QA status, current work-in-process (WIP) status, and finished product locations.

Real-time materials data is obtained from the process automation and management system in order to track material usage and status through the process. These records support the forward and backward genealogy of component raw materials for each lot of finished product.

The production tracking/tracing function can now be integrated to collect, organize, and analyze information for all units, raw materials, and products used in a batch process. Tracking can also include QA and maintenance repair information for defective materials or units. Tracking/genealogy reports can then be defined and generated to show raw materials usage, the complete as-built history, subprocess/subprocess relationships, QA information, yield data, and summarized results for individual batches.

VIII. GMP REGULATORY ISSUES

A. Good Manufacturing Practices

The Food and Drug Administration (FDA) is empowered by the Federal Food, Drug, and Cosmetic Act to enforce the federal regulations defined in Title 21 of the Code of Federal Regulations (21 CFR). Part 210 is entitled "Current Good Manufacturing Practice in Manufacturing, Processing, Packaging, or Holding of Drugs; General," while part 211 is entitled "Current Good Manufacturing Practice for Finished Pharmaceuticals."

B. Standard Operating Procedures

Written user SOPs must be available to operations for production and process control per 21 CFR 211.100 (3). In automated batch processes, these SOPs should be available online by request and possess functionalities such as dynamic scrolling as the batch procedure progresses. Some software systems allow the SOPs to serve as an electronic operator log with provisions for input of real-time operator comments during batch operation. The SOP, along with all operator comments, is then stored as part of the batch database and can be incorporated into the batch report. An online dynamic SOP feature gives the user the opportunity to look ahead to see what will occur in a batch and also provides a mechanism to allow documented semiautomatic operations to occur in conformance with established recipe procedures. This allows the batch recipe to drive the manual operations within the batch as required.

C. Recipe Version Control

Current automated batch control systems should have an object-oriented architecture approach to recipe procedure configuration. They should also conform to ISA S88.01-based master and control recipes containing sections on header, equipment requirements, formulas, recipe procedures, and other information.

To configure a recipe procedure, symbols are selected from a recipe configuration palette and placed on the recipe configuration screen. Each selected block is assigned its specific function in the recipe and then linked in the proper sequence to form the recipe procedure. The S88.01-defined hierarchy of recipe procedures (operations, unit recipe procedures, and batch recipe procedures) is then created in this manner.

These created recipe procedures are saved in a library of recipe procedures for future reuse in multiple recipes. Recipe configuration tools should support the creation of recipes that contain logic-based branching, recipe procedure synchronization, looping, and exception handling. Recipe manager functions should provide the user the capability to save combinations of phases, operations, and unit recipes that are organized to perform a task. This eliminates the need to reconfigure groupings of recipe procedures that are used in multiple recipes.

An important feature of any automated batch system configuration tool set is the ability to maintain and control recipe versions. Every recipe in the system should have a version number. Recipe revision data should be stored in a version history file that can be accessed by the user. If changes are made to any recipe, the version number must be updated each time a recipe is installed onto a control system for available use. The system should not allow a new or modified recipe to be saved under an existing file name or version control number. At the same time the version number is updated, the version history of the recipe can also be updated with appropriate comments annotating the revisions. This file should be available for viewing in the header section of the recipe.

Complete revision histories should be maintained for each recipe and equipment database file. Currently installed operational versions may be maintained independently of multiple versions stored off-line. Revision histories include time/date stamps, recipe author, and comments about the changes made.

D. Batch Data Collection, Records, and Reports

Current good manufacturing practices (CGMP) regarding batch processes are defined within 21 CFR 211, ''CGMP for Finished Pharmaceuticals.'' Specific sections referring to batch records include 211.186, ''Master Production and Control Records,'' and 211.188, ''Batch Production and Control Records.''

Capabilities of a batch process automation system should allow batch tracking and audit trails for GMP compliance. Comprehensive electronic batch records are possible through audit trail and genealogy documentation that is captured for all batch runs. This includes the collection of user-defined process data, batch event history, and SOPs. All data should be capable of being viewed on operator display terminals, organized into user-defined report formats and printed, or transferred to a relational database for more sophisticated documentation handling. Flexible data collection tools integrated with recipe procedures allow data collection to be synchronized with every recipe procedure block and automatically coordinated for the batch record (3).

An important part of any plant operation is the capability to document the manufacturing of a product. The process management and control system must allow the user to define not only what data to collect but also where in the recipe procedure the data collection should begin and end. This allows the user to specify when during the recipe it is important to collect data rather than to just collect meaningless data at all times. All data collected should be stored by batch identification number in a read-only, nonmodifiable batch database. This provides the user with the capability to archive, retrieve, and organize information based on the batch identification number. The required batch record can then be stored on a system such as a write once read many (WORM) drive for archiving.

The batch database capabilities should include the following:

1. An event history section that contains recipe start and end times, operator messages and responses, operator actions, system alarms associated with the batch, the SOP, and any user comments.
2. A key data section that contains a defined snapshot of the batch. This

could include information such as the batch ID, recipe name, maximum batch temperature, quantities of components added to a vessel, and summary data for materials used.

3. A periodic data section that consists of variables that have more than one value per batch such as the batch temperature profile and the batch pressure profile. These data must be time- and date-stamped.

E. System Configuration Documentation

A batch configuration reporter documents the entire equipment database, the recipe database, and batch report formats. The equipment database information includes a breakdown of the equipment, the version number of the equipment database, the recipe phases that can be run by each equipment unit, and the attributes of each piece of equipment.

Documentation of the recipe database includes information such as the type of recipe procedure, its version number, the parameters used in the recipe procedure, the lower-level recipe procedures used in this recipe, and the higher-level recipe procedures that use this recipe procedure.

This type of documented information generated by the system will simplify the validation efforts of that batch process automation system.

F. Security

Access to all functions within an automated system must be secured to allow only authorized individuals the ability to perform operations for which they are approved. The system should then have the capabilities to log an individual's activities on the system as events and include them in the batch record as necessary. In addition to the operational security functions, automated systems should have a means for addressing electronic signature requirements of current 21 CFR as amended by part 11, ''Electronic Records; Electronic Signatures'' (4).

Compliance with these regulations can be accomplished on a ''closed system''—''an environment in which system access is controlled by persons who are responsible for the content of electronic records that are on the system''—(4) by employing at least two distinct identification components. This can be accomplished through the use of user log-in password protection and a second means of identification such as an identification code, a bar-coded identification card, or a magnetic card for all operating personnel. With computerized batch process systems having configurable security levels such as operators, supervisors, and engineering, the system can allow for unique signature requirements with each level configured to access different system functionalities.

G. Validation

The ability to provide documentation and reports to meet CGMP requirements using the system itself is of great importance when executing the validation protocols. Reports providing process information from a computerized control system that has been properly qualified and validated can then be used in the validation of the process itself. System-generated SPC process capability studies can be used to provide the final documented evidence that the process is capable of operating within specifications both consistently and reliably (3).

IX. SUMMARY

Products manufactured in batches are dependent on three factors: raw materials, the quantity of each raw material, and the recipe procedure. Changes to any of these factors can alter the product produced. Multiple products can be produced using a single set of batch equipment. Process automation begins with the desire to optimize the production of an identified product. As the complexity of controlled equipment, connected input/output signals, recipe requirements, and batch record histories increases, more complex batch control systems are needed. Computerized process control systems allow the application of pertinent hardware and software for executing multiple recipes, controlling complex batch processes, and for storing and archiving data and information for GMP compliance.

Modular batch automation results in the creation of sets of control instructions that are reusable in creating multiple recipes. This is possible because these sets of control instructions are recipe-independent and equipment-specific.

In order to meet the needs of their customers in a timely manner, individual departments, groups, or organizations within an enterprise must communicate real-time information. Activities within the enterprise that are linked and dependent upon each other can be managed intelligently with the availability of this real-time information. In order to link batch systems to enterprise information systems, a strategic enterprise management plan is a prerequisite. Enterprise management systems can provide the means for rapid release of batch materials to decrease product time to market, identify potential problems before production interruptions occur, assure that product quality specifications are satisfied, and simplify GMP compliance issues.

When planning for batch process automation, the computerized process management and control system should include integrated functionalities to address regulatory requirements of the FDA's CGMP. An important part of any plant operation is the capability to document the manufacturing of a product. In automated batch processes, SOPs should be available online by request. A system configuration tool set should have the ability to maintain and control recipe versions. In addition, capabilities of a batch process automation system should allow batch tracking and audit trails as required for GMP compliance.

Comprehensive electronic batch records are possible through audit trail and traceability documentation that is captured for all batch runs by the automated batch process system. This includes the collection of user-defined process data, batch event history, and SOPs. All data collected should be stored by batch identification number in a read-only, nonmodifiable batch database. This provides the user with the capability to archive, retrieve, and organize information based on the batch identification number.

Today's computerized batch process automation systems provide the user with the ability to consistently and reliably manufacture products to specifications, limit security access to all functions within the system to allow only authorized individuals the ability to perform operations for which they are approved, provide documentation and reports to meet CGMP requirements, and integrate the process-level system with management systems to communicate current time information and documentation for optimizing enterprise operations.

REFERENCES

1. "Batch Control Part 1: Models and Terminology," ISA-S88.01, The International Society for Measurement and Control, 1995.
2. Code of Federal Regulations, Title 21 (21 CFR), Food and Drug Administration, Washington, D.C.
3. K. S. Kovacs, *Validation Assurance and GMP Compliance*, Elsag Bailey Process Automation, 1995.
4. 21 CFR as amended by Part 11, "Electronic Records; Electronic Signatures," Food and Drug Administration, Washington, D.C., March 20, 1997.

Index